Health policy and the National Health Service

SOCIAL POLICY IN MODERN BRITAIN

General Editor: Jo Campling

POVERTY AND STATE SUPPORT   *Peter Alcock*
HEALTH POLICY AND THE NATIONAL HEALTH SERVICE
    Judy Allsop
FOUNDATIONS OF THE WELFARE STATE   *Pat Thane*
THE ELDERLY IN MODERN SOCIETY   *Anthea Tinker*
SOCIAL WORK, SOCIAL CARE AND SOCIAL PLANNING   *Adrian Webb and Gerald Wistow*

HEALTH POLICY AND THE NATIONAL HEALTH SERVICE

Judy Allsop

LONGMAN
London and New York

Longman Group UK Limited
Longman House, Burnt Mill, Harlow
Essex CM20 2JE, England
and Associated Companies throughout the world.

*Published in the United States of America
by Longman Publishing, New York*

First published 1984
Sixth impression 1992

British Library Cataloguing in Publication Data

Allsop, Judith
    Health policy and the National Health Service.—
    (Social policy in modern Britain)
    1. Great Britain — National Health Service — History
    I. Title   II. Series
    362.1'0941   RA395.G6

ISBN 0-582-29599-8

Library of Congress Cataloging in Publication Data

Allsop, Judy, 1938—
    Health policy and the National Health Service.

    (Social policy in modern Britain)
    Bibliography: p.
    Includes index.
1. Medical policy — Great Britain. 2. Great Britain. Ministry of Health. I. Title. II.
Series. [DNLM: 1. Health policy — Great Britain. 2. Health services — Great Britain. 3.
Health services — Organization and Administration — Great Britain. 4. State medicine —
Great Britain. W 275 FAI A44h]
    RA395.G6A654   1984   362.1'0941   83-995

ISBN 0-582-29599-8

Set in 10/11pt Linoterm Plantin
Produced by Longman Group (FE) Ltd
Printed in Hong Kong

CONTENTS

PART FIVE. DOCUMENTS

EDITOR'S PREFACE

This series, written by practising teachers in universities and poly-technics, is produced for students who are required to study social policy and administration, either as social science undergraduates or on the various professional courses. The books provide studies focusing on essential topics in social policy and include new areas of discussion and research, to give students the opportunity to explore ideas and act as a basis of seminar work and further study. Each book combines an analysis of the selected theme, a critical narrative of the main developments and an assessment putting the topic into perspective as defined in the title. The supporting documents and compre-hensive bibliography are an important aspect of the series.

Conventional footnotes are avoided and the following system of references is used. A superior numeral in the text refers the reader to the corresponding entry in the list of references at the end of each chapter. A select bibliography is found at the end of the book. A number in square brackets, preceded by 'doc', e.g. [6, 8], refers the reader to the corresponding items in the section of documents which follows the main text.

In *Health Policy and the National Health Service*, Judy Allsop has brought together an analysis of policy issues and policy-making in the NHS since the 1940s, with a review of radical critiques of health policy which take as their starting point the social production of health and ill-health. The book highlights the challenges and paradoxes of contemporary health care and shows how the possibilities for change are constrained by the structure of power in decision-making. The book, as well as providing a theoretical framework for studying health policy includes an account of the 1982 reorganisation of the health service and the shift in emphasis brought about by the 1979 Conser-vative government. It therefore provides an up-to-date text for anyone concerned with the health service either as students, profes-

sionals or users. As a lecturer in social policy with an interest in health
and illness, and a member of a health authority, the author has both
practical and academic commitments to the health service, which add
considerably to the content of the book.

Jo Campling

AUTHOR'S PREFACE

This book has been written in an attempt to widen the field of study of health care in Britain for students of social policy and administration. Traditionally the focus has been primarily on health services provided through the NHS; their structure, distribution and purpose. This has reflected a generally held assumption that a national health service has solved the problem of dealing with ill-health. Clearly it has not. Recent critiques of contemporary health care have drawn attention to the social bases of ill-health and to its association with poverty. At the same time studies of policy-making have indicated that the NHS, for structural reasons, has been slow to respond to government policies which aim to meet new needs.

I have attempted to incorporate these perspectives together with an account of the changing policy emphases in the NHS, as a guide to those studying the NHS. I am conscious that criticisms of the NHS at a time of retrenchment from a commitment to existing levels of public expenditure may be used to support the case for a more 'mixed-economy of health care'. My own view is that the NHS is part of the infrastructure of health care, a civilised and civilising institution; the aim must be to make it more responsive to changing perceptions of need rather than follow policies which undermine its very existence.

Judy Allsop

LIST OF ABBREVIATIONS

AHA	Area Health Authority
ATO	Area Team of Officers
BMA	British Medical Association
CHC	Community Health Council
DCP	District Community Physician
DGH	District General Hospital
DHA	District Health Authority
DHSS	Department of Health and Social Security
DMT	District Management Team
ENT	Ear Nose Throat
FPC	Family Practitioner Committee
GDP	Gross Domestic Product
GNP	Gross National Product
GP	General Practitioner
HMC	Hospital Management Committee
IMR	Infant Mortality Rate
MOH	Medical Officer of Health
NHS	National Health Service
OHE	Office of Health Economics
RAWP	Resource Allocation Working Party
RCT	Random Controlled Trial
RHA	Regional Health Authority
RHB	Regional Hospital Board
PEP	Political and Economic Planning

ACKNOWLEDGEMENTS

My thanks are due to those at the Polytechnic of the South Bank who made it possible for me to have a sabbatical term at a time of economic uncertainty. This enabled a first draft of the book to be completed. My thanks, too, to Yvonne and Annette who helped to type early drafts, to the librarians at the Polytechnic and the King's Fund who were unfailingly helpful and to Judy Collingwood for her patience.

I have drawn heavily on the ideas of others who work in, or have done research on the National Health Service. They have added immeasurably to my understanding of the paradoxes and problems of health care.

My greatest debt is owed to my friends, who will be aware, each in their own way, of the contribution they have made, not least in reminding me of the multifaceted nature of health. Peter, Saul and Ellinor have my particular gratitude for their conviction that the book would be completed.

We are grateful to the following for permission to reproduce copyright material:

George Allen & Unwin Ltd for Table 12; the author, John Berger for Doc 30(2); Marion Boyars Publishers Ltd for Doc 32; Croom Helm Ltd for Fig 5; The Eugenics Society for Doc 24b; the author, Dr L. Fagin and the Controller of Her Majesty's Stationery Office for Doc 26; Heinemann Educational and the Controller of Her Majesty's Stationery Office for Tables 2a & b; the Controller of Her Majesty's Stationery Office for Docs 1–3, 7–12, 14, 16–19, 22–3, 24a, 27–29, Figs 2, 4, 6–12, Tables 1, 3, 5–9, 11, 14; Lexington Books/D.C. Heath & Co for Fig 3; Office of Health Economics for Doc 13, Tables 4, 10; Policy Studies Institute (formerly Political and Economic Planning) for Doc 6; Routledge & Kegan Paul Ltd for Docs 20, 25b; The Society of Authors on behalf of the Bernard Shaw Estate for Doc 30a; Social Science Research Council for Docs 21, 31; Times Newspapers Ltd for Table 13.

Part one
THE BACKGROUND

Chapter one
INTRODUCTION: POLICIES FOR HEALTH

Good health is the bedrock on which social progress is built. A nation of healthy people can do those things which make life worthwhile and as the level of health increases so does the potential for happiness.[1]

Health affects every aspect of life. Our ability to work, to play, to enjoy our families and to socialise with friends, all depend crucially upon our physical well-being. Serious illnesses create enormous pain and suffering, even minor transient ailments can be depressing psychologically as well as debilitating physically. And ill health which leads to death makes all other services of satisfaction irrelevant.[2]

These quotations underline the twin values which underpin intervention by modern governments in the pursuit of health policies. Good health is seen as a positive benefit to both the individual and to the collectivity and the provision of health services has been justified in terms both of fulfilling individual needs and as necessary for national progress. The development of health services and policies for health has in consequence been part of the growth of modern welfare states.

Beneath the surface of commitments to the improvement of health lie uncertainties and ambiguities as to what constitutes a policy for health and how this may best be implemented. Furthermore, health systems which have developed as a result of governmental policies reflect societies: their social structure, patterned inequalities, economic and political organisation and the distribution of power and influence in those societies. The reality of health provision may be far removed from the promises of health policies, and even further from actual improvements in a nation's health status. This book aims to explore some of these issues through the examination of health policies pursued by governments in Britain since the establishing of the National Health Service (NHS) in 1948. This is the focus of part two. Part three looks at the broader spectrum of health care needs and the social bases of ill-health which have been matters for contemporary debate. The major theme of the book is that there is now greater questioning, conflict and uncertainty over the role and purpose of health policies and about the tasks of governments in providing health services through the NHS, than at any time since the establishment of the service. We are in a period of change not only in relation to the structure of the NHS but also with regard to how health and ill-health and responsibilities for them, are perceived and understood. The following section of this chapter outlines the structure of the book and how it seeks to elaborate the theme of uncertainty and change before looking more closely at what is meant by health policy.

THE STRUCTURE OF THE BOOK

The aims, principles and structure of the NHS as it was established in 1946 are outlined in Chapter 2. The NHS is the main vehicle of health policy and the main provider of health services in Britain, so it is important to consider its scope. The 1946 Act which was the legislative foundation of the service sought to provide access to personal health and medical services for the people, free at the point of service. This included the cure and care of the ill and services for the prevention of illness. There was an implicit emphasis in the Act on the treatment of illness in the individual and the structure of the services reflected this. The structure itself was, of course, a consequence of an already existing division of labour and distribution of power in health care. These had developed around and centred on, the medical profession from the nineteenth century onwards and in many respects the NHS Act consolidated the position of the profession at the centre of a state-financed service.

An account of government policies in relation to the NHS is, broadly speaking, the purpose of Part two. The various chapters follow through particular policy themes which reflect successive governments' perceptions of the 'problems' in health care. The desire of the centre to control the health authorities at a lower level in the NHS, to ensure efficiency and effectiveness through a proper structure of organisation and management is discussed in Chapter 4, while the necessity to allocate resources appropriately to meet particular needs is the theme of Chapters 5 and 6. Policies to allocate resources to meet the health needs in different parts of the country on a more equitable basis developed during the 1960s, and form part of the discussion on resources in Chapter 5. Policies to give priority to the development of services for the elderly, the mentally ill, the mentally and physically handicapped, or as they are referred to in this book, dependent groups, are considered in Chapter 6.

A background to this part of the book is provided in Chapter 3 where it is argued that for most of the period, the NHS operated within a framework of political consensus. There was a tacit acceptance that the existence of an NHS had 'solved' the problem of dealing with ill-health by providing health services. The major objective of governments was a gradually expanding service to keep pace with demographic change and technological advance. Rising expenditures were accommodated by the historically high rates of economic growth in the economy as a whole. The mid-1970s marked an end of the period of consensus in relation to priorities in health policy and within the NHS. Since then, there has been a far greater diversity of views about the proper focus for health policy and the objectives of the service. This diversity, amounting at times and in relation to certain issues, to open conflict, has continued into the 1980s. It has been apparent in the NHS itself, in the diverging policies of the political parties and is reflected in the emergence of radical critiques of health policies and services. The greater uncertainty and conflict has led to talk of 'crisis' in the NHS. This sense of 'crisis' is due to a combination of factors which are intrinsic to the provision of health services in modern industrial societies, to factors which relate to the NHS itself, and to changes in the context in which it functions. Significantly, it is not only Britain which is said to have a crisis in its health care system, other countries have experienced similar dilemmas and tensions.

It is argued in Chapter 3 that it is the end of the era of high growth rates which has brought an end to the period of consensus in the NHS. Controls on NHS spending have been further tightened by the determination of the 1979 Conservative government to cut public expenditure. Economic policy has taken precedence over social policy and the consequent changes in health policy as far as the health service is concerned, are discussed in Chapter 7.

A factor which has increased a sense of crisis in the NHS is the structure of the service itself. Conflicts and problems are in many respects highly visible politically. As was pointed out at the beginning of this introduction, health services have an important place within modern welfare states. Health is an emotive area of care, it is concerned often with life and death. Furthermore, the structure of the NHS is highly centralised and thus the government is the employer of a large and complex labour force. The tensions between the state as employer and the state as the provider of health services, responsible for the well-being of its citizens, are played out in the public arena of the media with all contestants to disputes having a vested interest in generating a sense of crisis.

There are, however, more fundamental factors which have brought greater uncertainty about the proper focus for health policy and the purpose of health services in all health systems. On the one hand it has been acknowledged for some time that the demand for health care is capable of infinite expansion. In consequence it is recognised that there is no easily identifiable 'right' level of health service provision, or funding of expenditure on health care. This is a matter of what a country can afford, or what is politically acceptable, or what can be negotiated by the interests involved. On the other hand, the actual efficacy of health services in improving health has too come increasingly into question. During the 1970s and 1980s a broadly based radical critique of contemporary health care has developed and in relation to the NHS. It has been widely argued that the service is far too concerned with the treatment of illness and too little with the maintenance of health. Part three deals with these issues by examining the social bases of health (Chap. 8), recent policies for prevention (Chap. 9) and critiques of contemporary health care (Chap. 10 and 11).

A final factor which has served to increase the level of conflict in the NHS and to a degree in other health systems also, is the resistance of health systems to change. Governments in various countries have attempted to shift the direction of health policies by giving priority to particular groups in need, and by attempting to shift the emphasis from the treatment of acute illness towards the maintenance of health. However it has proved extremely difficult to implement changes and this reflects the power of particular interest groups in health care and the diffuse nature of decision-making in health care organisations. Those who make the decisions at the grass roots; in the hospitals, in the clinics, health centres and surgeries tend, ultimately, to determine both the overall quantity of, and the distribution of, resources.

These various factors which have led to greater questioning of health policies and the NHS, have led to what the American policy analyst, Aaron Wildavsky calls a sense of 'doing better and feeling worse'[3]; despite a growth in health care expenditure there is doubt about the benefits which have accrued. It is likely that this scepticism reflects a fundamental shift in attitude which marks a movement from a relatively simple one-dimensional objective of providing health services to cope with illness in individuals, towards the more diffuse and difficult goal of improving health.

The remainder of this introductory chapter will lay down the approach taken in this book to understanding the aims of health policy, the shift which has taken place in the policy paradigm and the existence of structured interest groups in health care.

WHAT ARE THE AIMS OF HEALTH POLICY?

The NHS in 1946 aimed to provide a preventive, curing and caring service. This apparent simplicity glosses over what are difficult conceptual and theoretical questions. There are problems in the definition of the core concepts with which health policies are centrally concerned: the maintenance of health, the treatment of illness, the care of the frail. There is no single satisfactory definition of health, illness or frailty, simply alternative approaches which contain particular ways of seeing, interpreting, giving meaning to these universal aspects of human existence. Definitions of health and illness are more fully discussed at the beginning of Chapter 8, but for our purposes here, the main point is to argue that in different times and in different periods, often for concrete historical reasons, governments have tended to emphasise one or other of two fundamental approaches to dealing with questions of illness and health in society. Either the major purpose of health policy has been seen to be the maintenance of health and the prevention of ill-health through the appropriate social and economic arrangements for ensuring physical fitness, and mental repose; a 'social model' of health or, alternatively, the approach in health policy has been to concentrate on providing access, for the ill, to treatment by professional healers. Health here is implicitly seen as the absence of illness in individuals, or more specifically in modern industrial societies, the absence of disease. This has been termed the 'medical model' as the treatment of illness and disease is seen as the preserve of the medical profession, whose expertise lies in the diagnosis and treatment of disease.

These two ways of approaching health and illness are of ancient origin. Their importance to us is that in the intervention of modern governments into health care, the two approaches have become central to particular policy paradigms.

Rein suggests that a policy paradigm is based on a particular view of the essential problem to be solved.

> It is a working model of why things are as they are, a problem-solving framework, which supplies values and benefits, but also procedures, habits of thought, and a view of how society functions. It often provides a guiding metaphor of how the world works which implies a general direc-

tion for intervention, it is more specific than an ideology or a system of beliefs, but broader than a principle of intervention.[4]

Rein goes on to suggest that policy paradigms are a 'curious mixture of psychological assumptions, scientific concepts, value commitments, social aspirations, personal beliefs and administrative constraints'.[4]

In mid-nineteenth-century England the dominant policy paradigm was a preventive approach to health. The nineteenth-century public health reformers were concerned to alleviate the appalling conditions in towns. Disease and illness were seen to be caused by poverty, and conditions of work and living which were conducive to the spread of infectious disease. Health policies were primarily concerned with maintaining health by removing public squalor. Chadwick had little but contempt 'for the bumbling pretensions and hopeless disputes of doctors and for the pathetically inadequate curative medicine of his time'.[5]

From the early twentieth century onwards, emphasis shifted towards a policy paradigm based on the improvement of health through the treatment of illness in individuals, and this itself reflected the rise of science and the expectations of what medicine could achieve. The struggle was for a health service providing access for the whole population to free health care. This policy reached its fullest expression in the National Health Service. The existence of the NHS has tended to obscure the importance of the maintenance of health in populations and the 1970s have brought a rediscovery and promotion of the preventive paradigm. This implies a shift in the structures providing health care and has been presented diagrammatically by Illsley. It is reproduced in the document section [doc 31].

WHO MAKES HEALTH POLICY?

There are two major approaches to looking at the question of who makes policy. One takes as a starting point government policies as statements of intent. This is the official and formal view of policy and its implementation at different levels of agencies and organisations. The second approach is to suggest that policy-making is what agencies actually do, policy is the outcome of a process of policy implementation.

Part two of this book takes as its starting point government policies in relation to particular themes in health care; policies concerned with resource allocation, with the management of the health authorities and the care of dependent groups. The initial assumption is that policy is what governments say it is going to be; that it can direct lower level authorities to carry out and implement its policies. On the surface the NHS looks like this. It is highly centralised. The Secretary of State for Social Services with the Department of Health and Social Security (DHSS) are formally accountable for all activities in the NHS. The reality of policy-making is rather different from this, and in the discussion of policy themes, an attempt is made to suggest the forces at work which modify and inhibit the implementation of policy in the health authorities. The 'policy as process' approach focuses on groups of 'actors' involved in the process of policy implementation, their assumptions, their interests and values. Policies may be implemented or fail to be implemented, for a variety of reasons depending on the interests of those involved in implementation. The forces supporting the maintenance of existing ways of doing things rather than innovation and change, have informed a number of studies of local and central government.[6] However, it is only recently that the process of policy implementation has been examined at a local level in the NHS, through the examination of the working of the health authorities.

Whether the study of health policy is made from the perspective of government policy or the process of policy implementation in health authorities and agencies, an understanding of the distribution of power and the structuring of interests is vital to an understanding of the forces influencing the articulation of *particular* health policies, rather than others, and of the modification of policies in the process of implementation. This book draws on the work of Robert Alford who, in *Health Care Politics*,[7] used the notion of 'structured interest groups' in health care to analyse the influence of particular interests on the scope, direction and implementation of health policies. These interest groups are briefly described below.

STRUCTURED INTEREST GROUPS IN HEALTH CARE

Alford suggests that interests in health care can be classified into three major groupings: the professional monopolisers, the corporate rationalisers and the community interest. These interest groups have particular aims and objectives and their power is structured in particular ways. The dominant interest group, he argues, contains the professional monopolisers; the doctors whose control of medical knowledge both explains and reinforces the dominance of the disease model of illness. Although numerically small, as compared for example to nurses, their definitions of health and illness tend to dominate health policy and provision. Alford comments:

> Physicians have extracted an arbitrary set from an array of skills and knowledge relevant to the maintenance of health in a population and have successfully sold these as their property for a price and have managed to create legal mechanisms which enforce that monopoly and the social beliefs which mystify that population about the appropriateness and desirability of that monopoly.[8]

The second major interest group is composed of 'the corporate rationalisers'. This includes the politicians, adminstrators, at central and local level, and some professionals whose main objective is to achieve greater co-ordination and integration of health services, and to achieve improvements in the planning and delivery of health services. Their interests lie in improving the efficiency and effectiveness of health services and making the best use of the health resources of the collectivity. Their influence has been enhanced as health care expenditures have increased.

The third interest group identified by Alford is 'the community interest'; the cluster of organisations and individuals which seek to represent a different order of priorities, alternative perspectives on health policy and perhaps a broader view of health care. In Britain there is a wide variety of pressure groups which lobby public and Parliament, and interests which find expression in the media. The Patients' Association, MIND, The Disability Alliance, Des Wilson's CLEAR, which aims to draw attention to lead pollution, are examples. These groups represent interests which are relatively submerged in the health policies of the NHS itself. Their focal point tends to be the national policy arena, rather than the local one which reflects the highly centralised nature of the NHS. Compared to the other two structured interest groups these groups are diffuse and tend to lack a power base in the NHS.

Alford's model of structured interest groups is based on an analysis of health care in the United States and although it is sufficiently generalised to have a utility in looking at the distribution of power and influence in other health systems, it does omit one interest group which has a structured base in the National Health Service, that is the NHS workforce. There are almost one million workers in the service, of which doctors are about 7 per cent. This workforce, an analysis of which largely falls outside the scope of this book, has rarely acted as a cohesive single group. It is composed of a variety of interests and the role of these in policy-making has been poorly documented.

However, the existence of such a large group of state employees has tended to act as a force for inertia against change and its existence underlines the corporate nature of the NHS.[9]

Since its inception the NHS has tended to be viewed by the majority of providers of health care and the public as 'outside' politics, as being a basic and uncontentious service. Critiques of health policy and the NHS and recent economic and social policies have shown that it is not. The context of health care, the interests involved in providing it, the dilemmas in striking a balance between competing claims and objectives are all highly political and contain judgements about value. It is the purpose of this book to illustrate the processes through which health policies are determined and health care provided.

REFERENCES

1. MINISTRY OF NATIONAL HEALTH AND WELFARE (CANADA), *A New Perspective on the Health of Canadians* (Chairman: M. Lalonde), Preface, Ottawa (1974).

2. LE GRANDE, J., *Strategy of Equality. Redistribution and the Social Services*, Allen & Unwin, London (1982), p. 23

3. WILDAVSKY, A., *The Art and Craft of Policy Analysis*, Macmillan, London (1980)

4. REIN, M., *Social Science and Public Policy*, Penguin, London (1976), p.103

5. LAMBERT, R., *Sir John Simon and English Social Administration 1816–1904*, MacGibbon & Kee, London (1963), p. 62

6. For example DEARLOVE, J., *The Politics of Policy in Local Government: the Making and Maintenance of Policy in the Royal Borough of Kensington and Chelsea*, CUP (1973), and HECLO, H. and WILDAVSKY, A., *The Private Government of Money*, Macmillan, London (1974)

7. ALFORD, R., *Health Care Politics*, University of Chicago Press (1975)

8. *Ibid.* p. 195

9. KLEIN, R., 'The corporate state, the Health Service and the professions', *New Universities Quarterly*, **31**, No. 2, 1977

Chapter two
ESTABLISHING THE NHS

The National Health Service (NHS) came into operation on 5 July 1948. This was in accordance with the National Health Service Act passed in 1946, and it marked the end of a period of argument and discussion about the shape of a national health service which had continued since 1942. The steering of the NHS Bill through Parliament, and the eventual agreement of the majority of doctors to join the service was a major political achievement for the Minister of Health of the 1945 Labour government, Aneurin Bevan. His success reflected a broad consensus of public and political opinion in favour of the establishment of a national health service, free at the point of service, to combat what Beveridge had called in his 1942 Report on National Insurance, the 'Giant of Sickness'.

The Act was of crucial importance in establishing the pattern of the present health care system in Britain. It rested on the principle of a collective responsibility by the state for comprehensive health services, to be provided on the basis of equal access for all citizens. This represented a radical new commitment. The Act too established a new structure through which health services were to be administered. This 'tripartite' structure remained for twenty-six years until the health service was reorganised in 1974. Less obviously but of equal importance the Act committed the state to a particular *kind* of health service. There was an emphasis on the provision of personal medical services through a set of institutions which gave doctors a decisive role in determining what these medical services were to be, and how they were to be provided. In this sense the Act was not new. The medical profession had important powers over the content and scope of medical care before the Act and retained them afterwards. The Act did not, either, immediately produce new or different health care. As Watkin puts it, 'there were no new hospitals, no new drugs or treatment. It did not even make available to the poor what had previously been available to the rich.'[1] What the Act did do was to commit the central government financially to funding a health service which rested on the principles of collectivism, comprehensiveness, equality and universality. Although these have proved difficult to realise in practice they remain intrinsic to the idea of nationalised health care.

This chapter begins by examining in greater detail the aims and intentions of the 1946 Act and the administrative structure which was established in 1948. As these were strongly influenced by the existing division of labour in health care and the history of state intervention in health services during the nineteenth and early twentieth centuries, the growth of the medical profession and state involvement in dealing with problems of health is then broadly sketched. The chapter concludes with a discussion of the factors which underpinned the compromise made between the state and the profession in 1946, and an assessment of the 1946 Act.

THE AIMS AND INTENTIONS OF THE NHS ACT

The collectivist principle

A central aim of the NHS Act was that the state should provide health care free at the point of service for those in need. This reflected the collectivist principle of state responsibility for its citizens. Thus the NHS Act was seen at the time by opponents and supporters alike as epitomising the social welfare and social service society of the future being rounded out by the post-war Labour government. Bevan saw the NHS as the hallmark of a civilised society. 'Society becomes more wholesome, more serene, and spiritually healthier, if it knows that its citizens have at the back of their consciousness, the knowledge that not only themselves, but all their fellows, have access, when ill to the best medical skills can provide'.[2] It was Bevan's view that the state should, through collective action, provide free access to medical services. In this Bevan saw little difference between the NHS and the railways – in the case of both, centralised state organisation should be used to provide a service which was equally accessible to all citizens in distress and provided on an equitable basis according to need.

The proposed NHS was not without its critics. To some such collective action was reminiscent of the fascist state. Less dramatically, but more importantly for the success of the service, large sections of the medical profession became, during the passage of the Act, deeply hostile to what was seen as an interference by the state into conditions governing that sacred area of medical care, the doctor-patient relationship. On the whole however there was widespread acceptance of the collectivist principle as the extract in the document section from the debate in the House of Commons on the issue illustrates [doc 1]. The Second World War had changed the whole mood of influential sections of the population to state intervention. Indeed in 1942, the British Medical Association (BMA), the body representing the interests of the profession, itself passed a resolution (by a small majority) in favour of a free medical service for the whole community with a full-time salaried general practitioner service under *ad hoc* health authorities which were also to run hospitals.[3] Although this consensus disappeared in the face of concrete proposals from the government for change it reflected the degree of underlying solidarity in the nation in the face of total war.

The principle of state provision agreed in 1946 meant that financial responsibility for health services and for health policy rested with the central government. The Ministry of Health and its ministers were responsible for the institutions providing health services and were thus the central pivot of health policy. The more so, as unlike other social services such as education and housing, there was to be no elected tier in the health service. Power it seemed, was to rest with the centre with Ministers and their departments to make policy decisions, to allocate resources and to administer the service.

The comprehensive principle

The Minister of Health, furthermore, was to have a general duty to 'promote a *comprehensive* health service for the improvement of the physical and mental health of the people of England and Wales for the prevention, diagnosis and treatment of illness'. A summary of the 1946 Health Service Bill is reproduced in the document section [doc 2]. Two important areas of health care were however excluded from the NHS Act. Health care for school children remained for the most part in the hands of local education authorities and the health care of the worker, the culmination of a variety of Factory Acts, was to remain the responsibility of the Department of Employment and the Health and Safety Executive.

The diagram in Figure 1 shows the tripartite structure of the health service agreed in 1946 and the services it was to cover. The hospitals which had developed in a fragmented fashion during the nineteenth century in a variety of institutional forms under voluntary organisations, local authorities, poor law authorities, a process which is described in detail by Abel-Smith in his book on *The Hospitals, 1800–*

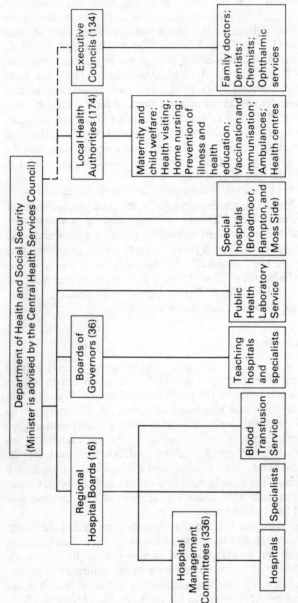

— Direct responsibility

‒ ‒ ‒ ‒ General supervisory powers

Fig. 1. Organisation of the National Health Service in England and Wales 1948–74

Note: The Ministry of Health became the Department of Health and Social Security in 1968.

1948,[4] were in effect nationalised. Each hospital or group of hospitals were to have an appointed Hospital Management Committee (HMC) composed of professional and lay members who were to receive their financing through the Regional Hospital Boards (RHBs), who in turn were responsible to the Minister of Health. The fourteen regions in England and Wales were to be responsible for co-ordinating and planning the provision of hospital services within their regions, again through a board composed of professional and lay members. Teaching hospitals were to have a separate status with Boards of Governors and direct financing from the Ministry. This was to protect their special responsibilities for teaching.

The local authorities, counties and county boroughs were to be concerned with providing domiciliary, environmental and preventive services under the authority of the Medical Officer of Health (MOH) in each area. They were also to provide ambulances.

General practitioners (GPs), and other professionals, dentists, opticians, pharmacists were under a separate form of administration. Executive Councils, rather similar to the then existing insurance committees were to be established over the same geographical areas as local authorities, and with a mixture of lay and professional people appointed to 'manage' the contractor services. GPs essentially continued to practise independently. They determined where and how they worked, from what kind of premises and within what kind of organisational structure, single-handed or with partners. Their only obligation was to remain within the terms of their contract with the NHS which was broadly concerned with providing care twenty-four hours a day, at practice premises or the patient's home. The 1946 Act sought to encourage the development of health centres, where the premises and management were provided by the local authority and where groups of primary health care professionals could practise together but this was not mandatory. Despite financial incentives health centres were very slow to develop. It was not until the 1960s with a new generation of GPs that the health centre movement gathered any momentum.[5]

The universal principle

As well as being collectivist and comprehensive, this new health service was universalist in principle. It provided a range of health services for the whole population, free at the point of use. It has been argued that the NHS therefore embodied a set of illness rights. The use of the term rights is however unhelpful. It is more accurate to say that health services were available without charge on the determination of need by professional service providers. This, nevertheless, in terms of what had gone before was a radical new departure. Since 1911, personal health services without direct payment had been available to the insured population, according to the terms of Insurance Committees established by the 1911 National Insurance Act. By the 1940s this covered only about half the population. In general manual workers, but not their dependants, were covered by national insurance, to which they contributed on a weekly basis along with their employer and the state. This population had access to medical care, according to their insurance record and the coverage provided by their particular committee.

The 1944 White Paper which outlined the government's intention to legislate for a broadly based health service described the universalist principle in the following way: 'the availability of necessary medical services shall not depend on whether people can afford to pay for them, or any other factor irrelevant to real need . . . to bring the country's full resources to bear upon reducing ill-health in all its citizens . . . money should not be allowed to stand in the way of providing advice, early diagnosis and speedy treatment'.[6] The White Paper described the deficiencies of the existing system and this is reproduced in the document section [doc 3].

The principle of equality

The NHS Act was overtly equalitarian in its approach. Bevan argued that 'we have got to achieve as nearly as possible a uniform standard of service for all – only with a national service can the state ensure that an equally good service is available everywhere'.[7] The tripartite structure was thus intended as an administrative structure which would ensure this uniformity throughout the country. The Regional Hospital Boards were to be concerned with the planning and co-ordination of the hospital and specialist services within their regions. In relation to the general practitioners, the Medical Practices Committee was to attempt to attain a more even distribution of GPs throughout the country by designating areas as restricted, intermediate and open and to prevent further movement of GPs to the 'over-doctored' areas.

The principle of professional autonomy

Although the NHS was explicitly based on the principles of collectivism, comprehensiveness, universality and equalitarianism, the principle of professional autonomy was also central to the structure and decision-making in the NHS. Bevan fully endorsed and supported the importance of the professions in both the decision-making and the running of the service and this meant a recognition of the centrality of the medical profession to health care. 'As I conceive it,' he argued, 'the function of the Ministry of Health is to provide the medical profession with the best and most modern apparatus of medicine, and to enable them freely to use it, in accordance with their training for the benefit of the people of this country. Every doctor must be free to use that apparatus without interference from secular organisations.'[8] The existence of clinical autonomy spelt out by Bevan meant that decisions about expenditure and therefore about resource allocation within the hospitals were in effect to be made by consultants within their specialisms and by GPs in primary health care. GPs were free to prescribe and refer for further specialist care at their own discretion with few limitations. The Medical Officers of Health in the local authorities, who were not concerned with the diagnosis and treatment of individual ill-health, operated within the financial constraints of local government where decisions frequently had to be made in competition with other services. They had less scope for the operation of clinical autonomy as they were largely concerned with public health matters or attempting to further develop the support services in the community for vulnerable groups.

Quite apart from the ability to make clinical decisions within very elastic financial limits, the profession was also well represented on the management and decision-making bodies in the NHS – the Hospital Management Committees (HMCs), the Regional Hospital Boards (RHBs) and the Executive Councils. Bevan had argued in the House of Commons in 1946, while steering the Act through Parliament, 'I believe it is a wise thing to give the doctors full participation in the administration of their own profession.'[9]

The consequences of functional autonomy and the place given to doctors in the structure of decision-making have been profound and well documented by a number of writers. Eckstein in *Pressure Group Politics*, a study of the BMA, in the 1940s and 1950s, MacKenzie in *Power and Responsibility in the NHS* and Pater's recent study, *The Making of the NHS*, have all highlighted the close relationships which exist between the elite of the profession, the political leaders in Parliament and civil servants at the Ministry of Health. These relationships exist formally through the representation of the leadership of the profession, from the example the Royal Colleges or the British Medical Association, on the network of statutory and advisory committees and informally through *ad hoc* consultation and discussion. MacKenzie goes so far as to argue that overlapping membership of such committees produces a group of sixty top doctors who have decisive influence and power.[10]

Where there are well documented sources as in the case of the 1946 Act, the evidence suggests that no significant policy change takes place in health care without widespread consultations with the medical profession. Gill indeed argues that the introduction of the state finance and central accountability for health care increased rather than reduced the degree of functional autonomy and freedom to practise enjoyed by the profession. The constraints on clinical judgement of the patient's ability to pay for medical care and treatment were removed, and a place for the profession assured at different levels of decision-making.[11] The NHS Act therefore consolidated the position of the medical profession. This was particularly the case with hospital medicine where the costs were highest and where, after the 1946 Act, the state was committed to what it did not anticipate in the 1940s, the rapid and consistent expansion of scientific and technological medicine. To understand the strength of the medical profession in establishing the form and structure of the NHS it is important to examine the development of the profession during the nineteenth century, and to this we now turn.

THE RISE OF THE MEDICAL PROFESSION AND STATE INTERVENTION IN HEALTH

The medical profession and the division of labour

The practice of medicine as an occupation in the nineteenth century had an organisational structure prior to the involvement of governments in any aspect of health care. This was a structure which was primarily concerned with safeguarding the interests of different groups of medical men who provided a service for individuals requesting medical attention. The state became involved during the course of the nineteenth century in what was essentially a private relationship by granting the right to medical men, through legislation, to establish a monopoly over their area of work. The 1858 Medical Act allowed a large degree of self-regulation to the profession in establishing qualifications and developing a register. The state was drawn further into health care during the course of the nineteenth and early twentieth century in three stages. First by becoming involved through the 1834 Poor Law in making provision for the sick poor; second, by responding to the growing concern for public health by establishing local agencies to deal with threats to health in the towns and cities; and third through the 1911 National Health Insurance Act which guaranteed access to medical care for manual workers. In the process of enacting this latter piece of legislation the state entered into negotiations with a, by then, highly structured and mature profession. This had undergone the transition during the century from what Elliot calls a pre-industrial status profession to a post-industrial occupation profession; from a profession which depended on patronage to one whose authority rested on the possession of a recognised body of skill and knowledge.[12]

Up until the first quarter of the nineteenth century what could broadly be called the practice of medicine was carried on by groups of doctors, each with a differing social status. The members of the Royal College of Physicians, established in the sixteenth century by Royal Charter, were at the apex of the pyramid. This thin top-layer tended to be Oxbridge-educated in the medical classics, with little practical knowledge of medicine. They typically provided care for the rich, primarily in London. Members of the more recently formed College of Surgeons (separated from the Company of Barbers in 1745) had a more practically-based training and tried to compete with the physicians in London, while in the provinces they practised where and how they could. Members of the Society of Apothecaries whose skill lay primarily in the provision of medicines, tended to be the poor person's doctor.

These different groups on the whole derived their status from the class of their patrons and they depended on their personal reputation with particular social groups to attract custom. Medical knowledge at this period still consisted of a variety of competing theories and ideas about the causes of ill-health and the treatment of illness. There were few predictably efficacious treatments and this factor too increased the dependency of the doctor on his client.

Industrialisation and urbanisation in the late eighteenth and early nineteenth centuries brought changes in most areas of social life, including medicine. First of all there was the gradual development of what has been termed hospital medicine which was to revolutionise the knowledge-base of medical practice by the end of the century. Equally important were the changes in social structure and the role of the state which led to an increased demand from various institutions and classes for medical care. Both factors combined to enhance the position and status of the profession and to consolidate its control over medical practice.

Waddington has traced the development of hospitals which began to function as centres for the development of a scientifically-based medical knowledge in post-revolutionary France, and somewhat later in England.[13] This new knowledge was based on the three pillars of 'physical examination, autopsy and statistics'. The hospitals were a focal point for the training of doctors and thus provided a foundation for the acquisition of the two basic ingredients of professionalism: a degree of technical skill based upon scientific knowledge and a wisdom derived from experience. Not that hospitals could provide much by way of therapeutic benefit to the patient until the last quarter of the century, when anaesthetics and antiseptic surgery began to be introduced. Indeed, the conditions in hospitals were frequently so poor that the risk of cross-infection was high. As Abel-Smith observes 'some of those who did not have fatal diseases when they entered hospital acquired them after admission'.[14] Partly for this reason hospitals tended to treat mainly the urban poor. Those who could afford it not unreasonably preferred treatment in their own home from a doctor, usually a physician or surgeon, who was also based at a teaching hospital.

The growth of hospital medicine had perhaps two main consequences. First, a division of labour was maintained between different types of doctor despite the existence from the middle of the century of the 1858 Medical Act which provided a basic medical qualification, and acted as a common denominator for all those who called themselves qualified. Those who practised in the hospitals retained a higher status than general medical practitioners. There was also a difference in outlook and practice between these two groups and doctors who worked as medical officers for the public authorities. The second consequence of the growth of hospital medicine was the change it brought in the doctor-patient relationship. The client or patron no longer dominated as the knowledge-base of medicine had developed and treatment had become more effective. Jewson comments 'the new occupational standing of the clinician was matched by the emergence of a new role for the sick man, that of patient. As such he was designated a passive and uncritical role in the consultative relationship, his main function being to endure and wait.'[15] As a consequence, although there were status differences and divisions among doctors, these depended rather more on professionally-determined criteria of qualifications and training, and rather less on the social standing of the patient.

The autonomy of the profession was also increased by the growing demand for more and better medical care from all social groups.

There was a particular demand in the community for dual-trained doctors, those whose qualifications combined the skill and knowledge of the apothecary and the surgeon; the forerunner of the general practitioner. Indeed the term first began to be used in the second decade of the nineteenth century. These general practitioners treated middle-class patients who could pay and also those who had a connection with the sick clubs and friendly societies which developed in the second half of the century within the trade union movement, or other organisations representing the interests of working men and women.

The state also played a role in increasing the demand for qualified medical practitioners. The 1834 Poor Law required the appointment of a parish medical officer to look after the sick poor. This was in part to distinguish between the sick and the able-bodied pauper, which was necessary in order to apply the principle of deterrence. It led to the provision of special facilities for the sick poor and educated a generation of medical practitioners in the connection between poverty and ill-health. Much of the material collected in the Victorian Blue books on social conditions drew on evidence from these public medical practitioners.

The establishment of an agreed qualification for doctors was fraught with many difficulties and the cause of much dispute throughout the century. The crucial step in consolidating the profession's monopoly over an area of work was, as referred to earlier, the founding of the General Medical Council under the 1858 Act. The Council among other things was licensed by statute to establish the requisite training for doctors. This enabled the profession to draw boundaries around itself by keeping a register of the qualified. Figures from the Census and the Medical Directories of the period give an indication of the success of the profession in reducing competition from the unqualified. The Census of 1841 showed 30,000 doctors while the first directories twelve years later listed only 11,000 qualified practitioners.[16] The establishment of a general qualification which reflected society's demand for medical care was quite compatible with status differences within the profession already mentioned. These status differences were basically about the degree of autonomy and remuneration enjoyed by the different groups and the location of their work. Hospital doctors, the physicians and surgeons, were likely to receive remuneration from the hospital or private patients. They were developing the scientific basis of medicine and were most socially and intellectually distanced from many of their patients. General medical practitioners relied on their ability to collect fees from the variety of different communities within which they practised and their degree of financial independence varied considerably. Public health doctors were employees of the public authorities. They were more like civil servants and were concerned with collective rather than individual ill-health. These differences in outlook, status and the type of medical work practised were reinforced by the 1911 National Insurance Act and the 1946 NHS Act. They still persist today and are one of the distinguishing characteristics of medical care in Britain.

A further special and persistent characteristic of British medicine, the referral system, was also established in the last quarter of the nineteenth century. An agreement was reached through the BMA and the Royal Colleges that hospital doctors would only treat patients *directly* in accident and emergency departments. In most circumstances, they would only treat patients *referred* to them by general practitioners. This was crucial in establishing a basic division of labour which was reinforced by subsequent legislation, enabling the GP, in effect, to hang on to the patient, despite the increasing specialisation in medicine and the importance of the hospital in the provision of individual medical care.

The 1911 Insurance Act: access to personal health services

The 1911 Health Insurance Act directly concerned GPs and consolidated their position. The Act provided a limited amount of medical care, initially to groups of working men earning under £2 per week but subsequently extended to cover other occupational categories. The scheme, a contributory one by state, employer and employee, entitled beneficiaries to free treatment and care by a GP – hospital services were not at first included. Sickness benefit, a sum to compensate for loss of earning power during sickness, was also paid. The 1911 Act is significant as a first attempt by the state to cushion a section of the working class from the costs of illness and provide for personal medical care. Parry suggests that 'the fact that doctors were well organised *prior* to the major entry of the State into the field of personal health care, was a crucial factor in the success of [GPs] in the negotiations with Lloyd George over the principles and administration of the National Health Insurance Act'.[17] GPs in essence were free to practise as they wished and received an income from the Insurance Committees. This was the position they were determined to maintain in their negotiations with Bevan in the next round of state intervention, the 1946 Act.

Preventive health policy: the nineteenth century

A quite different set of relationships governed state intervention in the area of preventive health as opposed to personal ill-health. Chadwick, in his *Report on the Sanitary Condition of the Labouring Population* in 1842 had propounded a theory of disease causation. The epidemic and infectious diseases among the poor were due, he argued, to atmospheric impurities generated by decomposing organic matter, itself the consequence of bad drainage, imperfect cleansing, inadequate water supply and defective ventilation. Chadwick's solution was to subordinate public health medicine to sanitary engineering. Medical Officers of Health were to be appointed under the Public Health Act of 1848 but their duties were primarily to implement sanitary reforms; they had to work closely with public health engineers. They were relatively isolated from other branches of the profession because of the very different orientation to health – and in public employment did not receive the financial rewards of other members of the profession. In terms of an improvement of general health, however, they undoubtedly achieved more than those practising the inadequate curative medicine of the time. This issue is discussed further in Chapter 8 but Chadwick's prescription for public health is reproduced in the document section [doc 4].

It was during the nineteenth and early twentieth centuries therefore that the functional autonomy of the medical profession was established, and the status divisions and interests within it. These were to be of major importance in the negotiations with the Government over the NHS Act in 1946 and on the final administrative compromise arrived at in 1948. This compromise reflected and protected the different interests of groups within the profession as they perceived them, and these perceptions were themselves a reflection of the profession's past experience. What still needs to be examined is the process by which this autonomous and independent profession agreed to a proposal by a Labour government that a National Health Service should be established.

We now turn, in the next section, to examine the factors which influenced public and political opinion in relation to health in the inter-war period and during the Second World War.

PERCEPTIONS OF HEALTH CARE PROBLEMS IN THE PERIOD PRIOR TO THE 1946 ACT

Rather as poverty is rediscovered, and sometimes redefined, so early death and unnecessary illness may be perceived as constituting a social problem at particular periods. This rediscovery, or redefinition becomes then, part of a political strategy for change in policy or provision, and various interest groups may attempt to put the issue on the political agenda. The concern for national efficiency in times of war has frequently been a mainspring for concern about the health of the working class. Anxiety about the state of health in recruits for the Boer War at the turn of the century caused concern for the viability of recruitment to the army. Document 5 reproduces contemporary material on this issue [doc 5]. The First World War also brought a concern about the high infant mortality rate. 'Public opinion is now keenly aroused on the existing deficiency and inefficiency of our public medical service, especially for maternity and infant welfare. There is widespread and insistent demand for improvement' wrote Lord Rhondda during the war. [18] Public opinion had been aroused too by the publication of 1915 of *Maternity, Letters from Working Women*. These had been edited by Margaret Llewelyn Davies from letters written to the Womens Co-operative Guild. The letters presented a picture of perpetual overwork, illness and suffering which was the experience of working-class women. 42.4 per cent of the mothers had had stillbirths or miscarriages. Davies, striking a curiously contemporary note, suggests that the main causes for the situation were: (1) low wages; (2) lack of knowledge regarding maternity services and of skilled advice and treatment; and (3) personal relationships between husband and wife. [19] The passage of the Maternity and Child Welfare Act in 1918 and the establishment of the Ministry of Health in 1919 show the level of concern for health in the period.

During the 1920s and 1930s there continued to be reports which revealed high levels of ill-health particularly among women which were commented upon in the reports of the Insurance Committees. The government mounted a 'Fitness Campaign' in the 1930s and the BMA issued pamphlets stressing the importance of 'positive health' and called for the prevention of disease through better housing, physical education and health education. Yet there was no agreement on whose responsibility it was to provide health services. Governments at this period were reluctant to take on any financial commitment to a more extensive system of health care. The Webbs in the Minority Report on the Royal Commission on the Poor Laws in 1904 represented the collectivist tradition. They saw a unified health service provided by local government as part of a general programme to alleviate poverty. This remained part of Labour Party policy between the wars although the two Labour governments had little chance to implement it.

The Council on Medical and Allied Services, chaired by a doctor, Sir Bernard Dawson, recommended in its report in 1920 that there should be a close co-ordination of preventive and curative services and spoke of 'the increasing conviction that the best means of maintaining health and curing disease should be made available to all citizens'.[20] It recommended a network of health centres in which services would be concentrated. The financing of such a system was not however tackled and during the latter half of the 1920s and early 1930s interest in administrative reform of health care waned. It needed a combination of circumstances, not the least of which was mobilisation for total war, to bring about the necessary public and political consensus to effect a radical restructuring of the health services.

In 1937, the influential and highly critical *Report on the British Health Services* was published by the independent research institute, Political and Economic Planning.[21] This drew together criticism of the existing pattern of health services and focused attention on the costs of ill-health to the country and to the inequalities in health status. The Report argued that the overall standard of health in Britain was low and cost the country over thirty million working weeks a year in terms of lost production. Moreover, ill-health was more serious and widespread in low income families than in the rest of the community. TB, for example, was twice as prevalent among the poor as the well-to-do. The infant mortality rate in Glasgow was 109 per thousand live births compared to 42 per thousand in Surrey. Existing health services were chaotic and fragmentary. GPs tended to practise where market forces guaranteed an income from private fees or through being included on the panel of an insurance committee or friendly society. Hospitals were provided by local authorities or voluntary bodies. Provision here reflected past philanthropy or civic pride. Document 6 reproduces the conclusion of the PEP Report [doc 6].

The inadequate nature of the health system was made very apparent to central government when planning began for the war. The first survey of hospitals undertaken since 1863 was carried out in 1938. It found that there were 78,000 beds in voluntary hospitals, 32,000 in local authority hospitals and 35,000 in isolation hospitals and tuberculosis sanitoria. These were estimated to be inadequate to meet the requirements to treat civilian war casualties and the sick and wounded from the armed forces. This survey and others revealed that the shortage of hospital beds was further compounded by an uneven distribution between different areas of the country. Even in the

London area, where many specialisms were concentrated, there were 'deficiencies in the quantity and quality in all types of accommodations in 1938'.[22] A Report on Sheffield and the West Midlands was more outspoken. 'We have seen far too many examples of dark, over-crowded, ill-equipped infirmary blocks in which the chronic sick drag out the last days of their existence with few amenities of civilised life.'[23] The PEP Report too had commented on the irrationality of the system. 'A bewildering variety of agencies, official and unofficial have been created during the past two or three generations to work for health mainly by attacking specific disease and disabilities as they occur.'

Efforts began to be made to provide appropriate facilities when in 1940 the Emergency Medical Service took over the organisation of all hospital beds as part of the war effort. Although there was no transfer of ownership the setting up of this agency was of great significance as it provided the Civil Service with the administrative experience of running a national health service and showed that such an endeavour was, in fact, possible.

The next important step forward in changing perceptions about the desirability and viability of a national health service was the Beveridge Report on Social Insurance and Allied Services in 1942. Beveridge proposed access to adequate medical care facilities as part of a comprehensive attack on the five giants standing in the way of social progress: Want, Disease, Ignorance, Squalor and Idleness. Such a broad policy approach would prevent ill-health and rehabilitate the sick after illness and so make the nation fitter and more productive. One of the stumbling blocks in discussions of proposals for an increase in state responsibility for health in the 1930s following the Royal Commission on National Health Insurance in 1926, had been the fear of the high level of public expenditure to which the central government would become committed. Beveridge however in his Report on National Insurance changed the nature of the debate. In Assumption B [doc 7] he argued that the burden and cost of ill-health on a society was born by the collectivity, irrespective of state provision of health care. It was therefore an intrinsic part of the purpose of any social security system to save the nation from these costs. 'Disease and accidents must be paid for in any case in lessened power of production and in idleness.'[24] The impact of a health service would be to reduce the overall costs of social security by making people healthier. A state-funded health service was therefore part of a package leading to greater rationality in public expenditure commitments *and* an increase in national efficiency.

Establishing the NHS

Following the publication of the Beveridge Report, the Coalition government announced acceptance of the principle of a national health service. This began what has been referred to as 'the war-time paper chase' to find a health service structure which was acceptable to professionals, politicians and other interests such as the voluntary hospitals and the local authorities. The most fundamental decision had already been taken by the early 1940s: that is that the provision of personal health services and national health service should be administered and financed by central government. The real arguments were now about the relationships between the medical profession and the state, and the extent to which different interest groups, within the profession, particularly the hospital doctors and the GPs, would accept becoming employees of the state in the interests of a unified health service administered by local government. When plans were in a general form, in 1942, there was a large measure of agreement, even from the British Medical Association. As discussions became more concrete so greater divisions of interest emerged. This was to lead to an abandonment of a unified system under local government in favour of direct accountability to the centre and a service divided into the tripartite structure described earlier.

THE SEARCH FOR A COMPROMISE

The various groups in the medical profession, the hospital-based doctors, the general practitioners and the public health practitioners had different interests. The Royal College led the specialists and consultants into the NHS and negotiations here proceeded with good will. By nationalising the hospitals, and moving away from a health service under local government Bevan won the co-operation of this section of the profession. Improvements in diagnostic and treatment techniques had, in the inter-war period, led to an increasing demand for expensive equipment. Many hospitals particularly in the voluntary sector were in a perilous financial position, so it was to the advantage of the consultants to secure a steady flow of finance and a system of regional planning. Furthermore, this group retained the right to continue with private practice, alongside NHS work. They also maintained a high degree of control over their conditions of work. Appointments, promotion and a merit awards system (which awards large salary increments on the basis of individual contributions to medicine) were controlled by this branch of the profession. The teaching hospitals too had a separate status as they were to be financed directly by the Ministry. This enhanced their position and the

27

autonomy of those working in them.

The local authorities and those who wanted an integrated service which combined curative with preventive and caring services provided under the Medical Officers of Health in the counties and county boroughs, lost out in the negotiations. This may have been due to the relative weakness of the public health doctors, as suggested by Gill[25], or, as Pater contends, a harmony of interests between the new Labour Government of 1945 and the consultants.[26] The public ownership or nationalisation of hospitals satisfied Labour Party philosophy while a stable source of finance satisfied the consultants. The voluntary hospital movement retained involvement through special boards of trustees and through lay membership of the hospital management bodies. The local government lobby was insufficiently strong to overcome these combined forces.

That left only the GPs represented by the BMA to be lured into the service. There was bitter opposition to a salaried service and organisation into health centres run by local authorities. Bevan conceded a method of payment by capitation fee for each patient and a considerable freedom to GPs to operate as independent contractors. The sale of practices was however to be stopped and a Medical Practices Committee was to be set up to attempt to get a fair distribution of GPs throughout the country. This was to be composed mainly of medical members. The role of local authorities was to be limited to building health centres where there were doctors who wished to practise from them. Negotiations dragged on however, long after the 1946 Act had been passed, and still, five months before the appointed day in 1948 there was doubt about whether the GPs would join the service. Then the trickle of those joining became a river and few, in the end, left the country to work in other health care systems. Pater comments 'there were histrionics on both sides, there were withdrawals and accusations of bad faith; but in the end, with what seemed trivial concessions the profession was persuaded to drop its intransigent attitude in what were, after all, not major questions and it was agreed to establish the service as it had been planned'[27] under the 1946 Act and the tripartite structure described in Figure 1.

AN ASSESSMENT OF THE NHS ACT

The NHS Act was undoubtedly a major political achievement. The co-operation of the medical profession had been bought at the cost of an integrated and salaried health service but this must not be allowed to cloud Bevan's achievement. His tactics of buying off the consultants and dividing the profession and gaining legitimacy through the passage of the Act through Parliament, where there was almost unanimous political support for an NHS, had paid off. An integrated health service had proved to be impossible because of the conflicting interests of parts of the medical profession and hostility to local government. A salaried service for GPs had also proved impossible to achieve because of its symbolic place in GPs' notion of their professional identity. Marmor and Thomas in an interesting study of the English, US and Swedish medical care systems argue that one of the limits of governments' power over medical care delivery is their inability to control medical payments methods.[28] Governments have to find ways around what they consider to be the disadvantages of particular payment methods to achieve their goals. In fact the capitation system of payment insisted upon by GPs proved to be to their disadvantage. In the mid-1960s they agreed to a package of basic and incentive payments which in effect guaranteed a basic 'salary'.

Although the NHS did embody radical ideas of universality, comprehensiveness, equality and collectivism it did so within a structure in which the functional autonomy of the medical profession was paramount. A DHSS Memorandum of 1970 put it in the following way:

> The health and personal social services have always operated on the basis that doctors and other professional providers of services have individual professional freedom to do what they consider to be right for their patients. Thus in each individual doctor-patient situation it is the doctor who decides on the appropriate objective and the appropriate priority. That is not to say that the department cannot impose overall constraints or influence behaviour, e.g. by the imposition of charges, but it is important to note that the existence of clinical freedom substantially reduces the ability of the central authority to determine objectives and priorities and to control individual facets of expenditure.[29]

The quotation succinctly sums up the nature of the compromise that underpinned the 1946 Act and which was to set the parameters of policy-making in the delivery of health care for the period covered by this book. It also neatly sums up the relationship between the state and the profession implicit in Alford's ideas of structured interest groups. The establishment of the NHS gave to the corporate rationalisers the responsibility and some power to determine the overall financial control of NHS spending and the determination of priorities, but made it difficult to achieve equality of access for the whole population, let alone equality of outcome of medical treatment for different classes, groups and regions. This, however, is to anticipate the discussion in subsequent chapters.

Health services as they developed after 1948 were to be primarily about the delivery of appropriate medical care. This was a consequence of both how health policy was generally perceived and of the centrality of the medical profession to decision-making. Despite the claims of the 1944 White Paper and the 1946 Act itself, 'curative' medicine has predominated. Although in the area of preventive health, vaccination and immunisation have been actively promoted, in other areas there has been greater timidity – in for example the fluoridation of water supplies. Factors *causing* ill-health such as poor nutrition and bad housing; types of personal behaviour conducive to illness such as smoking and alcohol abuse, have not been seen as central to the health service. Ironically the BMA itself in the 1930s had argued that the existing state care was a medical not a health service. This is a criticism which has continued to be made and is further discussed in Part three of this book.

The tripartite structure too made for difficulties in accommodating to the new demands on the health service which were to emerge during the 1950s and 1960s. The consultants were to dominate the hospitals, the Medical Officers of Health domain was the local authority health and welfare services while the GPs were primarily concerned with patients on their own list. This separation created problems for providing continuity of care particularly for the increasing numbers of elderly and those suffering from chronic and degenerative disease. This concern with the adequacy of the tripartite structure is discussed in Chapter 4.

REFERENCES

1. WATKIN, B., *The National Health Service: the first phase 1948–1974 and after*, Allen & Unwin, London (1978), Ch.1
2. BEVAN, A., *In Place of Fear*, MacGibbon and Kee, London (1961)
3. PATER, J. E., *The Making of the NHS*, King Edward's Hospital Fund for London, London (1981), Ch.2
4. ABEL-SMITH, B., *The Hospitals 1800–1948*, Heinemann, London (1964)
5. *Report of the Royal Commission on the National Health Service* (Chairman: Sir Alec Merrison), Cmnd 7615, HMSO, London (1979), Ch.7
6. MINISTRY OF HEALTH, *A National Health Service*, Cmnd 6502, HMSO (1944)
7. BEVAN, A., *Hansard* (House of Commons), 30 April 1946, col.45

8. BEVAN, A., *Hansard*, (House of Commons), 30 April, 1946, col. 52
9. BEVAN, A., *ibid.*
10. MACKENZIE, W. M., *Power and Responsibility in Health Care: the NHS as a Political Institution*, Oxford University Press, Oxford (1979)
11. GILL, D.G., 'The British National Health Service: professional determinants of administrative structure', *International Journal of Health Services*, **1** (4), 1971
12. ELLIOT, P., *The Sociology of the Professions*, Macmillan, London (1972)
13. WADDINGTON, I., The Role of the Hospital in the Development of Modern Medicine. A Sociological Analysis', *Sociology*, **7** (1973), 211–24
14. ABEL-SMITH, B., *The Hospitals*, *op. cit.*
15. JEWSON, N.D., 'The Disappearance of the Sick Man from Medical Cosmology 1770–1870', *Sociology*, **90** (1976), 225
16. GILL, D. G.,'The British National Health Service', *op.cit.*
17. PARRY, N. and PARRY, J., *The Rise of the Medical Profession*, Croom Helm, London (1976)
18. Quoted by BRIGGS, A., 'Making Health Every Citizen's Birthright: the road to 1946', *New Society*, 16 Nov. 1978
19. LLEWELYN DAVIES, M., *Maternity: letters from working women. 1915*, republished by Virago, London (1978)
20. CONSULTATIVE COUNCIL OF MEDICAL AND ALLIED SERVICES (Chairman: Sir Bernard Dawson) *Interim Report* (1920)
21. POLITICAL AND ECONOMIC PLANNING, *Report on the British Health Services*, PEP, London (1937)
22. These surveys are summarised in Nuffield Provincial Hospitals Trust, *The Hospital Surveys: The Domesday Book of the Hospital Service*, Oxford University Press, London (1946)
23. *Ibid.*
24. BEVERIDGE, W., *Social Insurance & Allied Services*, Cmnd 6404, HMSO, London (1942)
25. GILL, D.S., 'The British National Health Service', *op. cit.*
26. PATER. J. E., *The Making of the National Health Service, op. cit.*
27. *Ibid.*, Ch. 7
28. MARMOR, T. R. and THOMAS, D., 'The Politics of Paying Physicians', *International Journal of Health Services*, **1** (1), 1971
29. Quoted by *Report of the Royal Commission on the NHS*, *op. cit.*

Part two
POLICY ISSUES IN THE NHS

Chapter three

FROM CONSENSUS TO DISCORD: AN OVERVIEW OF
GOVERNMENT POLICIES, 1940s–1980s

This chapter seeks to provide a general background to the subsequent
chapters which develop the particular policy themes which have
persistently concerned all governments in the post-war period. Policies, taken initially at the level of statements of intent are a reflection
of government's perceptions of problems and issues to which a
response is deemed appropriate. They signify government's part in
the management of social change. However, problems of selection are
raised when looking at an issue as broad as government policies in
relation to health and the provision of health services. There is an
extensive range of policies which could be examined. Webb and
Wistow have attempted to handle the complexity by suggesting a
categorisation of issues into four different 'streams', governance
policies, resource policies, service policies and policies which attempt
to establish links and relationships with related policies in other social
service fields. This classification has influenced the order and selection of policy issues in the chapters following and needs to be
explained.[1]

Governance policies are those policies concerned with the role of
the state in general, central government in particular and the structuring of the relationship between governmental and non-governmental
bodies. They are also policies about issues relating to the organisation
and the management of such bodies. These aspects of the NHS are
dealt with in Chapter 4. Resource policies, which are those concerned
with the level and distribution of public funding, are considered
in Chapter 5. Service policies, that is policies concerned with the
identification of social need and preferred ways of meeting it, constitute the most diffuse and broad policy stream. However, governments
since the late 1950s have been particularly concerned to develop
policies to meet the needs of particularly dependent groups. These
policies are discussed in Chapter 6. Policies for dependent groups also

involve a discussion of what Webb and Wistow identify as the fourth policy stream, the relationship *between* policies in different service areas. The interconnections between the NHS and the personal social services and, indeed housing services, are particularly crucial to the effectiveness of care for dependent groups, particularly where these services aim to provide care in the community in a more domestic setting than the large acute hospital or residential institution.

The distinction made between different policy streams is, of course, only of use as a general analytical tool. In practice most policy makes implicit or explicit assumptions about the role of the state. Service policies always have resource implications, although these may be of secondary rather than primary importance. The idea of policy streams however provides a convenient shorthand to pinpoint the major thrust of a particular policy and the extent to which it is contradictory or compatible with other major policy objectives.

THE STUDY OF POLICY: THEMES OR CHRONOLOGY?

There is always a difficulty when deciding how to organise material relating policies which persist and develop over a period of time. There is a choice to be made between whether to pursue a particular theme through time which tends to lose sight of the way in which the social, economic and political climate in particular periods affects the broad spectrum of policy change, or whether to concentrate on examining the range of health policy in particular periods. For example, the unemployment of the 1930s and later the Second World War affected perceptions of problems to be solved, across the whole range of policy in those periods. Attitudes towards problems and of what was feasible or possible in terms of policy were affected across the board. However to look for the wider influences can fragment the following-through of themes over time, and the extent to which problems remain the same irrespective of the socioeconomic context in which they occur can be lost sight of.

The choice of approach is made easier in the case of the NHS as the period from 1948 to the late 1970s has been, in many respects, a period of relative consensus in relation to both health policy and the NHS. All governments and successive Ministers of Health have by and large worked within the same parameters. They have accepted as a given the NHS as established in 1948 with its emphasis on the centrality of professionally-provided personal health services. There has therefore been a consistency in the assumptions on which health policy has rested and a consistency in what have been seen as the major problems on the political agenda of Ministers of Health. A change has only occurred in the late 1970s. For this reason Part two of this book is organised around certain policy themes. There have however been 'phases' in the development of the NHS marked by a characteristic attitude or outlook and these are briefly sketched out in the next section, before examining the basis of the consensus.

PHASES IN THE DEVELOPMENT OF THE NHS

Hayward and Alaszewski, in *Crisis in the National Health Service*, suggest that a division can be made between the formative period, 1948–60, the managerial period 1960–68 and the period of reorganisation 1968–74.[2] Certainly the first years of the NHS were concerned with making the new service work. They were years of policy drift. The general direction of development in the health service whether in the hospital or local health services was the sum of local decisions which were influenced by the key service providers; the consultants in the prestige specialisms and the GPs in the community, the Medical Officers of Health in the local authorities. Ham's book on the Leeds Regional Hospital Board, *Policy Making in the National Health Service*,[3] is illustrative of this process at work in one area. The immediate concerns of the new service were seen at the time as financial rather than organisational. Successive Ministers were obsessed with the problem of rising expenditure, as it soon became clear that Beveridge's assumption that there was a fixed quantity of illness which would gradually reduce, leading to a levelling out of costs, was a fallacy.

Managerialism has tended to dominate the period from 1960–74. This was a time of expansion in terms of capital investment in new hospitals and the improvement of old; a time of the introduction of new technologies and increasing emphasis on the hospital sector. The centre, the Ministry of Health (from 1968 the Department of Health and Social Security) attempted to increase its control through measures to increase efficiency, irrespective of the political party in power. The strengthening of management was also seen as a key factor and the reorganisation of the service in 1974 was a strategy to achieve this. The bases of the managerialist ideology are spelt out more fully in Chapter 4.

In the late 1970s and early 1980s, however, there has been a marked change in government economic policy and in attitudes towards the role of the state in welfare which has affected policies in relation to the NHS and could be termed the 'period of discord'. These are discussed in Chapter 7 across a number of themes. These changes in attitudes may have profound repercussions on the NHS. Issues which a few years ago would have been unthinkable, such as an increase in privatisation and a change in the financing of the NHS now appear at least to be on the policy agenda. The next section therefore aims to examine the basis of the post-war consensus as a prelude to discussing the shift which has taken place in recent years.

THE POST-WAR CONSENSUS: 1948 TO THE LATE 1970s

The major factor in the post-war consensus in health policy was the acceptance of the NHS by the major political parties, by the structured interest groups in the NHS and by the electorate. Harold Wilson called the NHS at the beginning of the period, with quasi-religious imagery, 'the very temple of our social security system';[4] Alan Williams, a member of the Royal Commission of the NHS, referred to it in 1979 as 'the NHS we know and love'.[5] The principles on which the NHS was based, a centralised comprehensive service equally available to all in need and largely free at the point of delivery, were not seriously challenged and commanded widespread respect and affection.

This lack of political conflict served to insulate the NHS to a large extent from the vicissitudes of economic and social policies of particular administrations. Ministers of Health were thus relatively autonomous compared to Ministers of Education where, for example, differing political ideologies over comprehensive education brought greater Cabinet involvement, as well as greater changes in policy, with different governments. The relative insularity of the Ministry of Health from political controversy has been aided by its centralised structure and lack of a locally-elected tier. There was also an acceptance by decision-takers and the public alike of the importance and centrality of the hospital and acute services to health care and by implication emphasis on the medical or curative model of illness.

The persistence of policy problems in the NHS

Similar policy problems also concerned successive Ministers, in the period under review and to a large degree continue to do so. A major proportion of health service spending has always come from general taxation. 89 per cent of the national health bill in 1980 was met by the Treasury, compared to 9 per cent from NHS contributions.[6] All Ministers of Health have therefore been preoccupied with the funding of the NHS, with questions of efficiency, about how health resources are spent and whether resources are used effectively. Document 11 shows the profile of rising expenditure [doc 11].

This responsibility for funding has led to a second major preoccupation: the desire of the centre to control the periphery. Ministers and their civil servants at the Department have continually attempted to control the health authorities at grass-roots level. One of the central dilemmas of the NHS is to find the appropriate balance between centralisation and the need to be responsive to differing local circumstances. Or, put another way, the dilemma of reconciling efficient resource use and national standards of provision while reflecting differing local needs and aspirations has remained constant. Ministers in different periods have tackled the issue slightly differently but in general the trend has been towards a search for more effective controls at the centre because of the scale of NHS expenditure. In pursuing these governance and resource policies Ministers responsible for health have been beset by three major pressures identified by Crossman in 1972 as the pressures of demography, equality and technology.[7]

Since the Second World War there has been a marked transformation in the demographic structure of British society. The most significant factor as far as health services are concerned, apart from the impact of the rising birth rate in the early years of the health service with its consequences for the maternity and child health services, has been the increasing proportion of elderly people in the population. During the period from 1951 to 1981 the number of elderly people over the age of sixty-five rose by more than half,

Table 1. Estimated current expenditure per head £ cash 1979–80 for different age groups: Health and Personal Social Services (England)

	Total (all ages)	All births
Hospital and community health services	115	615
Family practitioners services	35	40
Personal social services	30	15
Total	180	670

Source: *The Government's Expenditure Plans 1982–3 to 1984–5*, Vol.II, Cmnd 8494 II, HMSO, London (1982), Table 2. 11. 4, p. 45

corresponding to a rise from 11 per cent to 15 per cent of the total UK population. Document 16 shows past and future trends [doc 16]. Elderly people are heavy users of health services accounting for about 36 per cent of NHS current expenditure during the year 1978–79.[8] Table 1, which shows expenditure per head on the Health and Personal Social Services for different age groups, indicates how heavily those over seventy-five dominate expenditure. The numbers in this age group are continuing to increase.[9] Policies to meet the needs of elderly people and other dependent groups have been emphasised by successive administrations and the attempts to establish priority for these groups are described in Chapter 6.

Inequalities in the distribution of health services have also perturbed Ministers of Health irrespective of party. The NHS came into existence with a geographical maldistribution of resources in relation to population distribution. This was a legacy from the past, of a combination of market forces, past philanthropy and civic pride. In relation to the distribution of GPs and other health care professionals, to hospitals and particular specialisms in hospitals, the south was better off than the north, the town than the country. Areas with a larger concentration of higher socioeconomic groups were better off than those with a predominantly working-class population. Specialist care for children, for the treatment of venereal disease, cancer and the practice of orthopaedics was virtually unobtainable outside London and the other large cities.[10] The 1944 White Paper had set the ideal 'every body in the country . . . should have equal opportunity to benefit from medical and allied services'. Yet existing inequalities proved difficult to eradicate and since the 1960s central government

				Age group
0–4	5–15	16–64	65–74	75+
120	50	65	220	545
30	20	30	45	80
45	40	10	45	160
195	110	105	305	785

policies have been concerned with attempting to achieve more even standards of provision nationally. These efforts are described in Chapter 5.

Crossman referred to the pressure of 'technology' and the consequences of technological change have been a further factor with which all governments have had to wrestle. This has led to a rising tide of demand for health care. 'There is virtually no limit to the amount of medical care an individual is capable of absorbing . . . the appetite for medical care *vient en mangeant*', wrote Enoch Powell in 1966 in *Medicine and Politics.*[11] He was not the first to point to this phenomenon. Dr Ffrangcon Roberts in *The Cost of Health* in 1952[12] had argued that Beveridge was wrong to assume that the demand for health care was finite and that it would fall as previously unmet needs were dealt with. Medicine, he argued, was expanding and new and more expensive methods of treatment were being developed. The result of this would not be the final conquest of disease but would only leave doctors more difficult problems to solve, those relating to the treatment and care of degenerative and chronic illness. These would be *more* prevalent as there was an increase in the numbers of people reaching old age. New and more sophisticated methods of diagnosis would also change ideas on the nature of disease and great costs would be incurred as doctors felt obliged to use all the techniques at their disposal to establish beyond doubt what their patients were suffering from. Powell's reiteration of the same point is important simply because as Minister of Health in the early 1960s his views were influential.

During the 1950s many new and potent drugs were being brought into use. The sulphonomides and antibiotics which began to be introduced in the 1930s were very widely used by the 1950s, when they accounted for half the ingredient costs of NHS prescriptions. Tranquillising drugs and new drugs to control chronic conditions such as diabetes mellitus and high blood pressure were also part of what has been termed the drug revolution of the 1950s. While these drugs could be used to keep people out of hospital other diagnostic, life-support and life-saving equipment were so capital-intensive that they could only be provided within a hospital setting. Surgical techniques were changing in relation for example, to the treatment of cancer in the 1960s; and to kidneys and hearts in the 1970s as transplant surgery developed. Chemotherapy and radiotherapy appeared to offer the hope of cure or at least the remission of symptoms in the treatment of cancer in the 1960s. Kidney dialysis had become routine treatment in the same period. Specialised diagnostic and support units were also being introduced. Pathology and x-ray units were extending the range and complexity of their services. Centralised sterile supply units developed to support surgery and other activities while intensive care units and post-operative recovery units provided a battery of equipment for life support in a variety of situations, from accident cases to premature babies. Nationally every hospital and every consultant wished to acquire the best and latest in up-to-date equipment.

Although the use of most of these services was professionally-determined their availability provided an essential ingredient to the process of raising public expectations about the contribution which medicine could make to the cure of disease, illness and disability. Advanced capitalist societies with their emphasis on work and productivity, their higher level of education, their consciousness that time spent being ill is time lost for work or leisure, have tended to place a high value on positive health. Medicine, in a sense, became a consumer good in the post-war period.

To sum up so far, it has been argued that the consensus of support for the NHS and similar perceptions of problems by ministers and their civil servants was responsible for the continuity in policy themes in health care from the 1950s to the late 1970s. These policies put considerable financial pressures on Ministers and their civil servants and policy goals were not always compatible. Decision-makers were frequently faced with a choice of striking a balance between equally desirable goals, for example between the maintenance of excellence in some medical establishments and the claims to equality of provision overall, between central control in the interests of efficiency and national standards and the need for flexibility in meeting local needs and interests. Furthermore, policies such as those concerned with meeting the needs of dependent groups or increasing financial efficiency were frequently hampered by lack of clarity in specifying objectives as well as formidable difficulties in evaluating progress. As a consequence policies were often intended to achieve some kind of accommodation with, and management of, problems rather than concerned with 'solving' them.

The second point which needs to be made in relation to the post-war consensus is a very fundamental one. This consensus rested on a rising economic growth rate for most of the period under review and a consequent general acceptance of a broadly Keynesian economic policy. Public expenditure going to the health service also steadily increased. This avoided any necessity to question the fundamental principles of the NHS. We turn now to examine the basis of the growth of public expenditure.

THE GROWTH OF PUBLIC EXPENDITURE

Judge argues that in most of the period from 1951 to 1979 Britain enjoyed historically high rates of economic growth and that this accounted for 75 per cent of the total increase in public expenditure.[13] The remainder was a result of increased taxation and a reduction in the proportion of public expenditure going to military spending. Total public expenditure increased by 15 per cent between 1951 and 1979, while social expenditure increased by 250 per cent. Table 2A below shows the share of GNP going to social expenditure, that is to

Table 2A. Expenditure and resources 1951–79 (at 1975 prices⋆)

Programme	1951 (£m)	*Share of* GNP (%)	1964 (£m)	*Share of* GNP (%)	÷ *1950* -64 (%)	1970 (£m)
Social expenditure	8,345	16.1	14,293	19.3	4.2	20,210
Defence	4,735	9.1	4,987	6.7	0.4	4,824
Roads and transport	755	1.5	2,318	3.1	9.0	2,520
Law and order	422	0.8	787	1.1	4.9	1,184
Total public expenditure	18,743	36.1	28,584	38.5	3.3	36,412
Gross National Product at factor cost	51,912	100.0	74,195	100.0	2.8	86,443

Notes: ⋆ Deflated by an index of total home costs
 ÷ Annual growth rate

Table 2B. Social expenditure 1951–79 (at 1975 prices⋆)

Programme	*1951* (£m)	(%)	*1964* (£m)	(%)	*Annual average* *1951 -64* (%)	(£m)
Social security	2,839	34.0	5,260	36.8	4.9	7,689
Education	1,880	22.5	3,837	26.8	5.6	5,300
Health and personal social services	2,068	24.8	3,063	21.4	3.1	4,384
Housing	1,478	17.7	2,040	14.3	2.5	2,586
Employment	80	1.0	93	0.7	1.2	251
Social expenditure	8,345	100.0	14,293	100.0	4.2	20,210

Note: ⋆Deflated by an index of total home costs
From: *Public Expenditure and Social Policy* (ed. A. Walker), Heinemann (1982) Table 2.1 and 2.2, pp. 28 and 30; CSO (1980)

social security, education, health and personal social services, housing and employment at different dates, and the average percentage annual growth rate between different periods. The highest average annual growth rate was between 1970 and 1974 when social expenditure rose by 6.8 per cent annually over the period. This had fallen to 2 per cent between 1974 and 1979.

The share of social expenditure going to the health and personal social services has also increased. Table 2B indicates that, aside from social security spending, which took the largest share of social spend-

Share of GNP (%)	÷1964 -70 (%)	1974 (£m)	Share of GNP (%)	÷1970 -74 (%)	1979 (£m)	Share of GNP (%)	÷1974 -79 (%)	÷1951 -79 (%)
23.4	5.9	26,327	27.3	6.8	29,118	28.3	2.0	4.6
5.6	-0.6	5,086	5.4	1.8	5.675	5.5	1.8	0.6
2.9	1.4	3,273	3.4	6.8	2,138	2.1	-8.9	3.8
1.4	7.0	1,553	1.6	7.0	1,814	1.8	3.2	5.3
42.1	4.1	44,478	46.2	5.1	46,815	45.6	1.0	3.3
100.0	2.6	96,368	100.0	2.8	102,717	100.0	1.3	2.5

1970 (%)	Annual average 1964 -70 (%)	1974 (£m)	1974 (%)	Annual average 1970 -74 (%)	1979 (£m)	1979 (%)	Annual average 1974 -79 (%)	Annual average 1951 -79 (%)
38.0	6.5	8,687	33.0	3.1	11,590	39.8	5.9	5.2
26.2	5.5	6,194	23.5	4.0	6,320	21.7	0.4	4.4
21.7	6.2	5,762	21.9	7.1	6,639	22.8	2.9	4.3
12.8	4.0	5,348	20.3	19.9	3,821	13.1	7.0	3.5
1.2	18.0	336	1.3	7.6	748	2.6	17.4	8.3
100.0	5.9	26,327	100.0	6.8	29,118	100.0	2.0	4.6

ing, health and personal social services took over from education as the second highest spenders in percentage terms in 1979. Furthermore these services have sustained a higher average annual growth rate than education since the mid-1960s: 6.2 per cent compared to 5.5 per cent between 1964 and 1970; 7.1 per cent compared to 4.0 per cent between 1970 and 1974 and 2.9 per cent as compared to 0.4 per cent between 1974 and 1979. Document 7 shows diagrammatically an increase in health and social service spending and the distribution between sectors [doc 7].

This favourable position of relative growth has helped to sustain support for the NHS. Conversely, the relatively lower growth rates in the 1970s together with other political and social factors have radically changed the context of health care policy in the late 1970s and early 1980s.

THE CONTEXT OF HEALTH CARE IN THE LATE 1970s AND 1980s

The slower growth rates since the mid-1970s have broken the dominant economic assumption of the post-war period which rested on the view that public expenditure could be manipulated, usually in an upward direction, to achieve economic and social progress. The high levels of inflation, the oil crisis of 1974 and the increase in the extent of government borrowing have helped to shift attitudes towards welfare spending. This has come to be seen as a public burden by, for example, Bacon and Eltis who argue that high levels of taxation and public borrowing have pre-empted investment in the private sector.[14] Monetarist as opposed to Keynesian economic ideas have been translated actively into public policy by the 1979 Conservative government although from the mid-1970s there were relatively ineffectual attempts by Labour governments to reduce public spending.

Conservative Party monetarists clearly see public expenditure as lying at the heart of Britain's economic difficulties. It is argued that growth rates must be improved before welfare services can likewise be improved. In its reply to the Select Committee on the Social Services in 1980 the Conservative government argued that economic policy must take priority over social policy. 'In a time of low economic growth there is an absence of resources . . . it is no use having a bleeding heart if you haven't got the money to pay for it.'[15] Thus the attainment of economic goals is given priority over social policy goals.

This explicit ranking of policy priorities has had repercussions on a variety of policies affecting the NHS – on the governance, resource and service policy streams. Private health care has grown with implicit central government support. Alternative ways of funding the NHS are being explored. A larger contribution from the voluntary sector is expected, particularly in relation to the care of dependent groups. Health is being increasingly defined as the responsibility of individuals and families rather than the state. There are signs of a retreat from aiming at national standards of provision in favour of delegating choices in the sharing of reduced resources to health authorities at the periphery, the new District Health Authorities (DHAs) and Family Practitioner Committees (FPCs). A fuller discussion of the implications of recent policies is given in Chapter 7.

The greater divergence of political attitudes towards public spending in the face of low or nil growth rates in the economy is just one aspect of the greater uncertainty in relation to the NHS. The largely curative approach of the NHS has come under attack, and greater stress has been placed on the need for prevention. The need for care as opposed to cure has also been emphasised. The debates about the causes of ill-health and critiques of health services in industrialised societies and the NHS in particular are discussed in Part three of this book. It is interesting however to turn to the Royal Commission on the NHS, written at the end of the 1970s, for this highlights three areas of increased uncertainty and concern.

THE GROWTH OF UNCERTAINTY: THE ROYAL COMMISSION ON THE NHS

The Royal Commission outlines the objectives of the NHS and it is instructive to compare these to those put forward in the White Paper of 1944. The summary of the NHS Bill in 1946 [doc 2] described the function of the Ministry of Health as being 'to promote a comprehensive health service for the improvement of the physical and mental health of the people of England and Wales and for the prevention, diagnosis and treatment of illness'. By 1979, the aims and objectives of the services were seen to be more complex and problematic, needing greater elaboration than simply the provision of a range of services.

The objectives are reproduced in full in document 8 but a shortened list of objectives is the following:

We believe the NHS should:
encourage and assist individuals to remain healthy;
provide equality of entitlement to health services;

provide a broad range of services at a high standard;
provide equality of access to these services;
provide a service free at the time of use;
satisfy the reasonable expectations of users;
remain a national service responsive to local needs.

The emphasis on providing services and improving access to them remains but there is a new emphasis on encouraging and assisting individuals to remain healthy.

The maintenance of health becomes not merely a technical question of providing services but of changing people's attitudes and behaviour. There is an implicit recognition that people's health may have something to do with the way they live and that they therefore have a role to play in the preservation of health. This touches on the vexed question of the degreee to which individuals have the ability to control their way of life and the environment in which they live and the responsibility of the state for ordering society in such a way that hazards to health are minimised. The argument is developed further in Chapter 9. The Royal Commission in this objective clearly seeks to highlight individual responsibility with the state playing an educative role in enabling the individual to become a more informed consumer. There is also a recognition in the Royal Commission's list of objectives that health needs may differ between regions, or groups of users and that simple provision of equal services, nominal equality, may be insufficient to meet these needs. Positive discrimination may be necessary to meet need but a careful elaboration of priorities and explicit and deliberate policy initiatives will be necessary to achieve this goal.

A second area of increased uncertainty which the Royal Commission identifies is the concern for efficiency and effectiveness in health services. Although it was argued earlier in the chapter that all Ministers for health have been concerned with this issue it becomes an even more pressing problem as resources are reduced in real terms compared to demands and needs. The Royal Commission points out that there is no simple summary measure of efficiency in the health service because of the fundamental problem of defining and measuring the outcomes of health care. There are crude indicators of efficiency, such as the average length of stay in hospital and the numbers of patients treated per hospital bed but these give little indication of the outcomes of health care.

Worsening industrial relations were also a matter of concern for the Commission and have continued to be so in the early 1980s.

During the 1970s virtually every group of workers in the health service took some kind of industrial action against their employers. The withdrawal of labour was also increasingly used as a bargaining strategy in disputes about pay and conditions of service. This, it could be argued, reflected a worsening of industrial relations in Britain generally. The effects on the NHS, however, if industrial action continued in the 1980s, could be profound. It is the largest employer in the country employing nearly one million workers. The NHS has been regarded as a great achievement for the values of community, equality and fraternity; therefore industrial action which underlines the dichotomy of interest between employees in the NHS and the care and treatment of patients must inevitably be damaging to the NHS as an institution. The Royal Commission points out that the visibility of strikes in the NHS is greater than other areas of public life because of the potential threat to life. In terms of the numbers of working days lost through industrial action, the only readily available measure of the success or failure of industrial relations, the NHS compares favourably with other workers generally. However the number of stoppages and days lost have increased markedly in the last decade.[16]

FINAL COMMENT

Worsening industrial relations are undoubtedly related to lower growth rates, inflation and government attempts at economic management. Wage freezes or ceilings at a time when living standards are perceived to be falling exacerbate divisions between groups of workers in terms of pay and conditions, particularly where freezes or ceilings appear to operate only at the lower levels. Trade union membership has increased in the NHS and all groups from consultants to ancillary workers have prepared to take industrial action.

The NHS has become more difficult to manage during the second half of the 1970s. Its relationship with government is more uncertain than at any time in its history. The worsening economic climate has exacerbated the difficulties of running the service and the radical reorganisation in 1974 and the subsequent reorganisation in 1982 have also created considerable uncertainty. This uncertainty is compounded by a greater diversity of views on priorities in health policy and radical critiques of health care. These changes in attitudes and ideology have had repercussions in all areas of policy and provision and will be taken account of in the discussion of policy themes in subsequent chapters.

REFERENCES

1. WEBB, A. and WISTOW, G., *Whither State Welfare? Policy and Implementation in the Personal Social Services, 1979–80,* Royal Institute of Public Administrators, London (1982), Ch. IV

2. HAYWOOD, S. and ALASZEWSKI, A., *Crisis in the Health Service.* Croom Helm, London (1982), Ch. 2

3. HAM, C., *Policy-making in the National Health Service. A Case Study of the Leeds Regional Health Board,* Macmillan, London (1981)

4. Quoted by BRIGGS, A., 'The Achievements, Failures and Aspirations of the NHS', *New Society,* 23 Nov. 1978

5. WILLIAMS, A., *Health Service Objectives,* Kings Fund Project Paper 10, Kings Fund Centre, London (1980)

6. OFFICE OF HEALTH ECONOMICS, *Compendium of Health Statistics 1981,* Office of Health Economics, London (1982)

7. CROSSMAN, R.H.S., *A Politician's View of Health Service Planning: 13th Maurice Bloch Lecture,* University of Glasgow, (1972)

8. OFFICE OF HEALTH ECONOMICS, *Compendium of Health Statistics, op.cit.*

9. *The Government's Expenditure Plans 1982–3 – 1984–5.* Vol. II, Cmnd 8494, HMSO, London (1982), p. 44

10. PATER, J.E., *The Making of the National Health Service,* King Edward's Hospital Fund for London, London (1981), Ch. 1

11. POWELL, E., *A New Look at Medicine and Politics,* Pitman Medical, London (1966)

12. ROBERTS, F., *The Costs of Health,* Turnstile Press, London (1952)

13. JUDGE, K., *The Growth and Decline of Public Expenditure* in *Public Expenditure and Social Policy. An Examination of Social Spending and Social Priorities,* ed. Alan Walker, Heinemann Educational, London (1982)

14. BACON. R., and ELTIS, W., *Britain's Economic Problems,* Macmillan, London (1976)

15. Reply by the Government to the 3rd Report from Social Services Committee. Session 1979/80, Cmnd 8086, HMSO, London (1980), p. 2

16. *Report of the Royal Commission on the National Health Service* (Chairman: Sir Alec Merrison), Cmnd 7615, HMSO, London (1979)

Chapter four

THE SEARCH FOR CONTROL: THE NHS AND ITS ORGANISATION

When Aneurin Bevan presented his plans for creation of the NHS it was opposed in Cabinet by Herbert Morrison the Lord President of the Council and a champion of local government. If the new regional and local management boards were to be subject to the Minister's direction in all matters of policy then they would be 'mere creatures of the Ministry of Health, with little vitality of their own'. Yet Morrison pointed out 'it is difficult under a state system to envisage the alternative situation in which in order to give them vitality, they are left free to spend Exchequer money without the Minister's approval and to pursue policies which at any rate, in detail, may not be the Minister's, but for which he would presumably be answerable'.[1]

This dilemma of control over both spending and policy in the NHS lies at the heart of the discussions which have taken place almost from its inception about the organisation of the service and raises issues of the 'governance' stream of policy, that is the relationship between the state, through central government, and the health authorities providing services. Bevan argues that although the new boards would be 'agents' of the Department

> . . . it is precisely by the selection of the right men and women to serve on these bodies that I hope to give them substantial executive powers, subject to broad financial control, and so prevent rigidity. Admittedly this is a field in which there is room for development in the technique of government, but the problem that will arise should not be incapable of solution.[2]

In the event, the relationship between the centre and the periphery in the NHS has been resolved with a different emphasis in various periods depending on the attitude and philosophy of central government. The 'techniques of government' have developed and changed during the evolution of the NHS. After an initial *laissez-faire* period, the general tendency has been for the Ministry of Health and later the

Department of Health and Social Security to attempt to increase its control over authorities at the periphery. The reasons for this have been consistent with the aims of Aneurin Bevan, the concern to achieve national standards of provision, more effective health services, to control the levels of expenditure and to achieve efficient use of resources. This chapter aims to deal with the first two of these issues while the third is discussed in the next chapter which deals with resource allocation policies over the period. There have been various strategies and policies adopted to improve standards of provision and to make health services more effective. Efficacy is a concept which has been used in different ways. Effectiveness in terms of value for money is explored in the next chapter, but during the 1960s and 1970s, the concern for a more effective health service centred on three main issues, the disadvantages of the tripartite structure, the need to plan the development of services and the need to improve the management of the service. We can begin by looking at the tripartite structure which was the result of the compromise reached between different groups of doctors and the state in the negotiations over the health service structure in the mid-1940s.

THE QUESTION OF UNIFICATION OF THE TRIPARTITE STRUCTURE

In 1948 England had been divided into thirteen regions with Wales as a region in its own right. The regions were of different sizes and shapes to accommodate the principle that each region should be linked to a university with a medical school. London was cut into four, extending outwards from central London to the coast and the Midlands. The Regional Hospital Boards (RHBs) were to plan for the hospital and specialist services in their area while the Hospital Management Committees (HMCs) were to run a large hospital or group of hospitals. There were 388 groups within the regions. The Boards were composed of professional and lay people from very different administrative backgrounds and experience, often from the voluntary or local authority hospitals. They had to learn to work together to run the new service. There were less dramatic changes for local authorities which continued to develop and fund from the rates the health and welfare services for which they had previously been responsible. GPs also continued to work much as they had done before the Act.

The greatest changes took place in the next decade in the hospital service. Each hospital was eager to acquire its own share of specialist consultants and the expanding medical technology. In the 1950s there was little or no attempt to plan or rationalise these developments by central government. The Minister and his civil servants allocated funds to the regions on the basis of expenditure in the previous year. The regions planned the service and allocated funds according to the dictates of local medical politics, a process which Ham has described for the Leeds region.[3] Teaching hospitals received separate funding and thus retained a privileged status. The share of NHS expenditure taken by the hospital sector rose consistently from the 1950s onwards as is indicated in Tables 2A and 2B.

A major problem was the lack of linkage between the three arms of the service which would of course have been avoided had they been integrated under local government control. As it was, the three branches of the service were administered according to entirely different criteria and policies. The boundaries of the Hospital Management Committees bore no relationship to those of the local health authorities in counties and county boroughs. This made for difficulties in maintaining operational continuities in patient-care particularly as local authorities ran the ambulances. Continuity of patient-care between the GP and the hospital and the GP and the domiciliary nursing, home help and social work services, rested almost entirely on personal initiatives of the professionals involved.

The weaknesses were discussed in the Guillebaud report in 1956.[4] The committee had been set up in 1953 to enquire into the costs of the NHS, and published their report three years later. Although some deficiencies were acknowledged, the committee as a whole felt it was not practicable to make changes in the organisation of the service at that stage. One member of the committee, however, Sir John Maude, expressed reservations. He attacked the tripartite division of responsibility as he believed that the administrative structure had a clear impact on the quality of service provision:

> The mischiefs to which the division of the service gives rise fall broadly under two heads (a) the administrative divorce of curative from preventive medicine and of general medical practice from hospital practice and the overlaps, gaps and confusion caused thereby and (b) the predominant position of the hospital service and the consequent danger of general practice and preventive and social medicine falling into the background.

His solution was the 'Morrisonian' one of transferring administrative responsibilities to local government – a view quite out of tune with the political thinking of his time and quite unrealistic given professional prejudices and the difficulties of financing the health service out of local rates.

However the argument that the health service should have a more unified structure persisted. The Cranbrook Report on the Maternity Services in 1959 was highly critical of the division of responsibility between the local authority and hospital maternity services. It saw the twin dangers of wasteful overlap as GP/hospital/and local authority carried out the same procedures or failed to provide ante- and post-natal care altogether as assumptions were made that services were being provided by one of the other agencies involved. This report was one of a number in this period which placed great emphasis on improving access to services and continuity in care as a way of improving their effectiveness. The Committee recommended an improvement in co-ordination of policies and co-operation between the three branches of the services and suggested particular procedures to facilitate this.[5]

The passage of the 1959 Mental Health Act made more urgent a structure which facilitated greater co-ordination of policies between hospital and local authority and encouraged co-operation between those providing care for the same individuals and families. The Act followed the Report of the Royal Commission on the Law relating to Mental Illness and Mental Deficiency which recommended the development of care in the community for the mentally ill as a more humane and cheaper alternative to care in a mental hospital.[6] Changes in methods of treatment had already altered the average length of stay in hospital for mentally ill patients quite dramatically. If community based services were to develop successfully, then planning and provision of services needed to take place between those running hospitals and those providing services outside, both in local authorities and general practice.

A change in the structure of services rested on the willingness of the medical profession to contemplate change and the Porritt Report of 1962 suggested that at least the leaders of the profession were sufficiently concerned about the problems of the tripartite structure to contemplate reforming it. The report was the work of a committee composed of representatives of the medical profession and conducted independently of the Ministry of Health. It suggested a form of unified administration of the three branches of the service under Area Health Boards. Although not worked out in detail, it did indicate that the profession accepted in principle the need for greater integration.[7] However it was to take another decade and another 'paper chase' to reach a compromise which was both feasible and acceptable to bring about the reorganisation of 1974.

THE AGE OF REFORM

Meanwhile reform was in the air. The 1960s was a period of rapid economic growth and there was an optimism about the possibilities for change and improvement of institutions and services. There were several major commissions and committees of enquiry which recommended radical changes in the structure of institutions. The Herbert Commission in 1960 led to the reform of local government in London. The Redcliffe-Maude Commission made recommendations for the restructuring of local government in England as a whole in 1968. The Seebohm Committee on the Personal Social Services was followed by the Social Services Act of 1970 which established the social service departments and centred social work in local government. The overhauling of the civil service followed the Report of the Fulton Commission in 1968.

Major constitutional change through the devolution of power to regions was also on the agenda. Reform of the NHS was part of this process of change, indeed it was planned to dovetail with changes in the organisation of social services and to coincide with the reform of local government. Both took place on 1 April 1974. There had also been a regrouping of departments and functions in central government to create a social service ministry, the Department of Health and Social Security, under Richard Crossman, in 1968. This was to be responsible for personal social services, health and social security.

Before looking at the reorganisation, however, it is informative to look at the other policy initiatives from the Ministry of Health in the 1960s and the attitudes and values which lay behind them, for in this period there was the growth of what has been called 'managerialism'. The more rapid rate of growth in the 1960s had led to the expansion of services fuelled by the pressures of demography, equality and technology referred to in the previous chapter. As the responsible Ministry the Ministry of Health became concerned to control and rationalise expansion. It introduced 'planning' into the NHS and in a number of ways attempted to improve management. The 1974 reorganisation was a logical extension of this process of increasing central control to ensure efficiency and national standards through greater integration, better management and planning. Managerialism amounted to what was described in the introduction as a policy paradigm, a set of assumptions about the way the world works and a guide to intervention.

What is 'managerialism'?

The common stock of ideas and assumptions on which managerialism was based included a number of characteristic ideas outlined by Haywood and Alaszewski in their book, *Crisis in the Health Service*:[8]

1. There was a belief that organisational change could be used as a

strategy for 'improving' service provision. Changes in structure would bring about improved access to better quality services because they would be better managed. Co-ordination of policies between different aspects of the service in hospital and community would facilitate co-operation between the different professions involved in care. The increase in specialisation in health care had, of course, exacerbated this problem.

2. There was an assumption that larger units of organisation would bring economies of scale and thus be more efficient. Efficiency was more important than easy access to services by patients or families.

3. The problems of managing local government, personal and social service departments, the NHS, hospitals, were believed to be similar to the management problems of any business organisation. Previously health care organisations had been seen as unique and totally different from other types of complex organisation. 'The absolute value given to the preservation of life, the presence of pain and death, the care rather than the cash relationship between provider and patient and the vocational element in employment were all seen to preclude managerial models.' This was replaced by the Brunel approach of ignoring the human aspects of organisation and concentrating on the mechanics. 'For our purposes the patient is not part of the organisation', they suggested.[9]

4. The principles of economic rationality were believed to be applicable to social service organisations, in terms of the efficient use of resources and a division of labour between management and the providers of professional services.

5. Planning was seen as a neutral tool. Targets could be set and progress made towards them. Parston suggests that planning was seen 'basically as a methodology, a set of procedures applicable to a variety of activities aimed at achieving selected goals by a systematic application of resources in programmed quantities and time sequences designed to alter the projected trends and redirect them towards established objectives'.[10]

These ideas which took a mechanistic approach to the organisation of health care were manifest in a number of policies during the 1960s and early 1970s. They were first applied in terms of attempting to plan for national standards and resource use in the most capital intensive area of the health service, the hospital service. This was allowed to expand rapidly during the period.

The Hospital Plan 1962

The Hospital Plan[11] laid down bed norms, a standard for the number of beds per population in the different sectors. The Minister of Health, who was then Enoch Powell, was concerned with the cost of hospital care. It was the area where costs were rising fastest, where provision was most uneven, both in terms of beds per population and the use of those beds, and where the element of capital investment was the greatest. Britain's hospitals were old and in a poor condition. Investment had been low, and limited mainly to additions to existing hospitals and the expansion of out-patient facilities. The belief was that beds could be used more efficiently by reducing the average length of stay and new buildings would ensure a better distribution of beds. The Plan was based on a region by region review of the country's hopsitals and on a series of estimates of the appropriate ratio of beds to population in the main specialties. The Plan envisaged a reduction in beds in most specialisms: acute medicine from 3.9 per 1000 to 3.3; mental illness 3.3 to 1.8 per thousand; mental subnormality remained constant and the numbers of maternity beds were to be increased from 0.48 to 0.58. The assumption was that by 1970 80 per cent of births would take place in hospital. The Plan proposed a massive new investment by building ninety new hospitals and modernising others.

The Hospital Plan did signal a hospital building programme which carried on until the 1970s although at a rate which was modified in the mid-1960s. New hospital building proved to be more expensive and slower than had been envisaged. David Owen was to write in 1978 'the hospital building programme in 1972/73, like so much expenditure in this country, was completely out of control. Even if Britain had been able to sustain the rate of economic expansion the forward planning of hospitals was completely unrealistic.'[12] These problems were partly due to inflation and partly due to the rigid and inflexible control which the Ministry of Health and later the DHSS kept over standards and costs in the building programme. The Hospital Plan provided a 'rational basis' for the development of the hospital service. It also reinforced the dominance of the hospital sector and therefore acute medicine in the NHS. The Plan affected too the funding of the new health authorities after 1974. The revenue consequences of the new building made it more difficult to implement the policy of resource allocation to the poorer regions discussed in the next chapter. It is politically difficult not to fully open and use new hospitals. The running costs of many of the new facilities were also to be very high, which was not forseen in the optimistic 1960s. It is more expensive to clean and heat a modern open-plan hospital, for example, than the traditional oblong ward with beds in serried ranks.

The concept of the District General Hospital

The concept of the District General Hospital (DGH) was also part of the move towards greater efficiency through larger units of operation. The Hospital Plan promoted a movement towards district general hospitals with 600-800 beds serving a population of 100,000 to 150,000 and providing treatment and diagnostic facilities for both in-patients and out-patients in *all* the commoner specialisms. This included both geriatric beds and some beds for the mentally ill. It was believed that there should be a greater integration of the mentally ill into the main stream of hospital provision as this would improve standards of care and help reduce the length of stay. However, most weight was given to the importance of bringing a wide range of facilities together in the interests of service *providers* both professional and administrative. It was believed that larger hospitals could bring significant economies of scale.

The committee on the functions of the District General Hospital (the Bonham Carter Report) in 1969[13] supported the view that larger hospitals covering all specialisms including a full complement of geriatric and psychiatric services should be developed. Again the report is interesting because it puts an emphasis on the needs of *providers* of health care. The assumption was that no consultant in a specialism should have to work on his own and that for each speciality there ought to be at least two consultants with appropriate supporting staff. This meant even larger hospitals than envisaged by the Hospital Plan. Hospitals with 1,000 beds and serving populations of about a quarter of a million people were proposed. Implicit in the notion of the district general hospital was the idea of self-sufficiency. The view was that people in each hospital catchment area should have access to a range of specialisms. This benefit was said to outweigh the disadvantage of longer travel for some patients and their visitors. As a result of the Hospital Plan and the Bonham Carter Report many small hospitals were to close and there was opposition to this over the years, in areas where communications were difficult or where there was a particular attachment to a local hospital.

During the 1970s there was a modification of the District General Hospital policy in the face of concern over escalating costs, a growing awareness of the disadvantages of overcentralisation and the greater emphasis on the convenience of patients. The idea of community hospitals, small local hospitals combining the facilities of a primary health care centre with accommodation for selected in-patients, out-patients and day patients, was developed and implemented in some areas. Community hospitals, as well as helping to bridge the chasm between hospital and community were thought to be particularly appropriate to rural areas. David Owen, as a junior Minister of Health in 1976 endorsed the development of community hospitals and ex-pressed the hope that they would be organised in old inner city hospitals as well. He introduced too the concept of the 'nucleus' hospital. This was based on the principle of developing hospitals in blocks or phases around a basic core.

Hospital planning has thus become less dogmatic and more flexible following the reorganisation of the health service and the waning of the influence of managerialism. Restrictions on capital spending and uncertain future growth in the 1980s has, perforce, brought a more pragmatic approach which is mirrored in the Consultative Document produced in 1980 by the DHSS on the Future Pattern of Hospital Provision in England.

The Health and Welfare Plans

Another excursion into planning in the 1960s was the Health and Welfare ten year plan. [14] Health and welfare services were of course at this time provided by the local authorities and the plans were simply an aggregation by the Ministry of Health and the local authorities' guestimates of what they thought they could achieve within the period. There was no attempt at the time to ensure any compatibility between the hospital and health and welfare plans. This had impli-cations particularly for the mental illness services where the reduction in beds was not compensated for in any coherent way by the local authorities' plans for more community-based care. Conversely local authority plans showed a planned increase in the number of com-munity midwives at a time when the hospitals were attempting to increase the bed provision for maternity cases.

Both the hospital and health and welfare plans were revised in the mid-1960s and the process was resumed following the Seebohm re-organisation and the establishing of the Social Service Departments in 1970. Local authorities were asked to prepare plans covering their personal social service capital and revenue programmes for the period from 1973 to 1983. The department's circular stated that their intention was to create 'both for the health authorities and the local authority services, arrangements for forward planning which would enable them to draw up their plans in relationship to one another and enable local government and central government jointly to review at regular intervals, the developments of the services and determine the best use of resources'.[15]

Webb and Falk argue that although this was the stated intention of the circular, this was virtually impossible in the short time given to produce the plans, from September until March.[16] The very detailed categories for which expenditure estimates were required precluded the calculation of other data. This resulted, in their view, in a set of 'feverishly concocted trend plans'. What was new about these plans was the inclusion of a set of guidelines for levels of provision. These, like bed norms, were based on a mixture of existing trends and views about good practice.

Planning for service development during the 1960s and 1970s led to a gradual improvement in techniques and although planning was a great deal less 'rational' an exercise than at first believed, it may have provided for a kind of 'social learning' in enabling the agencies providing health and social services to know more of the intentions and constraints operating within the different policy environments of health and social services. Rather than being an 'end' in themselves plans became the beginning of a process of dialogue about relative levels of provision at a local level.

Managerialism and the professions in the NHS

It began to be recognised in the 1960s and early 1970s that the workforce in the NHS was continuingly increasing in size and in complexity in terms of the division of labour. To illustrate, in 1949 the total number of staff employed in the NHS in England was approximately 400,000 but by 1980 there had been a two-fold increase to 822,390.[17] If Scotland and Wales are included then the NHS employed almost one million workers or 4 per cent of the population. It was, and is, the largest civilian employer in the country.

There has been since the 1940s an increasing division of labour within medicine and other professions into different specialisms. There are, for example, many more paramedical professionals employed by the NHS; speech therapists, occupational therapists, chiropodists, physiotherapists, radiographers, for instance. Nursing too has developed specialisation in particular kinds of work, some of which are based on different training, others on work experience. Nurses are by far the largest group of staff employed by the NHS and have grown steadily. Their numbers doubled between 1949 and 1979 and by 1980 they comprised 37 per cent of NHS manpower. [18]

One response to this increasing complexity and size of the NHS labour force on the part of governments and committees of enquiry, was to look to scientific management to provide a basis for organising the work of professionals and their relationship to each other. One of the early attempts at the managerialist approach was the reorganisation of nursing services in 1966, following the Report on Senior Nursing Staff Structure chaired by Brian Salmon, a businessman from Lyons, the food distributors. [19] This Committee recommended a division between managers and practitioners through the abolition of nurse matrons and their replacement by a hierarchy of nurse managers.

Under the changes brought about as a result of the Report, management became a specialist function in its own right. There were to be three levels of nursing management. The top-level managers were concerned with the making of policy while the middle and first-line managers were responsible for its execution. There was also to be a division between nurse managers and nurse teachers with the higher-ranking posts going to the former. Carpenter summarises the effect of the change:

> background and nursing knowledge are becoming less important compared with abstract managerial abilities that transcend local peculiarities and idiosyncracies. It is increasingly the case that nursing background is required less for its utility than to legitimise the position of managers over a workforce, many of whom have frustrated professional aspirations. The Salmon reform over-emphasised the importance of managerial changes in job content to the detriment of clinical changes. It created formal structures in which power, prestige and remuneration increased with distance from the point of patient contact. [20]

Carpenter also suggests that the emphasis on managerial values in nursing lies behind the increasing growth of union membership among nurses and the consequent pursuit of higher wages and improved conditions of work. On the other hand, had the changes following the Salmon Report not occurred, there would have been little preparation for the increased role in decision-making for nurse managers brought about by the reorganisation of the health service in 1974.

A similar attempt to create a managerial consciousness was made with the medical profession through the setting up of the Cogwheel Working Party which made its first report in 1967. [21] This was a committee composed of representatives of the Ministry of Health and consultants and the difference in approach between the implementation of this report and the Salmon Report is instructive. The committee represented the interests of the profession directly and was not chaired by a businessman. The strategy adopted for change was one of persuasion rather than an imposition of an entirely new structure as the case with the Salmon Report. There were two further Cogwheel Reports monitoring the degree of change and this was indeed gradual. By 1972 less than half of the large hospitals had introduced changes along Cogwheel lines.[22]

The first Cogwheel Report was concerned to encourage a more efficient use of hospital resources, greater co-ordination across specialisms and more planning of resource use over time. 'The hospital sector is the most complex, sophisticated and costly sector of the medical care services; problems of management proliferate in an organisation with many branches, many functions and many specialities: we believe that many clinicians fail to appreciate fully the importance of their role in management problems.'[23] In order to achieve greater involvement the Cogwheel Report recommended the grouping of clinicians into Firm and Divisions, with a representative Medical Executive Committee to make co-ordinative decisions in relation to the allocation of medical resources over the hospital as a whole.

The theory of the Cogwheel structure is clearer than the changes which have actually occurred as a result of it. Subsequent Cogwheel Reports suggest that consultants are reluctant to become managers of resources and studies of decision-making in hospitals carried out for the Royal Commission on the NHS in the mid-1970s indicate that individual consultants continued to make the key decisions on the use of resources. There is little evidence to suggest that these are modified to any great extent by the Medical Executive Committee.

The reorganisation of the NHS in 1974

The reorganisation of the NHS was the zenith of the managerialist phase. It was based on the notion of the essential unity of the NHS and designed to transform it into a more efficient and effective service through a change in structure, the strengthening of management and the introduction of a planning system. The process of planning for the change itself was lengthy and involved three different Ministers of Health (or as they became after 1968, Secretaries of State for Social Services) and what Watkin has called 'a sea of words'.[24] Two Labour Ministers, Kenneth Robinson and Richard Crossman, produced Green Papers in 1968[25] and 1970[26] and the Conservative Minister

Keith Joseph published a Consultative Document in 1971,[27] and a White Paper in 1972,[28] outlining the legislation which was to come into effect in 1974 to coincide with the reorganisation of local government. A number of themes run through the documents, and despite the different political persuasion of the Ministers involved, the similarities in approach are more apparent than the differences. This was in part due to a congruence of view between the different Ministers on the key issues to be tackled in the NHS and in part a consequence of the fact that any change in the NHS has to satisfy the major interest groups in health care.

There were five major objectives in the reorganisation. First, there was a wish to move away from the tripartite structure towards a more integrated service which would provide greater continuity of care and, in this sense, more effective services. Second, there was a desire to introduce greater control by the centre, the DHSS, to ensure both an efficient service and one which was effective in carrying through departmental policies, particularly in relation to evening out regional inequalities and giving priority to dependent vulnerable groups such as the elderly, the mentally ill and handicapped. Third, there was an intention to achieve an improved management structure with lines of accountability upwards to the Department and delegation of responsibilities and tasks downwards to the health authorities. Fourth, there was a concern to introduce a more democratic structure of decision-making and fifth, there was a commitment to introducing a planning system to ensure the forward planning of service provision to achieve DHSS goals and priorities at a local level. The Keith Joseph version of these intentions is reproduced in document 9.

This book does not aim to do more than sketch out the ways in which the reorganised structure sought to fulfil these objectives. Ruth Levitt has written a very detailed account of the structure in *The Reorganised National Health Service*[29] for those who wish for greater detail on the organisational arrangements. Figure 2 shows the structure of the health services after reorganisation and document 10 describes the functions of the different levels of health authority.

Administrative unification

The structure of Regional Health Authorities (RHAs) after reorganisation remained in very much the same form as the previous regions. There were still fourteen in England providing services over the same geographical areas, although their powers and responsibilities changed. They were to be responsible for the strategic planning of

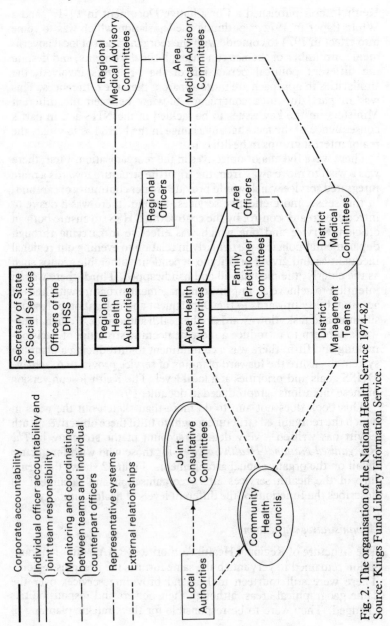

Fig. 2. The organisation of the National Health Service 1974–82
Source: Kings Fund Library Information Service.

community health service provision as well as the hospital services and related functions. An emphasis was thus placed on the planning for the distribution of specialist and other services for the region as a whole.

The Area Health Authorities (AHAs) were new. There were ninety of these, and in most cases their boundaries were coterminous with those of local authorities (the metropolitan districts and non-metropolitan counties) except in London. The areas were responsible for planning and providing a comprehensive health service, including hospitals, community and domiciliary care, the preventive and developmental health services. They were also responsible for identifying needs and managing within the resources provided for them by the RHA. They had a duty too, to provide the administration for, and collaborate with, the Family Practitioner Service, responsible for managing GPs. Thus, while the health services previously run by local authorities were taken over by the areas, the jurisdiction of the contractor services (the GPs, dentists, pharmacists and opticians) remained virtually unchanged. The Executive Councils became Family Practitioner Committees with a link at administrative level with the AHA. It had been impossible to devise a way of integrating the GPs into the new structure in England and Wales due to opposition from the professional associations representing GPs. This separation was avoided in Scotland where GPs come under the Area Boards.

The new structure sought to foster links between health and social services departments not only by making the boundaries of the health and local authorities coterminous but also by making collaboration in providing and planning for service provision mandatory. Joint Consultative Committees were established to ensure collaboration between the health and social services. Overall, the assumption of the reorganisation was that the AHAs with their broader span of responsibility would remove barriers to a 'comprehensive' view of health care.

Centralisation and priorities

Crossman had argued in the second Green Paper that reorganisation should 'ensure effective control over the money spent on the service . . . to ensure that maximum value is obtained from it'. This is a familiar theme and certainly the new structure was seen to be one in which the DHSS could control the spending of money more effectively and efficiently. It was also seen to be a structure in which the government's priorities in policy terms could be implemented. There were two major priorities. The first was the intention to reduce the extent of regional inequalities in health service provision, and the second the aim to develop 'the Cinderella' services, the services for the elderly, mentally ill and handicapped and the physically handicapped or 'dependent groups' as they have been termed in this book. In effect, this meant that the development of health services in the community for these groups was an implicit priority, in collaboration with the local authority social service departments.

The language of priorities implies that certain policies take precedence; that there is a political commitment to achieving change and that preference is to be given to the channelling of resources towards favouring some policies more than others. There were to be many difficulties in putting these priorities into effect which are discussed in subsequent chapters. The methods for achieving a shift in priorities were not developed fully until after reorganisation had taken place. The Regional Allocation Working Party (RAWP) recommended an increase in expenditure to the poorer regions at the expense of richer ones in 1976. The Priorities documents, Priorities for Health and Personal Social Services, 1976, and The Way Forward, 1977, recommended increases in expenditure on the Cinderella services.

The reorganised health service provided a framework within which the DHSS could lay down guidelines with the expectation that these would be implemented by the health authorities at the periphery; in other words it provided a framework for policy change. Crossman certainly saw the reorganisation as being primarily about social reform and he was influenced by his reading of the recent past in the NHS. In the hospital sector, the old system of Hospital Management Committees and Boards of Governors of Teaching Hospitals had done little to mitigate the unevenness in quality or quantity of health care for different regions or different care groups. There were hospitals which were very good and others which were extremely bad and Crossman's *Diaries* indicate his alarm and concern at the low level of care in some long-stay hospitals.[30] Barbara Robb's *Sans Everything* in 1967 had served to raise the level of awareness of the problem.[31] The Inquiry into Ely Hospital in 1969 revealed a horrifying story of inertia, 'an unduly casual attitude towards death and a continued acceptance of old-fashioned, unduly rough and undesirably low standards of nursing care'.[32] Other scandals and enquiries followed: Farleigh in 1971 and Whittingham in 1972. At Whittingham, the committee of enquiry accepted the allegations that troublesome patients received the 'wet towel treatment' (a wet towel was twisted round the patient's neck until they lost consciousness, and methylated spirits poured over patients' clothing and then set alight) were substantially true. The message seemed clear; there was too little public accountability and scrutiny. Standards were poor and so was management.[33] It was expected that a newly structured service with its improved management structure would complement the work of the Hospital Advisory Committee set up by Crossman to 'inspect' the long-stay hospitals, and improve standards of care.

Keith Joseph, who followed Crossman as Minister of Health, also put a heavy emphasis on management and the importance of accountability. His view was that centralisation with clear definition of tasks and roles at region, area and the operational level, the district, would ensure both efficiency, improved quality of services and a shift in priorities. He too was concerned about the Cinderella services. He commented when Secretary of State for Health and Social Services, 'This is a very fine country to be acutely ill or injured in but take my advice and do not become old or frail or mentally ill here'.[34]

Management

The new management and planning structure was to be the vehicle for achieving greater efficiency and a realisation of the government's priorities. Management teams in each authority, both region, and area, were charged with the responsibility of managing the services to meet the government's policies and guidelines. The principle was one of consensus management and was laid down in what was known as the Grey Book on 'Management arrangements for the reorganised NHS'.[35] There was to be no hierarchy in the management team. All members were to have equal status. The management team was composed of the major professional groupings in the service; the administrator, the treasurer, the nursing officer, the community physician, two elected medical representatives, a consultant from the Medical Executive Committee and a GP. At region and at area level the Area Management Team (AMT) was responsible to an appointed body of members, who were the formal executive body of the Authority. It was intended that members and the Chairman of the authority should concentrate on general policy-making and monitoring performance while the AMT had an executive and servicing role and was responsible for producing an area plan covering the separate districts.

At district level, the point at which services were actually provided through hospitals, clinics and the like, the role of the District Management Team (DMT) was rather more ambiguous. The DMT was collectively responsible for keeping district services under review, implementing area policies and its members were also individually responsible for their own sectors of work. The division of responsibility between area and district was muddled and confusing.

Planning

The planning system in the reorganisation was to be, according to the White Paper explaining the changes, 'the single most important influence for better resource allocation in the service'. It was to be the way of achieving a national strategy of objectives, standards and priorities.

The planning system had three key features. First, it was applied in a standard way throughout the country. Second, it included all aspects of NHS provision and third, it involved collaboration with local authority social service departments through the Joint Consultative Committees and the public, via the newly created Community Health Councils. Whereas guidelines on policy flowed down from the DHSS to the regional level and then the area level, the actual preparation of the plans, in terms of the guidelines was done first at district level, agreed with the area and on to the region and the Department. This was the planning cycle. It also included a short and long-term dimension, that is strategic and operational planning.

There were also Joint Care Planning Teams at district level which included GPs and representatives from the social service departments for specific 'need' groups, for example the elderly or mentally handicapped, to produce information about existing provision with proposals for change. The Joint Consultative Committees at area level too were to have planning teams for particular groups for joint planning of health and social service provision.

The planning system represented, *par excellence*, a belief in rationality. It was based on the assumption that problems could be analysed, future trends predicted and a policy developed to provide for future contingencies. Planning was seen as a neutral tool, as a way of directing resources to identified priorities and needs.

Democratic accountability in the NHS

As a counterweight to the centralisation and emphasis on management accountability in controlling activities and implementing particular policies, the restructuring of the NHS did involve changes in the type and extent of democratic involvement in policy-making and decision-taking in the service. Democratic involvement of various groups in the NHS was believed to be important by both Richard Crossman and Barbara Castle who was Secretary of State for Social Services when restructuring took place in April 1974. It was seen as a way of ensuring that an organisation as hierarchical and centralised as the NHS was responsible and accountable to local needs and interests. The restructuring aimed to achieve democratic accountability in three ways; through the membership of health authorities, through the appointment of Community Health Councils and through the setting up of certain internal management and advisory structures in the service. Two principles of democracy were involved, the representational and the syndicalist. Briefly, the former rested on the selection or appointment of individuals to represent groups or communities who used the service, while the involvement of the workforce in decision-making in the service reflected syndicalist views. Crossman had believed that the old health authorities were insufficiently representative and both he and Barbara Castle tried to increase the representation of local authorities on the health authorities. Members of the new area and regional authorities were still appointed by the Secretary of State but included more elected members from local authorities than originally proposed by Keith Joseph. The universities, and the main health professions were also represented. One doctor and one nurse had to be included although these it was argued were there primarily to make policy for the service rather than 'represent' interests as such.

Community Health Councils (CHCs) were a new innovation and their role was to represent the public interest. There were to be 207 of them, one for each district of the NHS. Half of their members were to be nominated by local authorities, one-third by voluntary organisations and the rest by the regional authorities. Their composition meant representation on the basis of geographical communities and for particular interest groups of consumers of health care so that voluntary organisations for the elderly, physically handicapped or mentally ill, could have a voice on the Council. The CHC itself was to have a role in acting as a spokesman *for* the public in the planning process and as a watchdog for the people in relation to health services. The CHC had limited powers, the right to information, to access to health service facilities to inspect them and the right to 'kick up hell' if their views were ignored. Their role is discussed further in Chapter 10.

Democracy of the syndicalist variety was reflected in the representation of the professions and the trade unions on the health authorities at regional and local level and within the management structure itself. First, a network of professional advisory committees was established so that the management teams could be advised of the views of the different professional groups. Second, the management teams themselves contained members of the *major* professional groupings so that decisions could be widely discussed and information disseminated.

THE LIMITS OF CONTROL AND INTEGRATION: GENERAL PRACTITIONERS

No discussion of the reorganisation of 1974 can be complete without some reference to the role of general practitioners. This remained something of an anachronism in the carefully planned and co-ordinated structure and we must turn back to the agreement reached with Bevan in 1948 to find out why. GPs had continued since 1948 to be self-employed practitioners under contract to provide services to the NHS. Although the overall co-ordination of the contractor services and the planning of health centres became the responsibility of the AHA in 1974, in effect this important area of primary health care remained outside the administrative control of the health authorities, and operated much as it had done before despite the importance of this aspect of health care to the broader spectrum of health services.

Most patients in the NHS are treated by general practitioners. While 3 per cent of patients are cared for as in-patients, 81 per cent are dealt with wholly by GPs. Almost the entire population is registered with an NHS GP and the average person visits their GP four times a year, as compared to admission to hospital once every ten years.[36] The implication of this is that GPs can be in touch with the needs of individuals in a way which few other health workers can. General practice, because it is organised around illness in individuals, families and communities, rather than body systems and illnesses, has the potential for embracing the curative and caring aspects of medicine.

One of the problems of the organisational structure of the NHS has been that as a consequence of the contractor status (within the limits laid down by the Medical Practices Committee), GPs are free to practise where and how they choose. There are few ways of ensuring that GPs practise efficiently in areas where they are needed or are accountable for what they do. There have been spontaneous changes over the years, there has been a steady decline in single handed practices and a growth in partnerships of four or more. In 1979 15 per cent of GPs in England practised single-handed, 43 per cent in partnerships of two or three and 42 per cent in partnerships of four or more.[37]

Health centres, which were Bevan's attempt to provide a setting in which a number of health workers could practise from the same premises, were initially slow to develop. This was despite a financial incentive; local authorities would provide premises and pay part of the management costs of health centres. By 1963 there were eighteen purpose-built health centres in operation in England and Wales. By 1969, 139 were in operation, and 300 by the end of 1971. This rate of increase has continued, so that by March 1977 there were 731 centres in use providing practice premises for 17 per cent of all GPs.[38]

Integration between local authority health services and GPs developed through nurse attachment and this helped to blur the distinction as far as the patient was concerned between health centres and the larger group practice. Reedy, in a survey carried out in 1974, found that 68 per cent of practices in England had at least one attached nurse. The larger the practice the greater the likelihood of attachment.[39] It was around the nucleus of group general practice with attached workers that the concept of the primary health care team developed. The Harding Committee (1980) defined it in the following way:

> the primary health care team is an interdependent group of general medical practitioners and secretaries and/or receptionists, health visitors, district nurses and midwives who share a common purpose and responsibility, each member clearly understanding his or her own function and those of other members, so that they all pool skills and knowledge to provide an effective primary health care service.[40]

The development of the primary health care team was first recommended by the Gillie Committee in 1963.[41] The Annual Report of the DHSS in 1974 suggested that these be developed as a way of 'facilitating co-ordination and mutual support in the planning and delivering of care'.[42] It was hoped that the 1974 reorganisation would facilitate the development of primary health care teams and greater integration of GP services by establishing structures and mechanisms for planning and co-ordination. More efficient and effective systems of service delivery could then be achieved through a division of labour around general practice.

This, like many other aspects of the reorganisation, proved to be overoptimistic. Changes in structure did not alter intrinsic difficulties. As independent contractors, GPs choose their own mode of operation, their patients and the geographical area over which they practise. Attachment, the primary health care team, brought GPs into relationship with the organisational structure of community nurses and raised questions of the management and the leadership of teams.

Nursing and other staff and doctors tended to operate in different social, professional and organisational worlds, so there were difficulties in establishing efficient ways of working.

There is little information on the working of primary health care teams or their effect on the delivery of care just as there is little information on the work of GPs in this respect. The Harding Committee did however find that, particularly in urban areas, nurses in the community have tended to return to a system of patch working to meet the needs of a particular population in a defined geographical area rather than around patients based on a particular practice. In one urban AHA it was estimated, for example, that 10,000 children out of a target population of 70,000 were not receiving visits when nurses were attached to GP practices.[43]

The difficulty of reconciling the different modes of organisation of health care professionals in primary health care and their varied relationship to the state remains one of the stumbling blocks in the way of operating a health service geared towards planning for, and meeting the needs of, the elderly, mentally ill and handicapped whose need for care is complex. Although different health ministers, and the 1974 reorganisation of the NHS, aimed to give priority to dependent groups and integrate the health service, general practice has remained largely autonomous. The fact that it has illustrates the capacity for survival of an existing division of labour and organisational structure and also the influence of the General Medical Services Council, a body representing the interests of GPs, and the BMA in maintaining a *status quo* in primary health care.

REORGANISATION AND ITS AFTERMATH

The years during and following the reorganisation of the NHS were years of upheaval for those working in the service for the process of reorganisation was not completed until the publication of the Priorities documents in 1976 and 1977. Yet barely two years after reorganisation a Royal Commission on the NHS was set up to enquire into the service. The Commissioners summed up succinctly the reasons for their appointment:

> We were appointed at a time when there was widespread concern about the NHS. There had been a complete reorganisation of the service throughout the UK in 1973 and 1974 which few had greeted as an unqualified success. The NHS had suffered a number of industrial disputes accompanied in some cases by at least a partial withdrawal of labour by ambulancemen, some ancillary staff, and hospital doctors and dentists. The then govern-

ment's decision to phase out private beds from NHS hospitals was being heatedly debated in the NHS, and was itself the occasion for some of the industrial action mentioned. In addition to all this, the NHS could not shelter from the country's chill economic climate in the mid-1970s, so that although it suffered no real financial cut-back it was denied the growth which it had come to expect to help it meet the rising demands made upon it.[44]

The Report of the Royal Commission, when it came in 1979 presented a different view of the NHS from the predominantly managerial model of the 1960s and 1970s. Not only was the NHS seen in a more 'organic' way but there was a shift away from the ideas of rationality in decision-making. Policy was tacitly acknowledged to involve more than the laying down of guidelines by central govern ment for implementation by the health authorities. Before examining these changes, policies for resource allocation and those for the care of dependent groups are discussed in the two following chapters. Policies in these areas were also influenced by managerialist ideas, changing ideas about priorities in health care, and the 'chill economic climate' of the mid-1970s.

REFERENCES

1. Quoted by KLEIN, R.,'Between central control and local respon-siveness: striking the balance', *British Medical Journal*, 9 Feb. 1980, p. 420
2. *Ibid.*
3. HAM, C., *Policy-making in the National Health Service. A case study of the Leeds Regional Hospital Board*, Macmillan, London (1981)
4. MINISTRY OF HEALTH, *Report of the Committee of Enquiry into the Cost of the National Health Service* (Chairman: C. W. Guille-baud), Cmnd 9663, HMSO, London (1956)
5. MINISTRY OF HEALTH, *Report of the Maternity Services Committee* (Chairman: Earl of Cranbrook), HMSO, London (1959)
6. *Report of the Royal Commission on the Law relating to Mental Health and Mental Deficiency 1954–1957*, Cmnd 169, HMSO, London (1959)
7. MEDICAL SERVICES REVIEW COMMITTEE, *A Review of the Medical Services in Great Britain* (Chairman: Sir Arthur Porritt), Social Assay, London (1962)
8. HAYWOOD, S. and ALASZEWSKI, A., *Crisis in the Health Service*, Croom Helm, London (1980)
9. Quoted in DRAPER, P. and SMART, T., 'Social Science and Health Policy in the United Kingdom', *International Journal of Health*

Services, **4** (3), 1974

10. PARSTON, G., *Planners, Politics and Health Services*, Croom Helm, London (1980)

11. MINISTRY OF HEALTH, *National Health Service. A hospital plan for England and Wales*, Cmnd 1604, HMSO, London (1962)

12. OWEN, D., *In Sickness and in Health*, Quartet Books, London (1976)

13. DEPARTMENT OF HEALTH AND SOCIAL SECURITY and WELSH OFFICE, *Report of the Committee on the Functions of the District General Hospital* (Chairman: Sir Desmond Bonham-Carter), HMSO, London (1969)

14. MINISTRY OF HEALTH, *Plans for Health and Welfare Services of the Local Authorities in England and Wales*, Cmnd 1973, HMSO, London (1963)

15. WEBB, A. and FALK, N., 'Planning the Social Services: the ten year plans', *Policy and Politics*, **3** (2)

16. *Ibid.*

17. OFFICE OF HEALTH ECONOMICS, *Compendium of Statistics 1981*, Office of Health Economics, London (1982)

18. *Ibid.*

19. MINISTRY OF HEALTH and SCOTTISH HOME AND HEALTH DEPARTMENT, *Report of the Committee on Senior Nursing Staff Structure* (Chairman: Brian Salmon), HMSO, London (1966)

20. CARPENTER, M., 'The New Managerialism and Professionalism in Nursing', in M. Stacey, *et al.*, *Health and the Division of Labour*, Croom Helm, London (1977)

21. MINISTRY OF HEALTH, *First Report of the Joint Working Party on the Organisation of Medical Work in Hospitals* (Cogwheel Report), HMSO, London (1967)

22. WATKIN, B., *The National Health Service: the first phase 1948–1974 and after*, Allen and Unwin, London (1978)

23. MINISTRY OF HEALTH, First Cogwheel Report, *op. cit.*

24. WATKIN, B., *The National Health Service, op. cit.*

25. MINISTRY OF HEALTH, *The Administrative Structure of Medical and Related Services in England and Wales*, HMSO, London (1968)

26. DEPARTMENT OF HEALTH AND SOCIAL SECURITY, *The Future Structure of the National Health Service*, HMSO, London (1970)

27. DEPARTMENT OF HEALTH AND SOCIAL SECURITY, *National Health Service Reorganisation: Consultative Document*, DHSS, London (1971)

28. HOUSE OF COMMONS, *National Health Service Reorganisation:*

England, Cmnd 5055, HMSO, London (1972)

29. LEVITT, R., *The Reorganised National Health Service* (Rev ed), Croom Helm, London (1977)

30. CROSSMAN, R., *Diaries of a Cabinet Minister*, Vol. 3, Hamish Hamilton and Jonathan Cape, London (1977)

31. ROBB, B., *Sans Everything: a case to answer*, Nelson, London (1967)

32. DEPARTMENT OF HEALTH AND SOCIAL SECURITY, *Report of the Committee of Inquiry into Allegations of Ill-treatment of Patients and other Irregularities at the Ely Hospital, Cardiff*, Cmnd 3975, HMSO, London (1969)

33. DEPARTMENT OF HEALTH AND SOCIAL SECURITY, *Report of the Farleigh Hospital Committee of Enquiry*, Cmnd 4557, HMSO, London (1971); DEPARTMENT OF HEALTH AND SOCIAL SECURITY, *Report of the Committee of Enquiry into Whittingham Hospital*, Cmnd 4861, HMSO, London (1972)

34. Quoted in MOONEY, G. H., RUSSELL, E. M. and WEIR, R. D., *Choices for Health Care*, Macmillan, London (1980), Ch.11

35. DEPARTMENT OF HEALTH AND SOCIAL SECURITY, *Management Arrangements for the Reorganised National Health Service*, HMSO, London (1974)

36. ARBER, S. and SAWYER, L., *Changes in the Structure of General Practice: the patient's viewpoint*, University of Surrey (1979), Vol. 1, Ch. 2

37. DEPARTMENT OF HEALTH AND SOCIAL SECURITY, *Report of a Study on Community Care*, HMSO, London. p. 92

38. DEPARTMENT OF HEALTH AND SOCIAL SECURITY, *Annual Report of the Department of Health and Social Security 1977*, HMSO (1978)

39. REEDY, B., 'The Health Team', in *Trends in General Practice*, Royal College of General Practitioners (1977)

40. DEPARTMENT OF HEALTH AND SOCIAL SECURITY, *The Primary Health Care Team. Report of a Joint Working Group* (Chairman: W. Harding) (the Harding Report) HMSO, London (1981)

41. MINISTRY OF HEALTH, *The Field of Work of the Family Doctor* (Chairman: A. Gillie), HMSO, London (1963)

42. DEPARTMENT OF HEALTH AND SOCIAL SECURITY, *Annual Report of the Department of Health and Social Security 1974*, HMSO (1975)

43. DHSS, *Primary Health Care Team* (Harding Report), *op.cit.*

44. *Report of the Royal Commission on the National Health Service* (Chairman: Sir Alec Merrison), Cmnd 7615, HMSO, London (1979)

Chapter five

EXPENDITURE AND RESOURCE ALLOCATION POLICIES
IN THE NHS

This chapter is divided into three parts. The first deals with the general financing of the NHS and the overall trends in expenditure and allocation to different sectors of the service. The second looks at the identification of priorities for NHS funds and the factors affecting those allocations, and the third examines the management and control of the allocation process at different levels of the health service.

THE FINANCING OF THE NHS

Before the NHS was created most people had to make choices about how much health care they would consume according to what they could afford. The 'nationalisation' of the service in 1946 replaced this with a service which in theory offered the best possible care to everyone. The 1944 White Paper stated that the Government:

> . . . want to ensure that in future every man and woman and child can rely on getting all the advice and treatment and care they may need in matters of personal health; that what they get shall be the best medical and other facilities available; that their getting these shall not depend on whether they can pay for them, or any other factor irrelevant to real need.[1]

The view was that the stock of ill-health would diminish and the proportion of GNP devoted to health would fall. There would therefore be no difficult choices to be made in health care between some areas of need and others. The only important question was the length of time necessary for the 'pool of illness' to reduce. In fact of course this has not been the case, needs have continued to expand and so has demand. Rationing mechanisms have developed either implicitly through, for example, queuing or waiting lists, and explicitly through the attempt to establish 'priorities'.

In the early years the NHS appeared to contemporaries to be in a state of constant financial crisis. Even Bevan commented, 'I shudder to think of the ceaseless cascade of medicine which is pouring down British throats at the present time. I wish I could believe that its efficiency was equal to the credulity with which it is being swallowed.'[2] Supplementary estimates wers raised in 1948/49 and 1949/50. Charges were introduced in 1951 on teeth and spectacles as part of Hugh Gaitskell's budget and this led to the resignation of Bevan and other Labour ministers. In 1952/53 the expenditure on the health service was £383 m. instead of the £170 m. estimated by Beveridge.[3]

The primary concern of policy-makers in the early 1950s was to contain the size of the NHS budget. In 1953 the Guillebaud Committee was set up to

> review the present and prospective cost of the NHS, to suggest means, whether by modifications in organisation or otherwise, of insuring the most effective control and efficient use of such Exchequer funds as may be made available; to advise how, in view of the burdens on the Exchequer, a rising charge upon it can be avoided while providing for the maintenance of an adequate service; and to make recommendations.

The Committee reported in 1956 and on the basis of work carried out by Abel-Smith and Titmuss found that far from being extravagantly high the cost of the NHS had *fallen* from 3.75 per cent of GNP to 3.25 per cent between 1949/50 and 1953/54 in real terms. Actual costs had risen but this was largely due to increases in the levels of salary paid to the NHS employees.[4] It was on the basis of these findings and their other investigations that the Guillebaud report recommended that there should be no change in the organisation of the NHS.

Cost containment however had been bought at the price of capital investment. Very few new hospitals were built or major modifications made. So the marked inequalities in the distribution of hospitals and beds, which had been a feature of the pre-war service, remained. 45 per cent of the hospitals had in fact been built before 1891 and were deteriorating rapidly. This led an American commentator on the English health services, Eckstein, to argue 'it is high time to let the health service go on a spending spree, instead of continuing to subject it to the miserly penny-pinching necessary in the immediate post-war period'.[5] This indeed occurred following the Hospital Plan, only to be cut back again in the mid-1960s. The *level* of NHS funding has always been a contentious issue, subject to criticisms of both overfunding and underfunding and we now turn to this issue, before pursuing the question of specific resource allocation policies up to the end of the 1970s.

Trends in NHS expenditure

The amount of money devoted to the NHS is ultimately a political decision as it is a nationally financed service. The sources of finance are three-fold. In 1981 around 89 per cent was derived from general taxation, 9 per cent from the national insurance stamp and the remainder from charges on recipients. In general a rising share has been paid for out of general taxation.[6]

It was explained in Chapter 3 that the NHS has taken an increasing proportion of GNP since the beginning of the 1960s and this amounts to a three-fold increase of real expenditure since 1949. Expenditure in 1980, in volume terms, was about £11,875 m. or £212 for every person in the UK. This can be compared to £9 per head at the start of the NHS. The share of GNP devoted to the NHS rose from 4.6 per cent to a record of 6.1 per cent in 1980.[7] Attempts have been made to cut the *rate* of growth in the NHS in recent years as shown in Table 3

Table 3. Current expenditure on hospital and community health services England: net of charge income; Survey 1980 prices

	Revenue (£m)	Revenue Growth (%)
1972–73	4,566	3.75
1973–74	4,737	4.75
1974–75	4,962	1.90
1975–76	5,056	0.39
1976–77	5,076	3.05
1977–78	5,231	2.55
1978–79	5,364	0.01
1979–80*		0.10†
1980–81		1.20
1981–82		2.10
1982–83		1.70‡

* Source: House of Commons, *17th Report from the Committee of Public Accounts, Session 1980–81. Financial control and accountability in the National Health Service*, HMSO, (1982) p. 111
† Supplied by the DHSS
‡ *The Government's Expenditure Plans 1982–3 – 1984–5*. Vol II, Cmnd 8494. HMSO (1982) Vol. II. This figure includes 'savings' for efficiency.

and public expenditure plans for 1982–83 to 1984–85 plan for only a very slight growth of 1.7 per cent. This assumes efficiency savings, does not cover the impact of demographic change nor technological innovations in medicine and it does not allow for the NHS having to meet part of the cost of salary increases above the level allowed for by central government in 1982 and subsequent years.

International comparisons and the adequacy of NHS funding

Compared to other post-industrial societies the UK devotes a smaller proportion of its GNP to health care. Table 4 shows the UK level of expenditure compared to other industrialised countries. UK expenditure at around 5.4 per cent of GNP is well below the Netherlands and France with 8.4 per cent and 7.2 per cent respectively and ranks low in comparison with most other industrial societies. It has the lowest level of spending per capita of population in the international league table. There is however a relationship between GNP per capita and health spending shown in Table 4. On the whole, the richer the country the more it spends on health care. This suggests that the relatively low level of spending on health care is related to the relatively low rate of economic growth in the UK rather than any other factor.

The way in which health care is financed appears to have little effect on health care expenditure. Critics of the NHS suggest that a move towards a system of private health insurance would increase the amount of expenditure on health but this may well be fallacious. Sweden spent just under 10 per cent of her national income on health care in 1975 while the equivalent figure for Britain was just over 5 per cent yet the proportion of publicly financed health care expenditure was almost identical, 91.6 per cent in Sweden, 92.6 per cent in the UK,[8] as Figure 3 illustrates. In both cases governments were responsible for different levels of funding. It is perhaps worth noting that the USA, with a large private sector, devotes a very high proportion of its national income to health care, but its government is concerned too with the cost explosion. It has, as a consequence of the private insurance financing of health care and the subsidies paid out to Medicare and Medicaid, few means at its disposal to control inflation of medical costs. A high level of spending on health care does not necessarily equate with good medical services as differences in percentages of national wealth devoted to health ·care are hard to interpret.

The NHS has been accused both of costing too much and of being underfunded. While recent governments have argued that the service

Table 4. Comparisons of health expenditure in selected countries

| | | *GNP*★★ | |
	per capita★ £	% increase ‡ over previous year
USA		
1976	4,451	11.3
1979	4,608	11.0
W. Germany		
1978	5,553	7.9
1979	4,350	8.5
France		
1978	3,988	11.9
1979	4,016	13.1
Japan		
1978	3,310	8.9
1979	3,918	7.3
Norway		
1978	4,631	9.7
1979	4,542	10.2
Netherlands		
1978	4.803	6.7
1979	4,169	5.4
UK		
1978	2,948	14.8
1979	3,419	14.7
Australia★★★		
1978	3,269	8.3
1979	3,656	12.4
Denmark		
1978	5,056	11.2
1979	4,621	10.1
Switzerland		
1977	5,729	—

Notes:
★ Due to fluctuations in exchange rates, figures for 1979 are not strictly comparable prices with previous year.
★★ At current prices.
★★★ Financial year.
† Excluding public expenditure.
‡ In local currency.
— Not available.
Source: Office of Health Economics, *Compendium of Statistics 1981*.
Office of Health Economics (1982)

Consumer Prices			Health expenditure
% increase ‡ over previous year	*% increase* ‡ over previous year	per capita* £	% GNP‡
7.6	6.9	389	8.9
11.3	12.5	405	9.0
2.7	4.9†	321†	5.8†
4.1	7.9†	280†	5.7†
9.1	12.5	323	7.2
10.7	14.1	327	7.2
4.2	11.7	142	4.0
3.7	10.0	171	4.4
8.4	14.4	373	7.8
4.7	7.5	356	7.6
4.1	9.9	402	8.4
4.2	8.6	357	8.6
9.0	13.6	141	5.4
13.3	15.3	162	5.4
7.9	13.2	254	7.8
9.1	11.3	278	7.6
7.5	—	372	7.4
7.6	11.7	345	7.4
—	—	394	6.9

Sources:
Health expenditure – private communications.
GNP – International Monetary Fund.
Consumer prices and exchange rates – CECD Main Economy

Fig. 3. Source of finance for health care expenditures: the mix between public and private in 1975 as a percentage of total

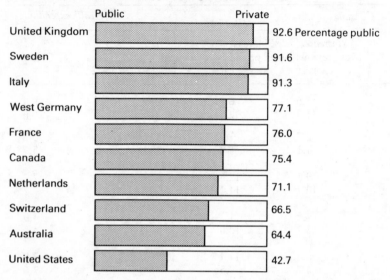

Source: R. J. Maxwell, *Health and Wealth; an international study of health care spending*, Lexington Books (1981) Table. 4.1

is costing too much, others argued that it is being starved of resources. The Public Expenditure Committee for example following an enquiry into the effect of cuts said categorically in 1974, 'It is the opinion of our committee that no government has ever provided sufficient money to allow the Health Service to function and to react to growing needs effectively. As a result of the inadequacy of finance, the service is grinding to a halt',[9] or again the BMA in its evidence to the Royal Commission on the National Health Service made the following comment: 'for some years now the money allocated by the Government for the service has been quite inadequate to meet the demands made upon it'.[10] However, levels of spending on health care say little about the efficacy of that spending. It could be that the NHS has been relatively successful in containing costs; a nationally financed service may be more efficient than services financed by other methods. Arguments about levels of funding, therefore, are largely meaningless.

One of the fundamental difficulties is that there seems to be no obvious link between the size of a country's health expenditure and the health status of its population. This is in any case difficult to measure by a single indicator. Mortality rates, infant mortality rates, life expectancy measure different things and themselves have limitations in what they measure. Sweden has the best mortality rates and the longest expectation of life in the international league table. It spends more of its GNP on health than the UK but less than the USA which has a worse mortality rate than either the UK or Sweden as the table in document 13 indicates. Another hypothesis could be that health status is affected by the way in which money is spent rather than the absolute amount. Both Sweden and the UK spend a large proportion of their health care expenditure on hospital services. Sweden the highest at 71 per cent and the UK at 63 per cent. Germany however with the same mortality statistics as the UK spends more on primary care and pharmaceuticals. Health status may have little to do with health expenditure and more to do with social and economic organisation, smoking, drinking or the introduction of seat-belt legislation and these issues are discussed further in Chapter 8. Maxwell, in *Health and Wealth: an international study in health care*, carefully explores some of these variables and concludes that it is impossible with the present state of knowledge to relate health expenditure to health status in any satisfactory way.[11] It is also difficult to argue therefore that increased expenditures will lead to improved health.

The Office of Health Economics in a recent publication argues that health care expenditures in all countries are likely to show a flattening of the rising curve in the near future and it may be that this is occurring earlier in the UK than other countries as it was one of the first to introduce a national health care system.[12] All governments are concerned with ever rising health expenditures, not only the UK. The need to provide care for dependency groups while not necessarily being cheaper, is changing the pattern of health care spending and increasing the need for other social services. The OHE suggests that the continuing development of new drugs may mean a second 'drug revolution' so that expensive hospital care can be replaced by less expensive chemotherapy. This is more controversial and begs many questions, not least the existence of entrenched interest groups with a concern for maintaining the level of functioning of existing structures and existing expenditure patterns. Whatever the future trends it is likely that all governments will continue to concern themselves with the *use* to which health expenditures are put, particularly in the UK where the system of financing is highly centralised and there is a political commitment to the reduction of public expenditure. The cost of the NHS and the use to which the money is put will remain of critical concern to governments.

EFFICIENCY, EFFECTIVENESS AND MEASURES OF PERFORMANCE

General problems of definition

The need to develop measures of efficiency and effectiveness in health care became increasingly pressing during the 1970s, so before turning to actual resource allocation policies the ways in which the performance of the NHS has been measured are examined. Unfortunately, although there are a great many statistics on the NHS they tend to measure activity rather than the efficiency or effectiveness of that activity. These two concepts are themselves of course elusive, and difficult to pin down. Efficiency can mean simply a service or procedure which costs less, irrespective of quality. However the term may be taken to mean at least the maintenance of a given standard of service at a lower cost or an improved standard at the same cost. Effectiveness presents more problems of definition as it necessarily includes criteria other than financial ones. It is essentially about an improvement in the quality of services or procedures which may be judged by social as well as economic criteria. These are difficult to measure even in crude terms. Furthermore there are temporal aspects to assessing effectiveness. It may be measured over a short or long term. Immunisation against typhoid may be effective for a limited period or a particular procedure may prolong the length of life for months or years. Cancer treatments, for example, tend to be measured in this way. Effectiveness at some stage may also have to be related to cost. Measuring the efficiency and effectiveness of the NHS as a whole is probably impossible although in theory at least, particular services and procedures could be evaluated much more rigorously than they are at present.

Measure of efficiency or performance

In the early years of the service total volume expenditure was used by governments as a very broad measure of efficiency as this was taken to reflect the containment of costs. Real difficulties arose when, in the more cost-conscious 1960s questions began to be asked about the performance and output of the health services.

There was and is as referred to earlier a plethora of figures on activity in the NHS; patients treated in different specialisms, as in-patients and out-patients; waiting times for admission; numbers of beds and their use; the length of stay in hospital; hospital equipment; numbers of staff employed. It is much more difficult to relate these figures to quality of provision or performance and there are still notable omissions from the data available.

Klein suggests that what is still missing is detailed information on the age and state of buildings in the NHS.

> There seems a strong case for a Domesday-book exercise, taking stock of the NHS's capital equipment. Even if it were impossible to provide complete information, it would surely be feasible to construct some indicators of the quality of the accommodation provided even rough and ready guides such as the proportion of patients in large wards or modernised wards, the availability of office space for doctors, the number of lavatories would be better than total ignorance.[13]

Such information might help establish targets for improvement and it might also provide a basis for comparing costs between different types of hospital. 'Minimum tolerable standards' have been established in the case of mental illness and handicap hospitals where a required ratio of consultants and nurses to patients has been laid down as well as standards for the provision of basic amenities. These can be used to indicate where particular hospitals fall below the norms and action taken to improve facilities.

Beds and lengths of stay in hospital

There is a good deal of information on numbers of hospital beds and length of stay in hospital for particular categories of bed and specialism. On the whole both have been falling. By 1979 there were 2,543 hospitals, 484 fewer than in 1959.[14] This has been due to the closure of smaller hospitals with a concentration of beds in larger units. The number of patients treated however has increased. The number of discharges and deaths, which are used as indicators of activity rates, have increased in Great Britain from 90.2 patients treated per 1,000 population in 1959 to 120.4 in 1979, an increase of over a third.[15] The number of cases treated per available bed (or throughput) has also increased. This reflects a shorter average length of stay in hospital. These changes which indicate an increasingly intensive use of facilities, can be taken as improvements in efficiency in the use of health care facilities overall.

The figures also indicate marked differences between the way beds are used by different consultants, in different hospitals, districts and regions. For example, the median duration of stay for the surgical treatment of septic ulcers under the care of surgeons in Scotland who treated at least twenty patients during the year varied from 6 to 26 days.[16] In 1972 the average length of stay in Britain for hernia treatment was 8.4 days.[17] This average concealed wide variations between different regions. In Manchester region the average length of stay was 9.5 days as against only 6.4 days in the Oxford region. Do these differences suggest inefficiencies in the use of resources? It is difficult to draw this conclusion as there are many possible factors involved. The length of stay may reflect the regimes and disposals of different consultants. It may reflect a desire to keep available beds filled, a hospital or ward with empty beds may face a threat of closure. Feldstein, in a study of hospital use in the 1960s, suggested that available beds tend to be filled and people who were admitted to hospital for a particular condition in one area were not in another, according to bed availability.[18] Length of stay may also reflect social conditions. A procedure which can be carried out on an out-patient basis in one area may be inappropriate in another with very deprived social conditions.

A major difficulty in assessing either the efficiency or the effectiveness of medical procedures is the lack of any adequate yardsticks to measure the optimum length of stay or treatment disposals for the handling of specific conditions in individuals. These, like medical diagnoses, are a matter of clinical judgement and have traditionally been left to the discretion of clinicians. However profiles could be built up of 'normal' or average lengths of stay, 'typical' treatments for particular conditions and used as part of a process of medical audit. Health care in the USA has developed along these lines and there are signs that the DHSS wishes to encourage similar developments in the UK. The setting up of the Körner Committee to enquire into information systems in the NHS is one step in this direction.[19]

However there are formidable obstacles in the form of professional practices and the politics of decision-making in the NHS which will have to be overcome in any search for greater efficiency.

The issue of beds and number of patients treated in them also has another dimension. Bed numbers have fallen, the numbers of patients treated has risen but so has the cost per head and the overall level of hospital expenditure. Klein, taking comparable figures between 1968 and 1973, suggests that while in-patient numbers treated rose by 8.6 per cent hospital expenditure rose by 14.5 per cent in the same period.[20] However, more recent figures for the 1980s show a reversal of these trends. The crucial element is manpower.

Increases in manpower – does more mean better?

Manpower represented two thirds of health care costs in 1974–75 (see Figure 4). By 1981 costs had risen to 70 per cent of expenditure. It

Fig. 4. The cost of health care in England 1974–75 (£m.)

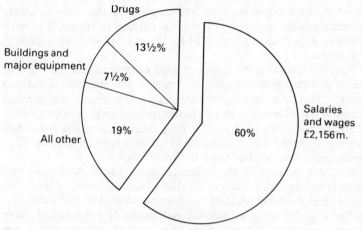

Drugs

Buildings and major equipment

13½%

7½%

19%

All other

60%

Salaries and wages £2,156m.

Total £3,596m.

Source: Great Britain. Parliament. *Annual Reports of the Department of Health and Social Security*, HMSO, London

is therefore an important input in the equation of efficiency. An increase in the numbers of health care professionals employed has often been used to suggest an improvement in services but again this is oversimplistic as can be seen from document 12 which shows the complex relationship between 'inputs' into health services in different countries and 'outcomes' [doc 12].

It has recently been argued that 'there is no longer any justification for assuming that an increase in numbers and expenditure on manpower can automatically be justified in terms of the extended service they provide'.[21]

There have been steady increases in most categories of manpower since 1949. Not only do manpower costs contribute a substantial proportion of overall costs but there is strong evidence that increases in wages and salaries constitute a major factor in increasing NHS expenditure. During the 1970s in particular wage increases had to be financed as well as meeting the costs of the increasing numbers of health care workers. The numbers of hospital doctors and particularly consultants have increased rapidly between 1949 and 1980 in England, an overall increase of 168 per cent or from 11,735 to 13,421. The numbers of nurses have increased by 161 per cent from 137,636 to 297,684 in the same period while the numbers of ancillary workers have remained relatively constant. This seems to suggest that those with the highest qualifications (and salaries) are also those which are increasing fastest in the NHS which is perhaps the opposite of what might be expected in a period where the attempt was being made to reduce costs.

Has, however, the increasing number of medical and nursing staff led to increasing productivity in terms of the numbers of patients treated? Haywood and Alaszewski suggest that overall, the increase in staff has *not* been matched by a parallel increase in patients treated. In the period from 1971 to 1977 hospital staff increased faster than patients treated both in terms of in-patients and out-patients. The percentage increases are shown in Figure 5 below.

A recent attempt by the DHSS to measure activity in acute hospitals is reported in a Study of the Acute Hospital Sector, 1981.[22] The study tries to relate numbers of patients treated in particular specialisms to the input of medical manpower. It has revealed major differences across the specialisms. For example, the number of hospital beds occupied by surgical cases has been falling slightly between 1969 and 1978. The number of patients treated has been slowly rising; but rising less rapidly than the number of consultant surgeons. This is not offset by a substantial increase in day surgery. This suggests a drop in productivity. Conversely in acute general medicine, there appears to have been a rise in productivity. More patients have been treated and there has been a broadly equivalent increase in the number of consultants. This was accompanied by fewer and shorter spells in hospital for patients, as more were treated as out-patients, so there has been a fall of 10 per cent in the number of beds in acute general medicine between 1969 and 1978.

The complexity of such an exercise becomes revealed by the look which the report takes at different specialisms. These differ widely in their patterns of treatment, some relying much more on out-patient and day care than the treatment of in-patients. Moreover the patterns of manpower 'input' varied with different ratios of types of staff (senior and junior registrars) to consultants. Neither does the amount of activity (i.e. patient throughput) necessarily measure workload. For example, although the productivity of ENT specialists appears to

Fig. 5. Hospital staffs, diagnostic tests and patients treated in England 1971–77

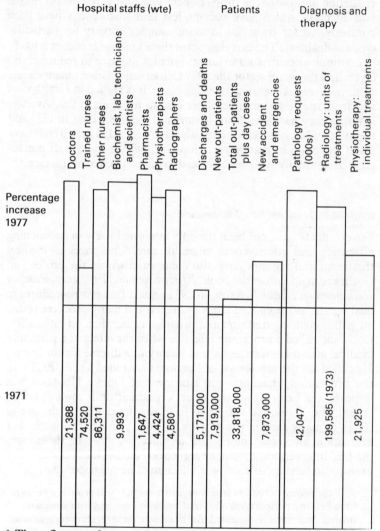

Hospital staffs (wte) — Patients — Diagnosis and therapy

	Doctors	Trained nurses	Other nurses	Biochemist, lab. technicians and scientists	Pharmacists	Physiotherapists	Radiographers	Discharges and deaths	New out-patients	Total out-patients plus day cases	New accident and emergencies	Pathology requests (000s)	*Radiology: units of treatments	Physiotherapy: individual treatments
1971	21,388	74,520	86,311	9,993	1,647	4,424	4,580	5,171,000	7,919,000	33,818,000	7,873,000	42,047	199,585 (1973)	21,925

Percentage increase 1977

* These figures refer to 1973–77 because of a significant change in units of measurement in 1973.

Sources: DHSS, *Health and Personal Social Services Statistics for England*, HMSO London; From Haywood and Alaszewski, *Crisis in the Health Service*, Croom Helm (1981), p. 105

have fallen (fall in patient numbers, a rise in medical staff), the reduction of some of the simpler operations for the removal of tonsils and adenoids which have become less fashionable, may have been compensated for by a rise in more complex surgery for particular types of deafness. The carrying out of these kinds of exercises is likely to continue as central government pursues its drive to reduce costs. Overall in the acute sector the 1979 Conservative Government claims to have reversed the trend of rising costs. It is argued in Health Care and its Costs (1983) that costs per case have begun to fall. Average length of stay has fallen from 10 days in 1976 to 8.6 days in 1981 and the number of cases treated annually has increased. These trends have offset increases in manpower. However, neither more staff nor increased productivity necessarily lead to more effective health care. [23]

Professional concern for effectiveness

Governments have not been the only interested party in questioning efficiency and effectiveness in health care. Challenges to medical treatment and regimes have also come from within the profession. Cochrane in an influential book, *Effectiveness and Efficiency, Random Reflections on Health Services*, in 1971 argued that few procedures in health care had been rigorously evaluated and many practices rested on habit, custom, tradition and privilege rather than on rationality. Cochrane called a procedure effective when the effect of a particular medical action altered the natural history of a disease for the better. He called for the greater use of Random Controlled Trials (RCTs) in the prevention, diagnosis and treatment of illness. His book was important in bringing about a more sceptical attitude towards health care in the 1970s. He also underlined the limitations in the use of RCTs as many areas of practice are not susceptible to this method of evaluation for social, moral and technical reasons. In these cases medical intervention should, he argued, err on the side of caution. For example in relation to adeno-tonsillectomies he suggested that

> . . . the present situation is very unsatisfactory. It will probably be some time before a perfect controlled trial, without bias, and with adequate medical treatment, is mounted. At the present there seems every reason to limit tonsillectomy to cases of obstruction. No case should be placed on a surgical waiting list but always referred for medical treatment, and only when this fails after a prolonged trial should the case be sent to the surgeon. This should reduce the number of tonsillectomies to about one-fifth of the present numbers. [24]

THE DEMAND FOR HEALTH CARE

All the discussion so far has centred on what are essentially methods of intervening in various ways on the supply side of health and medical care and the difficulties of ensuring that it is both efficiently provided and effective. The demand for health care has also been a factor with which governments have had to reckon.

The NHS began its existence with an open-ended commitment to meet needs and no specific resource allocation policies. Chapter 3 has outlined the general factors underlying the increasing demand for health care in the post-war period, the pressures of demography, equality and technology. However most demands for health care have been generated by service providers. Demand is professionally-led. Klein makes the important point that consumer demand has *fallen* during the years the NHS has been free at the point of contact. There are two points of entry to the NHS where the consumer can voice a demand; to the GP, who acts as a gatekeeper to the hospital service, or directly to the hospital casualty department. Klein argues that:

> Contacts between patients and GPs have fallen by an estimated 25 per cent or so, which means a reduction of 20 million or more in the number of annual patient 'demands'. In contrast, the number of patient visits to hospital accident and emergency departments has only risen by about 5 million. All this has happened in a period when the total population of potential consumers has risen by over 20 per cent.

What has increased dramatically is doctor-determined demand. Referrals from GPs for hospital services, both out-patient and in-patient numbers have increased.

> The major part of the increasing cost is due to technological changes in medicine – virtually every field of medicine. Among the consequences of these changes is the doubling of the professional and technical staff working in the hospital service between 1951 and 1968. During the same period, the number of requests for pathology multiplied by three, and x-ray units of work by nearly two. [25]

The same point is made by Figure 5 for the period 1971–77.

Doctors are important decision-making agents in the health service in another sense too. As well as determining by and large the quantity of demand, they also make rationing decisions about which consumer demand will be satisfied and in what way. Very little is known about the process or effects of this decision-making but an illustrative example can be given. A study on the choice of patients for renal dialysis and transplantation found that recipients were likely to be between the ages of 15 to 45, without other health problems, married with children, rather than single, others were likely to be refused treatment.[26]

Demand for health care does not of course equate with need. Many studies have indicated a 'submerged iceberg' of illness. Wadsworth, Butterfield and Blaney, in a study of a population in South London, found much unreported illness, some of it serious. Of the first 1,000 cases screened, only 67 were judged completely fit and 500 were referred to their doctor.[27] Need for health care has been primarily professionally defined at the pont of contact and translated into demands. At a higher level it has been translated by policy-makers into service policies or resource policies. It is to the latter that we now turn.

RESOURCES POLICIES: THE SIZE OF THE NHS BUDGET

The primary concern of policy-makers in the 1950s was to control the size of the NHS budget and not to question too closely how it was spent. The process of budget-formation, starting from the grass roots, proceeded in a number of stages. A budget was prepared by the local Hospital Management Committee (HMC) which related its planned *future* expenditure to recent *past* expenditure. Each October the HMCs were required to submit forecasts of the revenues they required to maintain services and meet 'urgent developments and improvements'. These were passed to the region which then put forward a total regional bid. The Ministry then decided on the growth rate. The total budget was then divided among the regions broadly in proportion to their expenditure in the last year for which figures were available. The regions then passed budgets to HMCs in two parts, one to cover the current costs of new developments, and the second to maintain existing services. The process was very imprecise and was based on the principle of 'What you got last year, and an allowance for growth, and an allowance for scandals'. This was the political environment of an implicit resource allocation policy. Its consequence was a maintenance or even an accentuation of inequalities in provision in different areas. There were attempts made by the Ministry of Health and later the DHSS to influence the health authorities through circulars and plans which were described in the previous chapters, but the main strategy employed to influence health authorities was one of advice and persuasion plus control over large capital projects.

The 1960s and early 1970s brought greater efforts by central government to control and review public expenditure as a whole and following the Plowden Report in 1961 a system of annual review was introduced. The Treasury presented a series of estimates for public expenditure in various areas based on its estimate of economic growth. However this did little to change the methods of allocation within the health service. Hospital and, after 1974, health authority budgets were still determined according to historic costs plus an allowance for growth. Any increase in expenditure due to pay and prices increases was covered by the DHSS in supplementary estimates. Supplementary estimates were allowed in 1974/75 and 1975/76. These were large as the reorganisation of the NHS itself had tended to increase expenditures. However it also increased the potential for greater budgetry control as up until this period, local authorities had determined the level of expenditure on the environmental and community health services. After 1974 overall hospital and community services expenditure could be controlled by the DHSS. Only the expenditure by the Family Practitioner Services, the amount spent on or by doctors, dentists, pharmacists and opticians remained, and still remains, largely demand-led. The most volatile element in this is expenditure by GPs on prescriptions, and referrals for further treatment. The latter of course create demands which reverberate through the rest of the health system. Attempts to curb GPs discretion in the exercise of their clinical autonomy have so far proved futile.

In 1976/77 however cash limits were introduced into health expenditures except in relation to GPs where these were 'demand-led'. Cash limits in simple terms mean that any overspending by a health authority is no longer met by the DHSS but is the first call on the next year's budget. Cash limits affected the size of the volume of funds to be distributed to the regions, for distribution to the areas, and it is by this method that the DHSS reduced the rate of growth in the health service. The total revenue available for distribution to health authorities is now based on the previous year's expenditure plus an allowance for the *actual* level of inflation in the previous year, with an additional factor, the Treasury's estimate for inflation for the forthcoming year. This latter element has tended to be set on the low side. Only 4 per cent was allowed for salary increases and 9 per cent price increases in 1982/83, for example. These low estimates are probably inevitable as higher allowances would tend in themselves to be inflationary. Table 3 shows the lower rates of growth in recent years as the 1979 Conservative government's priority for economic policy has affected resource allocation to the NHS. The effect of giving primacy to cutting public expenditure in the NHS is an increasingly tightly applied system of cash limiting. Should salary increases for NHS staff in 1982/83 for example be over 4 per cent then much of the cost of this will have to come out of the funds of the new district health authorities. A reduction in in-patient services seems inevitable unless savings can be achieved by a reduction in staff or through better house-keeping.

RESOURCE ALLOCATION POLICIES: THE EQUITABLE DISTRIBUTION OF RESOURCES

One of the factors which made the climate of expenditure controls of the 1970s so painful was the simultaneous attempt to redistribute resources according to new criteria of need. The reorganisation of 1974 and the subsequent Priorities documents were intended to bring about a reallocation of resources to poorer regions and to direct resources to develop services for dependent groups, and to primary health care. Priority in all cases implied relatively fewer resources to the better-off regions, less emphasis on patient groups other than the elderly, the mentally ill and handicapped, and less money for acute hospital care. This was a reversal of the implicit policies of the 1950s and 1960s when on the whole, regions which had a high level of services were allocated resources to run them, services for dependent groups were undeveloped and there was a steady increase in share of resources going to the hospital sector [doc 13]. The policy of regional reallocation was most clearly articulated in terms of an explicit policy while the other two policies were much less fully spelt out in terms of resource allocation, partly because they are not independent of each other. The development of services for dependent groups involves the development of community and primary health care. They are considered in the following chapter where the two main policy documents Priorities in the Health and Personal Social Services, 1976, and The Way Forward, 1977, are also discussed.

THE REALLOCATION OF HEALTH RESOURCES TO THE POORER REGIONS

A number of studies during the 1960s and 1970s had highlighted the regional inequalities in the distribution of resources in health care. These inequalities were to a large extent inherited from the past, but they had not been helped by the system of incremental budgeting and a failure to adjust to the movement of the population, from city centres to outer suburbs for example, or to other demographic changes such as the increasing numbers of elderly people. Cooper and Culyer, writing in 1972, found that not only were hospital beds unequally distributed but so were most other health care inputs.[28] GPs, hospital specialists, beds to population served, the range of specialisms, and out-patient facilities. In all, thirty-one indices were examined for different regions. In almost all of these the same regions or areas were relatively deprived. Sheffield, for example, came off particularly badly.

In all the thirty-one indices Sheffield was less well endowed than Oxford. Newcastle had twice as many gynaecologists per adult female as Sheffield; Birmingham twice as many consultants as Sheffield.[29]

Richard Crossman was the first Minister publicly to take on the problem of the relatively deprived regions, describing it as the most difficult he had to face as a minister. In 1971/72 when he was Minister of Health, the best endowed region had 41 per cent more resources than the regional average in terms of hospital expenditure per head of population, while the worst region had 23 per cent below. A formula was introduced in 1970 which attempted to weight allocations to regions on the basis of need. This was measured by numbers of beds and patient throughput to population. It was not until after reorganisation that the policy was fully developed through the reports of the Resource Allocation Working Party (RAWP) in 1975 and 1976 which devised a method of relating resource allocation to particular criteria of need. The introduction to the final report is reproduced in document 14.

RAWP aimed to provide a formula so that health resources could be distributed on the basis of need. The intention was that these extra resources would provide more health facilities and thus improve access to health services; equal opportunity of access to health care for people at equal risk. The assumptions were that needs for health care could be measured, that providing more resources would improve services, and that providing more services would improve access.

The final report of the Committee in 1976[30] developed the criteria for measuring relative needs in different regions of England, a separate report was prepared for Scotland and Wales, and this was used to establish a target budget for both *revenue* and *capital* allocations without reference to existing provision for each region. The budget was to cover the main areas of expenditure including all hospital-based services, ambulance services and community health services. The basis of the calculation was the size of the population served, weighted by appropriate combinations of age, sex, mortality (as an indicator of morbidity), fertility and marital status. These were used as measures of need for health services. There were then adjust-ments for such factors as cross-boundary flows of patients and the numbers of long-stay psychiatric patients. An allowance was made for teaching to compensate for the extra costs borne by hospitals with medical schools. This was called SIFT (Special Increment for Teaching). The components of the formula were then aggregated and the resources available nationally, divided to produce a revenue target for each region. Because immediate changes would be too catastro-phic, given the variations in budgets, there was to be a period of planned change over ten years. The actual allocations to regions would move gradually closer to the target budget, those with the greatest needs gradually receiving resources commensurate with their needs. Table 5 shows the result of the application of the RAWP formula. The London regions were to lose by the exercise while the northern regions were to gain. RAWP did not affect the total size of the NHS budget, but provided a principle for the equitable distri-bution of available resources. The intention was that regions would apply the RAWP formula to areas and districts within their boun-daries to bring about an equitable distribution of resources using the same approach.

The RAWP policy for reallocating resources to poorer regions was first applied in 1977/78 and aroused widespread criticism. Some of this was technical. It was argued, for example, that the data on which the formula was based were poor and the measures inadequate. In particular it was argued that measures of mortality did not give an indication of the amount of sickness 'morbidity', in a region. Nor did they take sufficiently into account disadvantageous social and en-vironmental conditions in particular regions. The RAWP calculations did not allow either for the availability of services which were com-plementary to care for which health authorities were responsible, such as primary care and personal social services. The unequal distribution of GPs is quite pronounced and so is that of local authority social services. Logically RAWP, it was argued, should have allowed for these factors in relating allocation to need. The working party did consider many of these points and for a variety of reasons did not move in these directions. There are, for example, no really adequate measures of morbidity, furthermore the health authorities could not really be expected to compensate through the health services for inadequate services or for wider social and economic inequalities, even though these might lead to worse health. These criticisms of RAWP are reminiscent of the debate about Educational Priority Areas in the 1960s, and ways of measuring deprivation. Both pro-

Table 5. RAWP Formula: Comparison of estimated targets, revised targets, proposed changes and actual changes

	Original target change	*Illustrative first year change for 1977/78*	*Revised target change*	*First year change as applied to 1977/78*
	(1)	(2)	(3)	(4)
North Western	14.2	4.1	16.9	3.2
Trent	13.8	3.9	15.3	2.9
Northern	9.7	2.8	15.2	2.9
Wessex	8.7	2.5	9.0	1.8
West Midlands	7.8	2.2	8.7	1.8
East Anglia	2.9	0.8	7.8	1.6
South Western	3.8	1.1	6.9	1.4
Yorkshire	9.2	2.6	6.1	1.3
Mersey	2.8	0.8	5.2	1.1
S. W. Thames	−5.6	0.0	−5.5	0.4
Oxford	−1.9	0.0	−6.0	0.4
S. E. Thames	−8.0	0.0	−10.8	0.3
N. E. Thames	−14.7	0.0	−11.8	0.3
N. Thames	−14.4	0.0	−12.8	0.2

Notes and sources: All figures are percentages of 1976/77 revenue allocations (excluding SIFT)

Col. (1)   DHSS figures underlying RAWP report calculations.
Col. (2)   Illustrative DHSS figures underlying RAWP report calculations: assuming 1.5% national growth rate.
Col. (3)   DHSS figures which, based on RAWP formula but updated and revised data, formed basis for determining allocation.
Col. (4)   DHSS *Letter to RHA Administrators*, 21 February 1977.

Source: Buxton, M, and Klein, R. E, *Allocating Health Resources: A Commentary on the Report of the Resource Allocation Working Party*, Royal Commission on The National Health Service, Research Paper No. 3, HMSO, London (1979) p. 26

grammes have in common the concern to increase territorial justice.

Other criticisms of RAWP were more overtly political. Those regions which stood to lose from the process were bitterly opposed to it. In particular opposition came from the Oxford and the Thames regions and the London teaching hospitals. It was argued that the Thames regions contained many centres of excellence in health care, internationally renowned research centres which were not specifically allowed for in the calculations. These provided a national service and would be crippled by lack of funds. The RAWP redistribution did indeed raise issues which brought about a clash of principles between geographical equity on the one hand and the maintenance of excellence to meet national needs on the other. It was also argued that extra resources would not necessarily be quickly transformed into facilities and services but that centres of excellence once lost could not be quickly replaced. It would be more efficient, it was suggested, to bring people to centres of excellence where there were beds, than create more beds in the areas of high population.

There is a similar kind of equity/efficiency conflict in relation to cross-boundary flows of patients from one region or area to another. It may be cheaper to allow patients to go to where the facilities exist rather than base services on regional or area self-sufficiency, and for this reason cross-boundary flows were partly allowed for in the RAWP calculations.

Implementation of RAWP

Despite the criticisms, and indeed active opposition in many quarters, the RAWP formula has been applied to regional budgets since 1977/78 and according to Maynard and Ludbrook writing in 1980, has been working quite smoothly.[31] The most deprived regions, North Western, Trent and Northern regions have made substantial gains in terms of both revenue and capital. This is despite the fact that RAWP has been applied in a period of slower growth in NHS expenditure. A closer examination, however, reveals problems in the process of implementation.

There have been special difficulties for regions where budgets are lower than they would have been had the RAWP formula not been applied. When budgets are falling relatively, cuts are not always made rationally but in the areas where they are easiest or least painful. This is unlikely to be in the medical service in acute hospital care as these are difficult to cut and are well defended. Studies of the Oxford region have indicated that community hospitals and 'social beds' are being cut, which in the long run may affect the health authorities' capacity to keep people in the community and undermine the aims and philosophy of the Priorities documents.[32]

Politically RAWP has been resisted, most publicly by Lambeth, Southwark and Lewisham AHA, which refused to implement economies in its three teaching hospitals. Members of the authority were suspended in 1979 but this was later ruled as illegal by the courts and the commissioners put in to run the service were replaced.

There seems to be considerable doubt too about the degree to which the RAWP formula is being used by regions to allocate resources to areas or districts within their boundaries. The North region has gained considerably from RAWP but only a small amount has been passed on to areas for distribution. Most have been used to support *regional* priorities. There seem indeed to be genuine difficulties in distributing growth money to compensate for the greater health needs of populations in the areas. Mooney suggests that 'it is all too easy for a health board or authority to become heavily engaged in *ad hoc* decisions on minor changes in resource allocation, in patching up deficiencies in individual services'.[33] This contention is supported by Haywood and Elcock's study *The Buck Stops Where?* which looked at accountability and policy-making in selected regions and area authorities in 1978–79. They found that change was difficult in the short term mainly because of the revenue consequences of capital projects already started. New hospital facilities begun can hardly be left standing unfinished or empty and therefore tend to take priority. They are funded at the expense of other AHAs without these developments and at the expense of non-acute services and services in the community. Also, the increasing numbers of very elderly people in some areas tended to generate an irresistible demand for acute beds. For these reasons Haywood and Elcock conclude that 'our health authorities frequently adopted budgetary policies which were intended to dilute, evade or even reject the reallocation policy set out by RAWP'.[34]

Perhaps the fundamental problem of RAWP is that it remains simply a mechanism for resource allocation and not an agent of radical social change. It cannot ensure, of itself, an improvement in access to services or in patient care. This would assume a control over the process of policy implementation which simply does not exist in the NHS. Further, RAWP cannot change quickly the result of years of unequal service development. As Klein and Buxton suggest even in societies where the supply of medical care is highly planned and controlled there are marked inequalities in service provision in relation to need. In a health service which, despite its centralisation, is as loosely controlled as the NHS, equality of regional provision according to need is likely to remain a goal to work towards. Despite these difficulties both the Royal Commission on the NHS and the Black Report on Inequalities in Health, endorsed the RAWP approach. The latter commented 'the RAWP formula is in fact a perfectly acceptable attempt to assess differences in need and to compensate for them'.[35]

In some ways it is too early to tell what the effect will be of RAWP policies. This depends on how vigorously they are pursued by the DHSS and by the regions. The strength of the decision-makers at the periphery in maintaining existing patterns of service has been demonstrated in a number of recent research studies described in Chapter 7. Moreover 'centres of excellence' where considerable research is carried on may develop strategies to maintain their flow of resources. Early indications are that in the face of a very low rate of growth the RAWP policy is being paced very slowly. It has been frozen for the 1982–83 budgets as the new district health authorities attempt to implement the 1982 reorganisation. The new structure places a heavy emphasis on the role of regions in rationing resources in various ways and the focus of attention at the DHSS appears to have switched to developing more effective techniques of overall cost control, leaving questions of resource use and allocations to health authorities at the regional level.

SUMMARY

Government resource allocation policies in the NHS since the 1950s have revolved around two major issues; the control of the centre over the level and use of NHS resources in the health authorities, and second, the attempt to bring about greater equity in resource distribution.

The chapter began with a discussion of the level of funding in the NHS and attention was drawn to the difficulties of establishing an appropriate level of expenditure given the intrinsic problems of measuring needs for health care. This same problem also explains the continuing search for measures of efficient and effective resource use by successive governments. Health care is expensive, demand is infinite; it is clearly important to ensure value for money yet accurate ways of relating health service inputs to outputs remain elusive. In the absence of such measures, the allocation of resources remains a question of sustaining existing services and ideological and political commitment. It must also be said of course, that just because the output of health services and their contribution to health status are difficult to measure, that the NHS has not contributed to improvements in the quality of life. The NHS remains a civilised and civilising institution which has reduced many of the uncertainties related to the handling of illness.

The second main objective of resource allocation policies has been the reduction of inequalities in the distribution of health service budgets to the regions. The policy has had a limited success in terms of overall regional budgets but has made little impact at an area or district level. Again this is not surprising. Structured inequalities in needs and provision, by their very nature, are reinforced by structured interest groups which slow down and modify the pace of change. Changes in the way health service budgets are allocated can hardly, by themselves, compensate for fundamental social inequalities which lie at the root of much illness. The RAWP formula may redistribute resources to regions which have more 'illness' but these resources need to be translated into services, and the services have in turn to reduce illness to ensure 'equality'. RAWP, though politically and morally important, inevitably remains a crude instrument.

REFERENCES

1. MINISTRY OF HEALTH, *A National Health Service*, Cmnd 6502, HMSO, London (1944)
2. Quoted by WATKIN, B., *The National Health Service: the first phase 1948–1974 and after*, Allen & Unwin, p. 30
3. *Ibid.*
4. ABEL-SMITH, B., and TITMUSS, R. M., *The Costs of the National Health Service*, Cambridge University Press, Cambridge (1956)
5. ECKSTEIN, H., *The English Health Service*, Harvard University Press, Cambridge, Mass. (1958) p. 62-3
6. OFFICE OF HEALTH ECONOMICS, *Compendium of Statistics 1981*, Office of Health Economics, London (1982) Table 1.5
7. *Ibid.*, Table 1.1
8. MAXWELL, R. J., *Health and Wealth: an international study of health care*, Lexington Books, Mass., Toronto (1981)
9. HOUSE OF COMMONS, Expenditure Committee (Social Services Sub-Committee), Fourth Report, Session 1974, *Expenditure Cuts in Health and Personal Social Services*, HC 307, HMSO (1974)
10. *Report of the Royal Commission on the National Health Service* (Chairman: Sir Alec Merrison), Cmnd 7615, HMSO, London (1979) p. 334
11. MAXWELL, R. J., *Health and Wealth, op. cit.*
12. OFFICE OF HEALTH ECONOMICS, *Trends in European Health Spending*, Briefing No. 14, Office of Health Economics (May 1981)
13. KLEIN, R., 'The National Health Service' in R. Klein (ed.), *Inflation and Priorities: social policy and public expenditure*, Policy

Studies Institute, London (1975)

14. OFFICE OF HEALTH ECONOMICS, *Compendium of Statistics 1981*, Table 3.1

15. *Ibid.*, Table 3.3

16. ABEL-SMITH, B., *Value for Money in Health Services*, Heinemann, London (1976) Ch.7

17. MORRIS, D., WARD, A. and HENDYSIDE, A. J., 'Early Discharge after Hernia Repair', *Lancet*, 1968, quoted by Maynard, A., 'Avarice, Inefficiency and Inequality: an international health care tale', *International Journal of Health Services*, 7 (2), 1977

18. FELDSTEIN, M. S., *Economic Analysis of Health Service Efficiency*, North Holland, Amsterdam (1967)

19. Steering Group on Health Service Information (Chairman: Edith Körner) established 1980

20. KLEIN, R., *The National Health Service, op. cit.*

21. OFFICE OF HEALTH ECONOMICS, *Doctors, Nurses and Midwives in the NHS*, Briefing No. 18, Office of Health Economics, Nov. 1981

22. DEPARTMENT OF HEALTH AND SOCIAL SECURITY, *Report of a Study of the Acute Hospital Sector*, DHSS (1981)

23. DEPARTMENT OF HEALTH AND SOCIAL SECURITY, *Health Care and its Cost*, HMSO, London (1983)

24. COCHRANE, A. L., *Effectiveness and Efficiency. Random Reflections on Health Services*, The Nuffield Provincial Hospitals Trust, Oxford (1972) p. 61

25. KLEIN, R., *The National Health Service, op. cit.*

26. Editorial, 'Selection of patients for dialysis and transplantation', *British Medical Journal*, 2 (1978), 1449–50

27. WADSWORTH, M., BUTTERFIELD, W. and BLANEY, R., *Health and Sickness: a choice of treatment*, Tavistock, London (1971)

28. COOPER, M.H. and CULYER, A.J., 'Equality in the National Health Service. Intentions, performance and problems in evaluation' in Hauser, M.M. (ed.), *The Economics of Medical Care*, Allen & Unwin, London (1972)

29. MAYNARD, A. and LUDBROOK, A., 'Budget Allocation in the National Health Service', *Journal of Social Policy*, Vol.9, Pt.3, July 1980

30. DEPARTMENT OF HEALTH AND SOCIAL SECURITY, *Sharing Resources for Health in England. Report of the Resources Allocation Working Party*, HMSO, London (1976)

31. MAYNARD and LUDBROOK, *op.cit.*

32. *Ibid.*

33. MOONEY, G., RUSSELL, E. and WEIR, R., *Choices for Health Care*, Macmillan, London (1980)

34. ELCOCK, H. and HAYWOOD, S., *The Buck Stops Where? Accountability and Control in the National Health Service*, Institute for Health Studies, University of Hull (1980)

35. DEPARTMENT OF HEALTH AND SOCIAL SECURITY, *Report of a Research Working Group. Inequalities in Health* (Chairman: Sir Douglas Black), DHSS, London (1980)

Chapter six

POLICIES FOR THE CARE OF DEPENDENT GROUPS

Policies in relation to the care and treatment of very dependent groups in the population have been one of the dominant policy themes within the 'service' stream of policy since the 1950s. It is however the most ambiguous and untidy area of policy provision to discuss because the conceptualisation of the major 'problem' which politicians have sought to meet has shifted over time and the policies themselves have been multidimensional and sometimes contradictory. In the early years of the health service it became apparent that the care and treatment of the elderly, the mentally handicapped and the mentally ill posed special difficulties. The strategy at this time was to develop policies and provision around each 'client' group through the publication of government sponsored Reports, White Papers, and consultative documents. These policy documents had a common policy theme, the importance of developing services in the community, rather than in institutions, whether these were run by health authorities or local authority social service departments. Governments in the 1970s sought to promote provision for these groups by establishing a 'priority' in terms of service provision. The implication was that the 'Cinderella' services were to receive extra attention as far as strategic thinking was concerned so that needs could be identified and policies developed and furthermore that preference was to be given in the allocation of resources.

This chapter is concerned with examining policies for community care and for giving priority to the 'Cinderella services' rather than the detail of service development for particular 'client' groups. A list of the major Reports, White Papers and consultative documents representing government policy statements for the mentally ill, mentally handicapped and the elderly is given in document 15 for the different groups. Before considering community care and priorities however, the question of why the treatment and care of groups such as the mentally ill and handicapped and the elderly should pose such special difficulties must be examined.

THE PROBLEM OF DEPENDENCY

The fact is, that it is not the membership of a particular group, as such, which creates a need for care, but the degree of dependency of many people who are mentally ill, handicapped, elderly, or chronically sick. Illsley has used the term 'dependency groups' to refer to 'individuals with impaired abilities to function independently. Their common characteristic is their resistance to curative treatment, their potential cost as long-term users of medical and social services and their multiple needs which are not the responsibility of a single profession.'[1] This broadens the category across other client groups such as the physically handicapped, the chronically sick, but highlights the features of care and treatment which are problematic. It is the dependency which creates the problem for society and which, if it is perceived as such by policy makers, is the real mainspring of policy initiatives.

The social care of the dependent poses particular difficulties for advanced industrial societies in general, because they are steeped in the philosophy of possessive individualism. Those who are not 'owners of themselves', who are unable to produce, create tensions and ambiguities. Care must be provided by others and although health and welfare services have developed to meet various contingencies, care for very dependent people remains very much the responsibility of families and neighbours. Who should provide what services raises fundamental questions of roles and responsibilities in society. Moreover as Abrams points out, there is a conflict of interest between the collectivity and the smaller group.[2] From a public point of view the provision of caring services is very costly and family or neighbourly care very cheap but from the point of view of the individual the situation is reversed: the costs of caring for others can be exorbitant while contributions to state welfare provision are relatively low, or at least unavoidable if they are spread through the tax system. The tensions between the roles and responsibilities of the state and of families have only recently surfaced as part of an active political and academic debate around the issue of the care of dependent groups.

DILEMMAS IN THE CARE OF THE DEPENDENT

The problem of the care of the dependent has become more apparent for a number of reasons. The 'burden' of dependency is seen to be growing. The policy of community care developed during the 1960s which appeared to have the twin virtues of both cheapness and moral worth, has been difficult to implement as it was too vaguely conceived and fudged the real issues of meeting need. Government policies to reduce public expenditure have exacerbated the difficulties by threatening to reduce health and social service budgets while at the same time the Women's Movement has created awareness of the 'burden' of social care for the dependent which, it is argued, falls mainly upon women.

The care of the elderly, mentally handicapped and ill also raises a further set of dilemmas for the NHS. Although as it was originally conceived the service aimed to provide facilities for cure, care and prevention, the NHS has become increasingly an 'illness' service centred on the curative model. The bulk of NHS resources are devoted to the hospital service and to the cure of acute illness as document 13 indicates. Groups which are by definition 'resistant to cure' and whose needs are primarily for care pose problems both organisationally and professionally to the NHS. Resource policies which give priority to services for dependent groups constitute a threat to resources for acute illness where they involve community care. They also create organisational problems in providing professional care outside the hospital and in devising ways of working in conjunction with other agencies which contribute to the social care of the dependent individual.

Government policies for the care of dependent groups therefore must be seen against the background of the diverse interests of individuals, groups and organisations involved in care-giving to dependent groups. Government policies themselves have sought to address the 'problem' of dependency but the implementation of those policies has been affected by the interests involved in the policy process. Difficulties of implementation have been compounded by the lack of clarity in the formulation of policy proposals and initiatives. In many respects this chapter is an account of the inadequacy of existing policies, however a clearer understanding of past failures may lead to more effective policies in the future.

THE GROWING BURDEN OF DEPENDENCY

'Social problems are what people think they are, and if conditions are not defined as social problems by the people involved in them, they are not problems to those people although they may be to outsiders or social scientists.'[3] Although the problem of the burden of dependency is relative rather than absolute in any concrete sense there is no doubt that governments since the 1950s have been concerned to respond to the increase in dependency which has been due to demographic and social factors.

There has been a dramatic increase in the numbers of elderly people since the beginning of the century. Although the total population has grown it has been at a slower rate than the growth of the numbers of elderly. Table 6 shows past trends and projections for the future.

Table 6. Population figures 1901–2001* – United Kingdom

	Total population (millions)	*% increase*	*Elderly† (millions)*	*% increase*
1901	38.2	–	2.4	–
1951	50.6	32	6.9	188
1977	55.9	10	9.6	39
1991‡	56.7	1	9.9	3
2001‡	57.5	1	9.5	-4

* Figures derived from *Social Trends*, No. 9, HMSO; London, Table 1.2 p.32.
† Males over 65, females over 60. ‡ Projected

What is also important is the structure of the elderly population. The numbers of very elderly, over seventy-five, have been a growing proportion of the elderly. Although the numbers of elderly are likely to grow less rapidly in future years the proportion who are very old is likely to continue to expand. Table 7 shows the trends and document

Table 7. The very old as a percentage of the elderly in the United Kingdom (1901–2001)*

	All elderly people† (millions)	*Elderly people 75 and under† (millions)*	*The very old‡ (millions)*	*Percentage of all elderly people who are very old*
1901	2.4	1.9	0.5	21
1951	6.9	5.1	1.8	26
1977	9.6	6.7	2.9	30
1991§	9.9	6.3	3.6	36
2001§	9.5	5.9	3.6	38

* Figures derived from *Social Trends*, No. 9, HMSO London, Table 1.2. p. 32.
† Males over 65, females over 60. §Projected.
‡ All 75 and over.

16 illustrates the picture graphically. The significant increase in the seventy-five and over age group is likely to continue to present a major challenge to health and the personal social services over the next decade. An increasing proportion of elderly people creates a challenge because the ageing process itself brings a larger amount of chronic and degenerative illness. For example, the incidence of senile dementia rises sharply in age groups from seventy-five onwards and so does the extent of disability and consequent handicap from chronic and de-generative illness due to arthritis, diabetes and heart disease.

The increase in the population has also brought an increase in the numbers of people with mental and physical handicap and in addi-tion, more children born with handicaps are surviving into adulthood due to the developments in medical science and rising living stan-dards. The Economist Intelligence Unit (1976) estimated that there has been an annual increase of 0.9 per cent in the numbers of severely disabled, an increase of 5,000 per year.[4]

As well as demographic changes in the incidence of disabling illness there have also been social changes which have brought a greater awareness of incidence of disability and chronic illness. The Chroni-cally Sick and Disabled Persons Act of 1970, for example, increased the extent of registration of the disabled while studies carried out for the DHSS in the 1970s collected accurate data on disability for the first time. An estimate of the numbers of disabled people in different age groups and with different degrees of handicap is given in Table 8. With knowledge of the extent of the problem comes political pressure to increase provision.

The growing incidence of mental illness has a more complex aetiology. The causes are likely to be due at least in part to the organisation of social life, to ways of living and awareness of the problem. Whatever the causes, the mentally ill make heavy demands on health services. It has been estimated that 600,000 people nation-ally receive specialist psychiatric services each year and a minority are long-term users of medical and social care.[5]

Not all elderly, handicapped or mentally ill people are dependent, or if they are, not for long periods. Among the elderly, for example, over 95 per cent live in their own homes, either alone or with spouses, while less than 4 per cent live in institutions.[6] However, the numbers of single elderly are likely to increase in the future, particularly the numbers of single elderly women. Changes in family structure may exacerbate the problem. Moroney and others have argued that there will be fewer carers available in the community as a consequence of social changes.[7] The higher incidence of marriage has reduced the

Table 8. Estimated and projected numbers of handicapped people living in private households, by age. Great Britain, 1968–2001 (Thousands)

Age group	Degree of handicap	1968–69	1981	2001
16–64	Very severe	42	42	44
	Severe	120	123	131
	Appreciable	215	220	233
	Total	377	385	408
65–74	Very severe	35	42	37
	Severe	99	123	108
	Appreciable	206	257	224
	Total handicapped	340	422	369
75 and over	Very severe	80	109	126
	Severe	123	170	197
	Appreciable	172	240	278
	Total handicapped	375	519	601
16 and over	Very severe	157	193	207
	Severe	342	416	436
	Appreciable	593	717	735
	Total handicapped	1092	1326	1378

Source: Wilson, J., *How many disabled people are there?* Disability Alliance 1980, based on Harris, A., *Handicapped and impaired in Great Britain*, HMSO (1971), Part 1 Table A11, *Population Projections* 1978–2018, HMSO (1980).

numbers of single women who were traditionally the carers while the smaller family sizes from the 1930s onwards has reduced the numbers of children in families to share the caring task. The increase in the employment of women, including married women, has also increased the opportunity-costs of caring. These factors are likely to add to the demand and need for state provided services over the next decades.

In the past governments have responded to these demographic and social changes through developing a variety of welfare provisions. Those in relation to the elderly and the disabled are discussed in other books in this series. However it is the impact of the problem of dependency on the NHS which concerns us here. The major policy response has been to develop policies for care in the community. This has involved seeking a close relationship with the personal social service departments of local authorities whose role is also to support the elderly, mentally handicapped and ill and their families.

POLICIES FOR COMMUNITY CARE

Community care eludes precise definition as it means different things to different professionals and agencies and has changed over time. A recent research Report on Community Care prepared for the DHSS suggests that community care can be viewed in two main ways; as a set of objectives and in terms of the provision of services. Their full explanation of the parameters of community care is given in the document section [doc 18].

The general overarching objective of community care has been to maintain individuals in their own homes whenever possible, rather than provide care in a long-stay institution or residential home. This was an objective which has been spelt out in the recommendations of most reports on dependency groups from the Phillips Committee's Report on the Elderly[8] in 1954, to the recent report in 1980 Mental Handicap: Progress Problems and Priorities.[9] The aim is put in a slightly different way in the White Paper on the Mentally Ill in 1975, where the emphasis is on normalisation. 'The aim is for people to be able to use the service they need with a minimum of formality and delay without losing touch with their normal lives . . . the philosophy is integration rather than isolation and the aim for the future must be to develop a much more locally-based service.'[10] The assumption here is that in the setting of everyday life treatment and care will have its maximum impact.

When we turn to the realisation of these objectives more problems of definition arise. Three distinct types of care can be considered to be under the general umbrella of community care: services provided *in* residential but relatively client-centred and open settings; services provided through the placing of professional and specialist personnel in 'the community'; and services provided *by* the community on a voluntary and quasi-organised basis. There has been a shift in emphasis over time. In the 1950s and 1960s the emphasis was more clearly on what Abrams calls community 'treatment' in either open or closed settings.[11] In terms of the health services this involved, for example, day hospitals, laundry services, chiropody, health visitors, district nurses, psychiatric nurses. For the social services, day centres, meals-on-wheels, aids and adaptations, social work support and home-helps. During the 1970s another dimension was added to community care; care *by* the community. Bayley in his work on the mentally handicapped pointed out that many dependent people need twenty-four-hour care which cannot be met by statutory or voluntary services but depends too on the informal network of support provided by family, friends and neighbours.[12] Further stimulus was given to this approach by the Aves Report in 1969[13] on the use of volunteers and by the Wolfenden Report on the Voluntary Sector in 1978.[14]

The Wolfenden Report drew attention to the 'mixed economy' of welfare. By showing that there were in fact a plurality of caring agencies the Report widened the discussion about community care so that more recent policy debates have been concerned with the respective roles of the statutory agencies, the commercial or private sector, the voluntary sector and the informal sector that is through family, friends and neighbours caring for the dependent in the community. In the recent Conservative government policy document, Care in Action, in 1981[15] the two latter categories are seen as the *primary* sources of community *care* if not community treatment, and statutory and private sources are seen as supplementing and supporting this provision. This marks a major shift in emphasis which will be discussed again at the end of the chapter.

In general terms the consistent support for community care policies has rested on two beliefs which are not necessarily consistent with each other and neither have they been validated. On the one hand it has been taken for granted that community care is morally better and more humanitarian than institutional care and on the other hand it has been assumed to be cheaper. The Guillebaud Committee on the Costs of the NHS in 1956 nicely incorporates both points. Policy it was suggested, 'should aim at making adequate provision wherever possible for the care and treatment of old people in their own homes. The development of the domiciliary services for this purpose will be a genuine economy measure and also a humanitarian measure enabling old people to lead the sort of life they much prefer.'[16] By happy chance the problems of demographic change and social aspirations could be maintained through a policy which was also more effective.

Other factors added to the arguments in favour of community care. Goffman had suggested in *Asylums* with both wit and insight that the organisation and environment of institutions diminished the quality of life for their inmates.[17] This message was forcibly brought home to the public in general by the scandals in the long-stay hospitals during the 1960s referred to in an earlier chapter. The Normansfield Inquiry of 1978[18] was a further indication that the large mental handicap hospital was fatally flawed in conception. Following the Jay Report on

Mental Handicap Nursing and Care in 1979[19] it has now become official policy that the mentally handicapped should be cared for wholly in the community. The only question that now remains is the speed of change. This is discussed in the most recent review, Mental Handicap: Progress, Problems and Priorities. There are to be no new long-stay facilities for this group and proposals foresee a gradual reduction in the existing long-stay population. Community Care, the DHSS Research Report of 1981, estimates that of the 15,000 mentally handicapped still in hospital, half could be discharged immediately if there were facilities available in the community.[20]

As well as the growing hostility to institutions in the 1960s there were developments in medicine which appeared to make a community care policy more feasible for some groups. Geriatrics was developing as a specialism. Its aim was to prevent the illnesses and diseases of old age becoming disabling and handicapping and where treatment was called for, returning the individual to a normal, active and self-supporting existence as soon as possible through active rehabilitation. The drug revolution of the 1950s also brought the possibility of dramatic changes in the treatment of mental illness. The average length of stay in hospital had been shortened for most new patients. Partly as a consequence of these developments there was an increasing awareness of the difficulties created by the division of function between hospitals providing acute medical care, and local authorities providing domiciliary services through their health and welfare departments. From the point of view of the hospitals an increase in domiciliary services and local authority residential care could lead to greater efficiency if it resulted in release of beds 'blocked' by long-stay patients. The reorganisation of the NHS in 1974 attempted to overcome the divide between health services in the community and hospital-based services, only to create another gulf in community care, between health and social services.

COLLABORATION BETWEEN HEALTH AND SOCIAL SERVICES

The restructuring of the health services aimed simultaneously to establish a priority for the development of what had come to be called the Cinderella services: services for the elderly, mentally handicapped and mentally ill. Health authorities were to be responsible for operating and planning the development of hospital and community health services *and* making arrangements for collaboration between the health and social services.

The Working Party on Collaboration between the National Health

Service and Local Government in 1973 made the case for collaboration. Health needs and social needs were seen to overlap and shade in to one another. Unless they were co-ordinated there was the possibility that people would get an unsatisfactory service or no service at all. It was also argued that the services were complementary, what was achieved in the hospital by way of rehabilitation of an elderly person, for example, could be undone if there were not supporting services in the community. Conversely domiciliary services could prevent hospital admission. The Working Party saw collaborative working as bringing improvements in efficiency and effectiveness in resource use.

The planning system introduced in 1974 was seen as the main method of developing collaboration between health and social services. The idea was that the setting of objectives and the working out of strategies in drawing up plans, should be carried out jointly between health and local authority social service departments. 'The real objective is not to achieve the joint consideration of plans which have been prepared separately by the two sides and brought together at a late stage to see how well they match up, but to achieve joint planning from the initial stages.'[21] So much importance was attached to joint planning that a special mechanism was established to ensure that it occurred. A Joint Consultative Committee made up of members of both health and social services authorities was to be established in each Area Health Authority and backed by a team of officers. Furthermore, in the Priorities document of 1976, Priorities for Health and Personal Social Services[22] a sum of money was earmarked by the DHSS for the financing of joint projects between health and social services. If schemes based in the community could be shown to reduce the costs of the NHS they were eligible for joint-financing. 60 per cent of the capital cost and part of the initial running costs were to be paid for from joint-financing while the subsequent running costs devolved on the local authority. Hostels for the mentally handicapped or a nightsitting service for the elderly could be developed in this way. There was a clear recognition that social service development could save the NHS money.

The Priorities document of 1976 and The Way Forward, 1977[23] completed the process of according priority to the Cinderella services begun by the 1974 reorganisation, by outlining a scheme for preferential growth for these services for the period up to 1979/80. Services used mainly by the elderly were to grow by 3.2 per cent a year, services for the mentally ill by 1.8 per cent, services for the mentally handicapped by 2.8 per cent a year; services for families with children 2.2

per cent; acute services by 1.2 per cent, while hospital maternity services were to receive 1.8 per cent *less* money each year. Current expenditure on the personal social services was to rise by 4 per cent and the NHS by 2.6 per cent for 1976/77 and slightly less in subsequent years. The documents gave priority to particular client groups and to the development of services used heavily by them, so extra resources were to go to the primary health care services and to the community health services, particularly health visiting and home nursing. This appeared at the time to be a positive step towards developing the services for dependent groups, for despite the emphasis given by successive Ministers in policy directives, local authority domiciliary services had developed in a very uneven way, and despite the establishment of the Hospital Advisory Service the conditions in long-stay hospitals still gave cause for concern.

The Way Forward suggested that the figures for growth indicated a general change in direction rather than an absolute prescription; 'they are not specific targets to be reached by declared dates in any locality'. There was nevertheless an intention to achieve a reallocation of resources from acute hospital services to the Cinderella services. It was certainly interpreted as such at the time. An editorial in the *British Medical Journal* thundered the hostility of the medical profession. They advocated increased spending on acute hospital buildings, renal dialysis, renal transplantation, brain-scanning equipment; the contribution of medicine to the treatment of coronary thrombosis, stroke, lung, bowel and breast cancers, and degenerative arthritis was praised; 'By putting people before buildings and by giving practical expression to the public sympathy for the old and the handicapped, Mrs Castle has, perhaps, allowed sentiment to overrule intellect.'[24]

COMMUNITY CARE POLICIES: AN ASSESSMENT

Although policies for community care for dependent groups remain central to government objectives in health care in Britain, there are difficulties in assessing their impact on services. These relate to (1) the multifaceted nature of the objectives; (2) the diversity of channels through which policies are being pursued; (3) the lack of clarity about what is meant by 'a priority'; (4) the degree of uncertainty about the level of needs to be met and (5) the extent to which these are changing with demographic change.

The Priorities document and The Way Forward sought to achieve a number of objectives, the most crucial from the point of view of this discussion was the attempt to promote the shift in resources towards services for the elderly, the mentally ill and the mentally handicapped. A second objective was to achieve a faster rate of development in services in the community provided by the health authorities and the local authorities. The difficulty is that each of these objectives is extremely broad, there is no ranking order of priority between different groups, nor are ways of achieving objectives specified. There is a degree of contradiction between the first and second set of objectives. For example the elderly are heavy users of acute medical care. In some hospitals the elderly occupy more than half the acute beds. Spending more in the acute sector *may* mean spending more on the elderly.

These difficulties are compounded by variations in need locally, differences in levels of provision and lack of information on needs. For example, although there are data on demographic trends in relation to the numbers of single-elderly nationally, these are lacking at a local level. Similarly there is little information about the extent to which needs are being met by local services, particularly through services from the voluntary and informal sector, the 'social carers'. Again although such data have been collected in national surveys by, for example, Audrey Hunt in the 1978 OPCS Survey on *The Elderly at Home*,[25] or through Nissel and Bonerjea's 1982 small scale survey *Family Care of the Handicapped Elderly: Who Pays?*,[26] these do not give any clear picture to local or health authorities of patterns of need, or the shortfall of services for dependent groups in their own areas. The availability of social care also varies considerably from area to area depending on a number of factors: local employment markets, local housing policies, the extent and organisation of voluntary agencies. The pattern of provision of health and personal social services has been developed in various ways in different areas as legislation in the sphere of community services has tended to be permissive. The structure of families, social and neighbourhood networks too are crucial in determining the level of demand and need for publicly provided care. There is little data of this kind available,[27] although unless such information is collected, neither local health authorities nor social service departments can rank priorities objectively. Provision, at best, is therefore likely to grow incrementally as a response to local pressures or political visibility.

The Priorities documents too lacked clarity in spelling out how the reallocation of resources was to be translated into action by the health regions, areas and districts. The Report of the Royal Commission on the NHS in 1979 commented that it was difficult to judge whether the newly introduced planning system had been effective in bringing about development of the Cinderella services as there were no clear guidelines about how allocations were to be ear-marked at a local level.

> Even after listening to the careful explanation by representatives of the DHSS about the way in which the needs of particular priority groups are taken into account in the allocation of resources to health authorities, we remain mystified. We are bold enough to think that this is because there is cloudiness in the department's thinking about these matters, which are as important as anything in the department's care.[28]

COLLABORATION AND JOINT PLANNING BETWEEN HEALTH AND LOCAL AUTHORITIES

It is also clear from the work done by Booth,[29] and Wistow,[30] that collaboration between health and local authorities is inherently difficult and that planning has not developed in the areas which these authors studied in the joint way that was intended. Local authorities and AHAs have tended to plan separately according to their own perceptions and priorities. Both are micro-political systems which operate in a particular environment with their own organisational imperatives, system of financing and professional and political perceptions of priorities. Change tends to occur only at the margins as most expenditure in health and social services is already committed. The balance of influence in the local political system may also have a stronger effect on policy choices than directives from the DHSS on priorities. Joint-financing has aided collaboration although the use of monies has tended to be *ad hoc* and incremental rather than part of a larger scheme of planned growth and development in a particular direction.

One inherent problem is that community care tends to mean different things to the local authority and the health authority. To the former it may mean a reduction in the amount of residential accommodation while to health authorities the existence of residential accommodation or high-intensity care substitutes, such as sheltered housing, increases the opportunity to discharge patients from hospital. Community care may then mean simply getting patients out of hospital and releasing 'blocked beds'. Booth's studies found that social service departments frequently perceived the AHA as trying to offload their problems on to social services, leaving little room for bargaining and reciprocity. Hospital consultants may for example reduce the length of stay, or discharge patients, without reference to social services or their ability to cope with very dependent people.

Nevertheless there have been positive effects from reorganisation *and* the arrangements for collaborative working. Joint-financing has benefited particularly the elderly and the mentally handicapped, 40 per cent of joint-financing has gone to develop services for the elderly, and 33 per cent for the mentally handicapped.[31] Joint collaborative machinery, Booth suggests, would have been largely redundant without incentive of joint-financing money to oil the wheels.[32] (This amounted to £416 m. in 1981). At a field level, collaboration over planning and for co-ordinating services operationally remains essential and recent planning guidelines following the 1982 reorganisation stress the importance of the *process* of planning in building up relationships between health and social services on a flexible basis. This is more important than the production of detailed and time-consuming plans.

Has a shift in priorities been achieved?

Despite the problems outlined above has there in fact been a shift in resources to dependent groups and a development of services in the community? There is no definite answer to this question although there is some information available. The Royal Commission on the NHS in 1979 commented that the number of in-patient treatments had fallen while the number of out-patients or day-patient treatments and day hospital attendances had increased for the elderly, mentally-ill and handicapped. This could be taken as indicative of an increase in community care. Furthermore, in spite of an increasing population of very elderly people, the numbers of patients in geriatric departments has remained constant. Conversely, this may simply reflect a lack of beds. It may also be that the population cared for in local authority residential accommodation and sheltered housing is becoming increasingly frail. With a lack of detailed data it is difficult to judge.

The research report Community Care in 1981 suggests that there have been steady increases in staff and facilities in some community services. The number of GPs has been rising steadily at 1.5 per cent a year. Most groups of nurses in the community have also increased. Between 1949–79 the numbers of community nurses rose by 238 per cent from 9,529 to 32,162. There was a particularly sharp rise between 1967–71, that is, *before* the Priorities documents. However in 1979 there were still ten nurses in the hospital compared to every one in the community. There have also been increases in the numbers of day-centre places and in home helps.[33] The home help service is particularly crucial in allowing the elderly to remain in their own homes and the elderly make up 90 per cent of the home help case-load.

What is not known from this data is whether the increase in manpower has fully kept pace with demographic and social change. Almost twice as many pensioners lived alone in 1971 as compared to 1961. Furthermore very little is known about how some groups of professionals spend their time or how effectively. Does an increase in GPs mean that they work *more* with elderly people, for example, or that this enables them to remain in the community when they otherwise would not have done? Like many other aspects of health care it is easier to obtain measures of service input than outputs, or measures of effectiveness of service provision.

Increases in manpower and facilities do not by themselves give any indication as to which priority group has benefited most from the increase. The research Report on Community Care however does conclude that there has been a significant shift in the way in which the mentally handicapped are cared for. In 1969 the numbers of mentally handicapped adults and children in hostels were 7.8 per cent and 21 per cent respectively of those in public care. By 1977 these proportions had risen to 19.3 per cent and 36 per cent.[34] The DHSS Report, Mental Handicap: Progress, Problems and Priorities in 1981 agreed that there had been progress but that a considerable number of mentally handicapped remained in hospital because there was no alternative provision in the community.

The position of the elderly is less clear and services for this group appear to have been affected particularly by recent cuts in public expenditure. They are a very much larger group and their needs are more various. Webb and Wistow conclude that the proportion of expenditure devoted to the elderly is declining marginally within local authority budgets, although this is contrary to national policy guidelines from the DHSS. Meals-on-wheels have hardly grown in volume and have failed to keep pace with the growing numbers of elderly people. Day-care places have similarly fallen in proportion to the population over seventy-five since 1979/80 and additionally, between 1976 and 1980, expenditure on aids and adaptations has been reduced. The evidence suggests that numbers of frail or chronically ill elderly occupying acute hospital beds have not diminished and the level of frailty of the elderly occupying local authority residential homes and sheltered housing has increased. Community care it seems has not kept pace with demand.[35]

The resistance of the NHS to a change in priorities

The lack of coherent strategy in central government priorities has not been the only factor constraining the implemention of policies to develop services for dependent groups. The NHS is itself highly resistant to change. One of the factors which inhibits change is the extent to which most expenditure in the NHS is already committed to on-going programmes. 'For hospital and community services current expenditure needs to grow at about 1 per cent a year merely to allow for demographic change and to make some provision for the spread of improved medical techniques without detriment to standards in other parts of the services.'[36] The logical consequence of Priorities documents is therefore that some areas of provision will have to lose for others to gain. This exercise becomes extremely difficult in an organisation where the political reality is that crucial decisions made by the clinicians at the grass roots are frequently more concerned with protecting their own specialisms than in making choices between them. Mechanisms for enforcing government priorities simply do not exist and managers in the health service have been seen as facilitating clinicians and other professionals to carry out their jobs, rather than implementing government policy. This follows from the Bevanite principle of reliance on professionals running the health service and on the notion of clinical autonomy. The principle was indeed re-iterated in 'Patients First', the consultative document on reorganisation in 1982.[37]

Studies by Haywood and Alaszewski,[38] R. G. H. Brown,[39] and David Hunter[40] on decision-making have suggested that policy-making in health authorities has tended to revolve around the influence of clinical interests and commitments to existing projects and expenditure. Authorities on the whole were not willing or able to make changes in allocations unless monies were made specifically available. In management in the health service there has been what Hunter calls a high 'puzzlement' factor, managers have often been uncertain about how to change in line with central government policies. Moreover as there have been no sanctions on defaulters, central government directives have on the whole, been treated as rhetoric and ignored. The activities of the health authorities at the periphery have therefore been of crucial importance in affecting the implementation or non-implementation of central government policy. This matter is pursued further at the end of the next chapter.

CARE IN ACTION: A CHANGE OF EMPHASIS

Care in Action is the successor to the Priorities documents and out-lines the 1979 Conservative Government's policies and priorities for the health and social services.[41] As far as policies for dependent groups are concerned the emphasis is much the same. Priority *groups* are identified as the elderly, mentally ill, mentally and physically handi-capped, priority *services*, that is those in the community, are widened to include the maternity services, reflecting concern to reduce infant mortality and a then rising birth rate. The primary care services and services for children are also singled out for mention. However these priorities are not ranked in order and neither are they linked to resource allocation targets so the difficulties of implemen-tation already discussed still apply. Some of the tensions are acknow-ledged, such as the demand by elderly people for acute beds, although no attempt is made to resolve them. Overall the document pays lip service to the commitment to community care made by previous administrations.

There are however changes of emphasis which mark a retreat by central government from its responsibilities in caring for dependent groups through the provision of extra resources. The main priority in effect has become the reduction in public expenditure and this means a reduction from present expenditure levels in the personal social services and very low growth in the health service. The strategy to achieve the meeting of social needs is what Klein calls a 'non-strategy'.[42] It relies on two factors, the careful husbanding of NHS resources to achieve savings and the 'innovative' use of the informal, voluntary and private sectors in care. Patrick Jenkin, the Secretary of State for Health, outlined his approach in 1980: 'we cannot operate as if the statutory services are central providers with a few volunteers here and there to back them up. Instead we should recognise that the informal sector lies at the centre with statutory services and the voluntary sector providing expertise and support.'[43] This shifts the emphasis of policy-making still further to the periphery of the NHS and to the social service departments; the role of central government is limited to providing overall financing, albeit at a reduced level. The shift in responsibility is illustrated by the extracts from Patients First and Care in Action reproduced in the document section [docs 18 and 19].

In relation to the care of dependent groups there is further sugges-tion for a change of emphasis in government strategy which implicitly limits the commitments of central government. Attention is focused on the need to support 'boundary' groups rather than providing services for care groups as a whole according to need. The research Report on Community Care defined boundary groups as 'those groups whose need put them at the margins of different forms of care, that is, those who require some degree of continuing care because of a combination of dependency, frailty and social circumstances'.[44] The danger is that a definition of what constitutes membership of a 'boundary' group may prove to be elusive. Boundary groups may be taken to be those whose needs the health and social services department can afford to meet rather than those who need support and care.

The Report on Community Care quite rightly draws attention to the costs to informal carers of community care for 'boundary groups', arguing that 'the effectiveness of a package of community care depends greatly on the presence of informal care' and the cost effectiveness of community care depends on 'not putting a financial value on the contribution of informal carers who may in fact shoulder considerable financial, social and emotional burdens'. Care in Action makes no comment on this issue, beyond suggesting the need for further consultation. It is hard to avoid the conclusion that this latest consultative document while continuing to mouth the rhetoric of meeting the needs of dependent groups, has seized upon community care in conjunction with the Wolfenden Report concept of the mixed economy of welfare, to reduce the 'burden' of care on the state. The emphasis is no longer focused on the importance of meeting the needs of dependent groups for humanitarian reasons but on the economic imperative to reduce state expenditure.

Responsibility in Care in Action has been shifted in two ways. First, it is to be the responsibility of health and local authorities at the periphery to devise strategies for community care. However, no special funds have been earmarked in allocations for this purpose. The Select Committee on Social Services in their report on the public expenditure White Paper in 1980 stressed this point when they commented:

> We are struck by the apparent lack of strategic policy-making at the DHSS and the failure to examine the overall impact of changes in expenditure levels and changes in the social environment across the various services and programmes for which the department is responsible . . . Community care of the elderly and disabled demands financial commitment . . . there is strong evidence to suggest that the need to make short term savings in Personal Social Services budgets may be obstructing the shift to community care.[45]

It is unlikely that authorities in the field will be able to fulfil their responsibilities to dependent groups in view of the pressure to reduce existing budgets and the costs of the reorganisation of the NHS in 1982. Authorities may however take the blame for failing to do so. Care in the Community, the 1981 consultative paper for sharing resources between health and local authorities urges a more flexible use of resources but does not provide extra money for this purpose.[46]

Care in Action and subsequent circulars shift responsibility by emphasising the role of the informal and voluntary sectors. The capacity of these sectors to cope mush be in doubt. Webb and Wistow, among others, have shown the extent to which the voluntary sector relies on the state sector for subsidy for providing services and in order to organise volunteers.[47] The care of dependent groups is therefore likely to continue to mean what it has primarily always meant, unpaid community care by women, and as the numbers of dependent people grow, and opportunities in the labour market decrease, a de-skilling of women.

The Equal Opportunities Commission study, Who Cares for the Carers? comments:

> The expectation that a women will provide the necessary care within the family whatever the cost to herself, still underpins the reality of community care. Cuts in health and social services and cash benefits intensify the demands placed on carers, they mean there are less physical resources to aid them, less alternatives to relieve them, and less money to support them. Savings in public expenditure increase the cost to carer in terms of her social life, her employment prospects and ultimately her physical and mental well-being. These costs are borne individually and do not figure in any public expenditure account. The price paid is the restriction placed on women's opportunities.[48]

Nissel and Bonerjea's study in 1980 suggests that women who give up work altogether to care, lose on average £4,500 a year while those who reduce their hours of work lose on average £1,900 a year. Carers also bear considerable indirect costs in loss of employment-related benefits, while the emotional costs of carers have also been shown to be high. Government policies have placed responsibility for caring on individuals[49] and it is they who will have to accept blame for being unable or unwilling to meet them.

FUTURE COLLABORATION BETWEEN HEALTH AND SOCIAL SERVICES

The Joint Finance circular of 1983[50] represents a watering down of the 1981 consultative document. It aims to provide pump-priming money to give impetus to community care. Health authorities may offer lump-sum payments to other agencies to take over the care of people previously in hospital and the period of time for which joint financing money is available for schemes is extended to ten years. There is thus a recognition that organisations are 'self-interested' and must be paid to work together. What remains in doubt however is the ability of social services or voluntary organisations on whom the burden of care will eventually fall, to cope with very dependent people at less cost.

REFERENCES

1. ILLSLEY, R., 'Problems of Dependency Groups: the care of the elderly, the handicapped and the chronically ill', *Social Science and Medicine*, Vol. 15A, No. 3 (Pt. II), 1981
2. ABRAMS, P., 'Community Care: some research problems and priorities', *Policy and Politics*, **6** (2), (Dec. 1977)
3. MCINTYRE, S., 'Old Age as a Social Problem', in R. Dingwall *et al.* (eds), *Health Care and Health Knowledge*, Croom Helm, London (1977)
4. ECONOMIST INTELLIGENCE UNIT, *Care With Dignity: an analysis of the costs of care for the disabled*, National Fund for Research into Crippling Diseases, (1973)
5. DEPARTMENT OF HEALTH AND SOCIAL SECURITY, *Better Services for the Mentally Ill*, Cmnd 6233, HMSO, London (1975)
6. EQUAL OPPORTUNITIES COMMISSION, *Caring for the Elderly and Handicapped. Community Care Policies and Women's Lives*, Equal Opportunities Commission (1982)
7. MORONEY, R.M., *The Family and the State: considerations for social policy*, Longman, London (1976)
8. MINISTRY OF HEALTH, *Report of the Committee on the Economic and Financial Problems of the Provision for Old Age* (Chairman: Sir J. Philipps), HMSO, London (1954)
9. DEPARTMENT OF HEALTH AND SOCIAL SECURITY, *Mental Handicap: progress, problems and priorities. A Review of Mental Handicap Services in England since the 1971 White Paper*, DHSS (1980)
10. DEPARTMENT OF HEALTH AND SOCIAL SECURITY, *Better Services for the Mentally Ill, op. cit.*
11. ABRAMS, P., 'Community Care', *op.cit.*
12. BAYLEY, M., *Mental Handicap and Community Care: A Study of Mentally Handicapped People in Sheffield*, Routledge & Kegan Paul, London (1973)
13. AVES, G.M., *The Volunteer Worker in the Social Services*, Allen &

Unwin, London (1969)

14. WOLFENDEN COMMITTEE, *The Future of Voluntary Organisations*, Croom Helm, London (1977), Ch. 1

15. DEPARTMENT OF HEALTH AND SOCIAL SECURITY, *Care in Action: a handbook of policies and priorities for the Health and Personal Social Services in England*, HMSO, London (1981)

16. MINISTRY OF HEALTH, *Report of the Committee of Inquiry into the Cost of the National Health Service* (Chairman: C. W. Guillebaud), Cmd 9663, HMSO, London (1956)

17. GOFFMAN, E., *Asylums*, Penguin, London (1968)

18. DEPARTMENT OF HEALTH AND SOCIAL SECURITY, *Report of the Committee of Inquiry into Normansfield Hospital*, Cmnd 7357, HMSO, London (1978)

19. DEPARTMENT OF HEALTH AND SOCIAL SECURITY, *Report of the Committee of Inquiry into Mental Handicap Nursing and Care* (Chairman: Peggy Jay), HMSO, London (1979)

20. DEPARTMENT OF HEALTH AND SOCIAL SECURITY, *Report of a Study on Community Care*, DHSS, London (1981)

21. DEPARTMENT OF HEALTH AND SOCIAL SECURITY, *Report from the Working Party on Collaboration between the National Health Service and Local Government on its Activities to the end of 1972*, HMSO, London (1973)

22. DEPARTMENT OF HEALTH AND SOCIAL SECURITY, *Priorities for Health and Personal Social Services in England. A Consultative Document*, HMSO, London (1976)

23. DEPARTMENT OF HEALTH AND SOCIAL SECURITY, *The Way Forward*, HMSO, London (1977)

24. Editorial, *British Medical Journal*, 3 April 1976

25. HUNT, A., *The Elderly at Home*, OPCS, HMSO, London (1978)

26. NISSEL, M. and BONERJEA, L., *Family Care of the Handicapped Elderly. Who Pays?* Policy Studies Institute, London (1982)

27. One such study has been undertaken by the London Borough of Hammersmith, *The Elderly at Home in Hammersmith and Fulham*. Report of the Research Project on the Needs of the Elderly (1981)

28. *Report of the Royal Commission on the National Health Service*, (Chairman: Sir Alec Merrison), Cmnd 7615, HMSO, London (1979)

29. BOOTH, T. A., 'Collaboration between the Health and Social Services, Part I: A case study of joint care planning, Part I and II', *Policy and Politics*, **9** (1), (1981) and **9** (2), (1981)

30. WISTOW, G., 'Collaboration between Health and Local Authorities: Why is it necessary?', *Social Policy and Administration*, **16**, 1,

Spring 1982
31. BOOTH, T.A., *op.cit.*
32. *Ibid.*
33. DEPARTMENT OF HEALTH AND SOCIAL SECURITY, *Report of the Study on Community Care, op.cit.*
34. *Ibid.*
35. WEBB, A. and WISTOW, G., 'The Personal Social Services: incrementalism, expediency or systematic social planning' in A., Walker (ed.), *Public Expenditure and Social Policy*, Heinemann, London (1982)
36. *Report of the Royal Commission on the NHS, op.cit.*
37. DEPARTMENT OF HEALTH AND SOCIAL SECURITY, *Patients First. Consultative Paper on the Structure and Management of the NHS in England and Wales*, HMSO, London (1979)
38. HAYWOOD, S. and ALASZEWSKI, A., *Crisis in the Health Service*, Croom Helm, London (1980)
39. BROWN, R.G.H., *Reorganising the Health Service*, Robertson, Oxford (1979)
40. HUNTER, D., 'Coping With Uncertainty: decisions and resources within Health Authorities', *Sociology of Health and Illness*, 1, No.1, 1979
41. DEPARTMENT OF HEALTH AND SOCIAL SECURITY, *Care in Action: a handbook, op.cit.*
42. KLEIN, R., 'The Strategy Behind the Jenkin Non-strategy', *British Medical Journal*, Vol. 282, 28 Mar. 1981
43. JENKIN, PATRICK, Speech to the Association of Directors of Social Services
44. DEPARTMENT OF HEALTH AND SOCIAL SECURITY, *Report of the Study of Community Care, op.cit.*
45. SELECT COMMITTEE ON SOCIAL SERVICES, Third Report, Session 1979–80, *The Government's White Papers on Public Expenditure: The Social Services*, HMSO, London, 1980, HC 702.1
46. DEPARTMENT OF HEALTH AND SOCIAL SECURITY, *Care in the Community*. A consultative document on moving resources for care in England, DHSS, London (1981)
47. WEBB and WISTOW, *op.cit.*
48. EQUAL OPPORTUNITIES COMMISSION, *Who Cares for the Carers?*, *Equal Opportunities Commission (1982)* ch. 4.
49. NISSEL, M., and BANERJEA, L., *op.cit.*, Ch. V
50. DEPARTMENT OF HEALTH AND SOCIAL SECURITY, *Health Service Development. Care in the Community and Joint Finance* HC(86) 6, DHSS, London (1983)

In April 1982 the NHS was reorganised once more. The Royal Commission on the NHS which reported in 1979 had highlighted again the perennial dilemmas which face those responsible for providing health services in Britain, the achievement of greater efficiency in the service, the implementation of priorities for the care of dependent groups and the alleviation of regional inequalities. It also identified the weakness of the 1974 structure and recommended a simplification of the organisation.

Some of these recommendations were incorporated in a consultative document, 'Patients First' in 1979, and circulated by the then Conservative administration, later that same year.[1] The 1980 Health Services Act enabled the government to introduce administrative changes in 1982. Patients First, and the subsequent handbook on Policies and Priorities, 'Care in Action',[2] reflect a subtle change of emphasis towards the role of government in relation to the NHS. Although the priorities in Care in Action superficially remain similar to those in previous governments, the strategies have changed. The two documents must be seen against a background of the government's commitment to economic policies outlined in Chapter 3; for the first time in its history the NHS is facing a period of low or no-growth and the new District Health Authorities are being looked to, to achieve both economies and a change in priorities simultaneously. Central government has become the stern parent primarily concerned with the overall level of public expenditure. This is in marked contrast to the approach of the Royal Commission which remained within the Bevanite tradition of the proud and understanding father.

This chapter, after briefly outlining the approach and major emphases in the Royal Commission Report, will describe the approach taken in 'Patients First' and 'Care in Action'. The remainder of the chapter will look at the characteristics of policy-making at a local level in the NHS to assess the possible impact of the new strategies.

THE ROYAL COMMISSION ON THE NHS

The 1974 reorganisation of the NHS had been an ambitious attempt to increase the efficiency of the NHS by increased planning and central control while at the same time introducing more 'democracy'. It had attempted to make the provision of the health services more equal by establishing criteria of equity in resource allocation. It had tried to meet the consequences of social and demographic change by developing policies to meet the needs of dependent groups. The effect of the reorganisation on those working in the NHS was traumatic and the years following were associated with industrial disputes, general disorganisation and loss of financial control. The Royal Commission was set up as a response to the tensions in the NHS and its terms of reference were 'to consider the interests both of patients and those who work in the National Health Service, the best use and management of financial and manpower resources of the National Health Service'. Implicit in these terms of reference was the view that the NHS was a social institution which was part of the basic fabric of British society, and that the interests of those who worked in the service were as important as those of patients. The Commission's approach was very much an organic one, ultimately better patient services could be achieved only through more harmonious working together of staff.[3] The Commission accepted collectivist ideas about health as part of the Welfare State and confirmed and updated the principles and objectives of the 1946 Act [doc 8].

The Commission's task was explicitly to manage what was seen as a 'crisis' in the NHS and in pursuing this the Commissioners collected a great deal of evidence, conducted surveys and commissioned research. The Report and its Appendices contain a wealth of information about how the NHS works and its discussion and recommendations contained something for everyone. There is sympathy for the consequences of reorganisation on groups working in the service. Reorganisation involved

> An immense amount of administrative work in preparation for the new
> machinery; disruption of ordinary work, both before and after reorganisation caused by the need to prepare for and implement changes; the
> breakdown of well-established formal and informal networks; the loss of
> experienced staff through early retirement and resignation; the stresses
> and strains on some staff of having to compete for new jobs.[3]

These consequences, it was suggested were due to the long drawn-out period of consultation leading up to reorganisation, yet the lack of real preparation of top management for their tasks in the new structure. Reorganisation involved a very large number of people, many of whom had a sense of confusion about their new roles in the service. The Report examines each group of workers in the service in turn, and their grumbles and grievances are dealt with. Their value, contribution and importance to the NHS is underlined. Patients too are brought to the fore. Their attitudes and opinions of the service are surveyed, Community Health Councils are appraised and an extension of their role suggested. The inadequacy of complaints procedures is criticised, and implementation of the Davies Committee Report on complaints procedures urged.

The mechanistic managerialist approach of the 1974 reorganisation is implicitly criticised by the Commission. On a number of issues it had become apparent that the 1974 changes had attempted to substitute structural or technical solutions for what were ultimately questions of relationships and values. One aim of reorganisation, for example, had been to achieve integration between agencies providing different aspects of health care, health and social services, and the various professional groups providing them, through a planning system and a system of consensus management. In this the Report suggests reorganisation failed. Integration had not been achieved and where it had, it was at the cost of 'additional work, uncertainty and frustration'. Kogan's paper on 'The working of the NHS' Research Paper I was critical of the 'unitary fallacy' of consensus management and the planning system.[4] This tended, he suggested, to slow down decision-making, brought too much concentration on trivial issues, and could not gloss over the fact that providing health care involved questions of values; about which services should be developed, or which cut back. Over such issues there were, inevitably, conflicts of interest and opinion and these ultimately political questions needed to be aired and discussed in order to be resolved. However there was often insufficient or inadequate information on which to base decisions, and consequently there were fundamental difficulties in implementing the government's priorities.

Overall the Commission's recommendations covered four major areas; issues relating to patient care, to the NHS and its workers, to the NHS and other institutions, to management and finance. In relation to patient services there was strong emphasis on prevention, particularly on effective screening programmes. Legislation on the compulsory wearing of seat belts was recommended and the importance of the fluoridation of water supplies and health education was stressed. On the second set of recommendations, those concerning the NHS and its workers, the most central were those relating to the importance of industrial relations and of a simplification of the management structure so that there were clearer lines of responsibility. Third, an improved health service was seen to rest fundamentally on good working relationships within the service. The Commission was critical of the relationship between the NHS and the local authorities. Their view was that great benefits could be derived from joint-planning, in collaboration with the social service departments, although fundamental thinking needed to be done on the respective responsibilities of health and social services in this respect. As for the fourth area, management and finance, the Commission recommended an abolition of the area tier and the integration of Family Practitioner Committees into the main management structure to strengthen primary care. This, in particular, would bring greater collaboration between the GPs, and other community health services. There was an overriding concern to strengthen responsibility for providing services which met local needs. The view was that local responsibility and flexibility to meet different local circumstances was fundamental to the service.

PATIENTS FIRST, AND THE 1982 REORGANISATION

'Patients First', the consultative document which followed, took its title from the spirit of the Royal Commission's Report, and incorporated some of the Commission's main recommendations on the structure of the service. Document 18 reproduces the introduction [doc 18].

The view that the 1974 reorganisation had been 'too ambitious, was in some ways ill-conceived and created a number of undesirable side-effects'[5] was widely shared. 'Patients First' aimed to simplify the structure and move responsibility for making decisions closer to the locality for which health services were being provided. It was argued that the Area Health Authorities were too remote from (a) local service providers; (b) patients and (c) the local community.

Large areas, especially those containing more than one district, it was suggested, should be broken into smaller District Health Authorities (DHAs) typically serving a population between 200,000 and 500,000. The new authorities should be centred on localities, taking into account social geography, the focus of the district being the District General Hospital or Hospitals and associated range of community services. The 'natural community' (i.e. hospital community) was it was argued a *more* important factor in drawing up boundaries than co-terminosity with the local authorities, the implication being that collaboration was not the highest priority.

'Patients First' recommended that the District should become the key accountable body in the new structure, responsible for *providing* services as well as *planning* for them. The locus of decision-making would then move downward. The DHA would be able to make decisions to meet local needs with a tighter system of management and a more loosely-constructed and simplified planning structure. There was less emphasis on integration in the document, for not only did coterminosity with local authorities take second place to hospital catchment area but, contrary to the Royal Commission's recommendations, Family Practitioner Committees who were responsible for managing the contracts of GPs were for the time being to retain their existing status. This latter recommendation confirmed the political reality of the separateness of GPs. Patrick Jenkin, indeed, in the introduction to Patients First, emphasised the plurality of organisations providing health care rather than their unity. 'I believe it is wrong to treat the NHS as though it were or could be a single giant integrated system, rather we must try to see it as a whole series of local health services serving local communities and managed by local people.'

'Managed by local people' was somewhat ambiguous but Patients First appeared to use this in two senses. The first was a representation of local interests through membership of the authorities. The new DHAs were to be similar in composition to AHAs in terms of a combination of professional and lay membership, though smaller. Members were to be from local authorities or appointed by the Region. Despite the emphasis on local people however local *authority* membership was to be reduced on the grounds that *all* members would be concerned with local needs. Earlier research studies had in fact indicated that few local authority members had sufficient time to devote to health authority work.[6] The membership of the DHA was to be about twenty, instead of over thirty, and four members were to be representatives of the local authority. There was to be a consultant, a GP, a nurse, a university nominee, a Trade Union member and the remainder were to be 'generalists'. All members were to be chosen for their personal qualities and the individual contribution they could make to the service. Paradoxically, despite emphasis given to the involvement by local people Community Health Councils were threatened with extinction in Patients First on the grounds that with more locally-based membership of DHAs they would be unnecessary and duplicate its work.

The second aspect of 'managed by local people', was the change of emphasis in the running of the service. Instead of the stress on the hierarchical accountability which characterised the 1974 reorganisation the health authorities at the periphery were to have greater flexibility in managing and administering the service to reflect local circumstances. Each DHA was to be serviced by a District Management Team, including a consultant, GP, nurse, medical officer, treasurer, and the administrator. This was to be responsible for managing, co-ordinating and planning the service by a consensus of the members. Lines of responsibility were simplified by the abolition of the area tier. Units of management were to be established and a team of three, administrator, nurse and medical representative were to manage the units. The nurse manager and administrator were also responsible to the district administrator and nurse respectively. Collaboration with local authorities was to remain, with arrangements for Joint Consultative committees although this would clearly be more complex where a new health authority spanned two or more local authorities.

Districts were to be responsible to Regional Health Authorities and the Minister in broadly the same way as in 1974. Regions did not alter their boundaries, nor was any major change in their functions recommended by Patients First.

THE 1982 REORGANISATION

On the 1 April 1982, 192 DHAs and 9 special health authorities were established in England based on existing districts or an amalgamation of districts. Figure 6 shows the new structure.

Community Health Councils survived the consultation to be reconstituted on the basis of the new districts while Family Practitioner Committees were to become fully autonomous bodies based by and large on the previous area boundaries, and therefore in some cases covering a number of DHAs, as soon as legislation was passed.

The reorganisation was broadly along the lines proposed in Patients First and laid stress on decision-making in the locality rather than at the centre. One example of delegation of responsibility has been the freedom to set up units of management which best suit local circumstances. These may be based on institutions such as hospitals and community services or on 'care' groups such as the elderly or mentally handicapped who need both hospital and community care or on a

Fig. 6. The organisation of the National Health Service 1982–

—————— Corporate accountability

⎫
⎬ Individual officer accountability and
⎭ joint team responsibility

⎫
⎬ Monitoring and coordinating
⎭ between teams and individual
    counterpart officers

—————— Representative systems

– – – – – External relationships

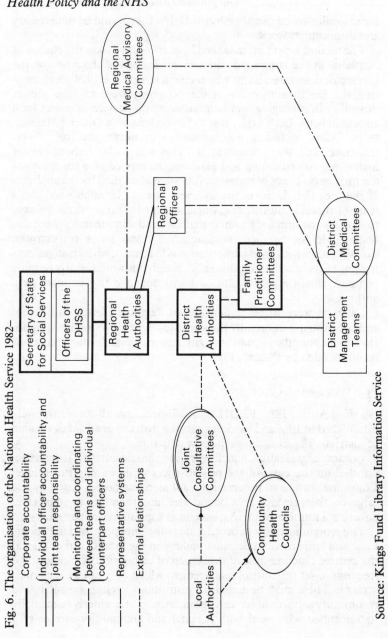

Source: Kings Fund Library Information Service

combination of the two. Given this discretion there is likely to be wide variety of different patterns of management in different health authorities.

Regions in the new structure have the task of planning the development of specialisms within the region. This is clearly intended to prevent a return to the pre-1974 policy drift and maintain both efficient ways of working and a dovetailing of specialist services provided by different districts.

CARE IN ACTION AND THE MIXED ECONOMY OF HEALTH

The changes proposed in Patients First must be seen in conjunction with the Conservative government's Policy and Priorities Document, 'Care in Action', which plans for service development into the 1980s. Although this maintains much the same priorities as previous governments there are changes in emphasis and changes in strategy. The service priorities remain similar. There is emphasis on the need to develop services for dependent groups, particularly through community care and in conjunction with local authorities. There is an emphasis on the importance of prevention which is discussed in Chapter 9. The importance of primary care is stressed, and so is maternity care. There is to be an increase in these services, reflecting the rise in the birth rate which has occurred since the last Priorities documents in 1976 and 1977.

The major priority however is contained in the preface to Care in Action: a restatement of the government's commitment to a reduction of public expenditure. Patrick Jenkin writes in the foreword, 'I'm sure you do not need reminding that the Government's top priority must be to get the economy right; for that reason, it cannot be assumed that more money will always be available to be spent on health care.' The strategies put forward rest on the assumption of very low or nil growth in the NHS. In these terms a major difference between Care in Action and the earlier Priorities documents becomes explicable. There are no attempts to put resource planning targets on specific services. There are no norms or targets about desirable levels of provision. David Owen warned in 1976, 'Governments must be prepared, if they award priority to say where the money is coming from.'[7] The warning has not been heeded so the statements in this document are clearly intended as exhortations or 'guidelines'. The implicit strategy is to place the responsibility on the new DHAs to follow government guidelines as best as they can. It is they who will have to determine local needs and pursue health policies which reflect local priorities. The suggestion of Care in Action is that they may find the money for growth for these services from efficiency savings, not in the area of acute medicine but from housekeeping economies such as energy savings, stock control, more cost effective storage, etc. New developments in acute medicine, the document suggests, will have to be found from within that sector by 'weighing the claims of developing services, such as renal services, against the continuation of patterns of expenditure elsewhere'. This again leaves the determination of development to the field level of health care, this time to the consultants in the hospital sector. There is no explicit suggestion that cuts in acute services should be used to develop those in the community. This choice is left to the Districts. 'The government are confident that entrusting responsibilities to the health authorities will be the best means of ensuring that resources are planned and applied in the most effective way.' The strategy is to diffuse responsibility for policy change to the periphery.

The NHS in the 1980s is clearly facing a situation of relatively static resources and the implications are evident in recent reports on the state of health of the nation. Although Secretary of State, Patrick Jenkin accepted the general finding of the Black Report on Inequalities in Health that inequalities between the health status of different classes were probably increasing, he argued in the preface to the Report that the government could make no financial commitment to improving health services in the worst off areas.[8] The same order of priority is reflected in the government's reply to the Short Report on Perinatal and Neo-natal Mortality, 'Improvements in social and living standards, including improvements in health services, are highly dependent on the prosperity of the economy.'[9]

A second plank of the strategy for handling low growth is also concerned with diffusing responsibility for health and social care. Care in Action looks to the voluntary and informal sector to take the central and major role in the care of dependent groups, through care in the community; and to the private sector to meet 'excess' demands for care in the acute sector. Thus the responsibilities of the State are reduced in what is seen as a 'mixed economy of welfare'.

The implications of this approach for the care of dependent groups has already been explored in the previous chapter where the increased emphasis on the role of the voluntary sector was explained. Care in Action in health as well as the social services draws attention to the importance of voluntary efforts in the acute sector of health care also. It is argued that voluntary contributions in cash and in kind could give greater financial flexibility to the NHS at the margins. There is seen to be a greater role for local fund-raising, in appeals for public contributions for special projects and it is again authorities at the local level which will have the responsibility for organising such activity.[10]

Care in Action also puts a new emphasis on the contribution of the private sector. This is seen as complementary to the NHS. 'Past governments have too often neglected or ignored the opportunities for co-operation between the private and public sectors' it is suggested. There could be a productive partnership between public and private sectors as private facilities could be used to supplement state provisions in shortage areas both for acute conditions and the care of those who are chronically ill. At this point it is worth describing the relationship between the state, the NHS and the private sector established in 1948 to provide a context for the Care in Action proposals and the other measures which have been taken by the Conservative government since 1979 to encourage the growth of this sector.

THE PRIVATE SECTOR

The definition of private practice is not easy. The Royal Commission on the NHS lists five different aspects of private practice,[11] but for our purposes two aspects of private care are important. First there has always been the right for private treatment by a private doctor in a private hospital to exist in the UK; financed by private health insurance or direct payment. Second, Bevan came to an agreement with consultants to make available a number of 'pay-beds' in NHS hospitals for private patients. Consultants were furthermore allowed to hold part-time contracts with the NHS so they could maintain some private practice. Pay-beds and part-time contracts constituted a half-way-house between private and public care.

The NHS and private care

In 1965 pay-beds amounted to 1.25 per cent of total beds in NHS hospitals. This number has subsequently fallen slightly and in 1980 there were 2,533 pay-beds. These beds were for many years heavily subsidised by the NHS but recently this subsidy has been reduced substantially.[12]

Barbara Castle when Secretary of State for Social Services, established the Health Services Board in 1976 to oversee the phasing out of pay-beds and to introduce controls over the development of private hospitals. The pay-beds issue had become the centre of political controversy in the mid-1970s. This, and Mrs Castle's plan to change consultants' contracts to encourage full-time commitment to the NHS, had caused considerable disruption to the service.

In 1980, the Health Services Act brought about a reversal of these policies in line with Conservative thinking. The Health Services Board was abolished, controls over private hospital development relaxed and co-operation between the NHS and the private sector explicitly encouraged through urging health authorities to contract-out to the private market for services where this was cheaper. It was suggested that laundry or catering or cleaning services, for example, were possible areas. The sale of NHS land to private medical interests was allowed. Negotiations with the profession were undertaken to allow a full-time contract with the NHS which would leave some time for private practice.

Private medical insurance

Partly as a result of the increasing cost of pay-beds, and partly due to other market forces, the take-up of private medical insurance has increased dramatically in the second half of the 1970s and privately run medical facilities have grown. The Royal Commission on the NHS estimated that 3 per cent of the total expenditure on health care in 1976 could be attributed to private health care but this may now well be an underestimate.[13] In 1981 around 3.5 m. people or 6.4 per cent of the population had some form of private health insurance. Ann Shearer estimated that if this rate of growth continued, in five years time some 20 per cent of the population would be insured to opt out of what the NHS provides.[14] The present government has suggested 25 per cent as a target.

The growth of private health insurance is attributable to two main sources of demand. The majority of subscriptions are taken out by employers for their employees as fringe benefits, and latterly, Unions have increasingly begun to take out subscriptions on behalf of their members. The second factor is demand from individuals who may be influenced by a desire to cut waiting times and to ensure what are perceived to be better facilities in private wards or hospitals. Many minor but irritating conditions such as hernia operations or hip-replacements, or varicose veins are dealt with by the private sector, as are 50 per cent of abortions. Recent fiscal policy through tax concessions to employers making contributions for their employees with incomes under £8,500 has been aimed at increasing subscriptions to private insurance.

The provision of private medical facilities is growing to meet the demand although accurate information is difficult to obtain. Goldie has calculated that in 1980 there were 5,400 beds in independent surgical hospitals with an additional 31,000 if the beds in small private nursing homes, typically for the elderly chronically sick, were included.[15] These latter facilities are of course not normally provided in the cover of private insurance. There is a considerable expansion planned for the 1980s of independent surgical hospitals and this is attracting foreign investment. It is in fact seen as an export earner.

Government policy in the private sector: an assessment

The present government has been considering alternative ways of financing the NHS through some form of public health insurance and has been examining the operation of some European health systems which are financed in this way. No decisions have yet been made on the issue. There is considerable doubt about the political, administrative and economic viability of such a move and the medical profession has indicated its hostility to such a fundamental change.

Care in Action's main contention is that the development of the private sector would be complementary to the NHS but this may be an erroneous assumption. This is not the place to examine the merits and demerits of private practice and insurance as a whole, it is done elsewhere.[16] However on the specific issue of complementarity, it must be pointed out that the two systems of care, public and private rest on two entirely different sets of assumptions. The NHS aims to provide for the totality of care; short and long stay, in hospital and in the community. It teaches health care professionals, to produce the next generation of health workers as well as treating patients. The DHSS plans for the national provision of health care. The private sector has much more limited functions: to provide independent surgical hospitals where there is a demand supported by private insurance or direct payment and to provide care for the old and chronically ill for those with sufficiently high incomes.

The private sector could have a distorting effect on the NHS if it develops beyond a small and minor element in the total system of health care. One of the major problems facing the NHS in providing a national service has been the unequal provision of health facilities in different parts of the country. The private sector exaggerates these inequalities in distribution, as most private health care is available in the south-east which is already well endowed with NHS care. Furthermore there is direct competition between the NHS and the private sector for trained staff. This affects the ability of hospitals to retain and attract staff, again particularly in the London area. Perhaps the most serious effect of the further development of the private sector is the diffusion of commitment to the NHS and the development of a two-class service, one for the poor, the elderly and chronically ill, and the very seriously ill who need complex, time-consuming and expensive treatments, and one for the better off who seek care for the acute conditions of the immediate present.

Care in Action by stressing the mixed economy of health care through the contribution of the voluntary, informal and private sectors, moves away from the mainstream of government policy operating since the establishment of the NHS in 1948 and represented by the Royal Commission Report on the service. The NHS faces low growth; whether this is inevitable or a consequence of government economic policy, is a matter of debate, but the government's response is clear enough; to diffuse responsibility for health to a wider health care system through the policies developed in Care in Action. At the same time the 1982 reorganisation devolves responsibility for making difficult choices over priorities to the District Health Authorities, to local authorities in relation to the social services, and to the Family Practitioner Committees which face new responsibilities as a consequence of autonomy. Blame is being diffused together with responsibility and this has been implicit in ministerial speeches. The key decisions, like the early period of development of the NHS in the 1950s, are to be made by the health authorities at the periphery where the politics of local decision-making is likely to play a major part in determining the outcomes of government policy.

It has been argued that this simply reflects the reality of decision policy-making in the NHS. Government policies, it is suggested, have created an illusion of change as the key decision-takers are at the grass roots. The service providers, particularly doctors at the field level, determine what health policy actually is. A number of studies have been carried out in recent years which have examined decision-taking at the local level in health care and although they relate to the period from 1974, they provide an account of power in the local health system. It is to these we now turn as they provide some empirical basis to an assessment of the possible outcomes of Care in Action and Patients First.

THE POLITICS OF POLICY-MAKING AT A LOCAL LEVEL IN THE NHS

Interest in policy-making at a local level in the NHS is of comparatively recent origin and this is probably a consequence of the centralisation of the service, the consensus surrounding health policy and the acceptance that the professionals providing care were the 'natural decision-makers'. It has become something of a truism to suggest that local politics in the NHS are medico-politics, that doctors' preferences dominate decision-making. Studies by Kogan[17] and Perrin[18] carried out for the Royal Commission and more recent work by R. S. G. Brown,[19] Haywood and Elcock,[20] and Haywood and Alaszewski[21] explain how this occurs and suggest that it is the consultants with their ability to define needs within their own specialism and therefore commit present and future capital and revenue expenditure, who determine the pattern of service and present and future resource allocation. This power to affect policy derives from the reality of clinical autonomy, the right to make decisions in relation to the treatment of patients.

Perrin in his study for the Royal Commission comments that after reorganisation the locus for decision-making frequently lay outside the management team altogether and lay with individual consultants. He suggests that 'clinicians may be so formidable as to dominate decisions about resource use . . . the exercise of clinical autonomy should not be allowed to extend to a veto on the reallocation of resources to cope with changes in need . . . and what would be in the best interests of health in the area'. He concludes that there is often uncertainty between clinicians and administrators and planners about the boundaries between individual decisions and public policies. The decisions of clinicians frequently have wider reverberations on resource use of which they are unaware. (Two examples of this are given in document 20.) In other areas as discussed in Chapter 5 the revenue consequences of on-going capital schemes frequently took all development monies, leaving little room for manoeuvre. This suggests that the priorities put forward in Care in Action, as they are exhortations rather than commands, stand little chance of changing the *status quo*.

There were certainly great difficulties in implementing priorities in relation to dependent groups following the earlier Priorities documents. R. G. S. Brown in an analysis of the first set of local plans confirms the failure of the DHSS to shift resources from acute services:

> In general, nobody is opposed to the development of services for the elderly. It is therefore easy for members of AHAs and other bodies to pass resolutions saying that it is their intention to improve services as and when circumstances and resources permit. It is quite another thing to accept

that, within a limited budget, the development of these services implies a cost to alternative objectives. The same authorities which passed pious resolutions in support of services for the elderly committed themselves to other developments which in effect made it impossible to achieve their objectives for the elderly.[22]

The underlying problem is that there are few objective criteria by which to measure the costs and benefits of alternative policies in health care, to evaluate the respective benefits to the elderly of, for example, increasing the number of beds for orthopaedics as opposed to providing more nurses in the community. Frequently the reality of medico-politics is continued funding of on-going projects and what growth money is available is allocated to those who shout the loudest. Perrin refers to 'allocation by decibel' or, as it is put less kindly, allocation by 'shroud waving' as consultants mount media campaigns to protect or develop their own specialisms. Planning, which was to have been 'the single most important influence in better resource allocation in the service' and which was seen in the reorganisation as a tool of management and a technical process, has proved on the available evidence largely to be an opportunity for bargaining and negotiation between doctors.

The inability to control clinical decisions has certainly been one of the factors which has weakened the authority of the management teams. Again the evidence from Kogan and Perrin suggests that because the teams were intended to manage by consensus, conflicts which involved a clash of interests were tacitly avoided. Trivial matters frequently took up considerable time while more crucial issues went by default. Administrators, as R. G. S. Brown comments, found their best survival strategy after 1974, as before, was to find out what doctors wanted and then find ways of getting it. They had no power or authority to work against medical interests. The 1974 reorganisation therefore, which was intended to strengthen management, shows little sign of having done so. Both management teams and area and regional authorities appeared powerless to act in a conflict with clinical practice. Klein cites the Normansfield Inquiry as illustrating the vacuum in management which existed. The Health Authorities concerned totally failed to come to grips with the maladministration at this mental handicap hospital despite being aware for a number of years of the problems. Neither was this an isolated incident.[23] Inquiries into the affairs of Solihull AHA and Rochdale criticised the ineffectiveness of management teams and the lack of monitoring and accountability.

CONCLUSION AND PROSPECT FOR THE 1980s

Patients First and Care in Action would seem to do little to change the influence and power of clinicians to commit resources. Indeed Patrick Jenkin in the launching of Patients First argued:

> I believe that doctors and other professional people in the NHS are trained to take professional decisions off their own bat, and do not need the torrent of advice to which in recent years they have been subjected. It is doctors, dentists and nurses and their colleagues in the other health professions who provide the care and cure of patients, and promote the health of the people. It is the purpose of management to support them in giving that service.[24]

However, this emphasis on clinical autonomy sits uneasily with the 1979 Conservative government's commitment to financial restraint. The Government Expenditure White Paper published in March 1982 implied a growth rate of 2.5 per cent in NHS services during 1982–83 of which 0.4 per cent was to be financed from efficiency savings. It is likely in a climate of tight resources that clinicians will look to savings from administration, even though these costs, in the context of other health services, are low, while managers may look to savings from clinicians. Certainly if services for dependent groups are to grow even in line with demographic trends, savings will have to be found from somewhere and unpleasant choices will have to be made at a local level, with those who can shout loudest, being, as in the past, the most successful.

The policy of tight central government control of overall resource allocation has been paralleled by efforts to monitor the performance of the regions and districts in terms of their efficiency and the degree to which they are following DHSS policy guidelines. There are notorious difficulties in measuring performance which are discussed in Chapter 5, but during the early 1980s further attempts have been made to devise methods of achieving greater value for money and to establish some development for the Cinderella services.

There is now a system of annual review by regions of districts within their area and regions will in turn be annually accountable to the DHSS through a system of review. Performance indicators covering clinical activity, staff, finance and estate management have been tested in the Northern Region. These have revealed enormous variations in costs. The total cost per in-patient case, for example, can vary by as much as 50 per cent and the cost of medical support services by 100 per cent.[25] These developments may create a new vocabulary for local policy-making and new possibilities for argument, negotiating and compromise. This development suggests that the comments of the two House of Commons Select Committees; the Public Accounts Committee on Financial Control and Accountability in the NHS and the Social Services Committee are being taken seriously. The latter Committee argued in 1980 that the DHSS should 'give a high priority to developing a comprehensive information system that would permit this committee and the public to assess the effect of changes in expenditure levels or patterns on the quality and scope of services provided'.[26] This theme was reiterated in subsequent years by both committees.[27]

During the early 1980s the major concern of central government has been to tighten the reins of financial control. This has been done by increasing the control of regions over the performance of districts and of the DHSS over regions. The effects in terms of the output of services or the quality of those services is largely unknown.[28]

A second objective has been to push the responsibility for making choices about spending decisions and policy to a more local level. The responsibility for resolving conflicts inherent in health care has been left to the District Health Authorities. Blame for any deteriorating health services or failure to meet demands for cure or care has been diffused to the districts. Much will therefore depend on the commitment and ability of those appointed to the service to bring about a more effective and efficient use of health resources. Many have learnt valuable lessons about the extent and limits of change from the period between 1974 to 1982. Operating on a smaller canvas may increase the ability of DHA members to identify and be involved in the key policy decisions. However DHAs lack the legitimacy of being elected authorities, and health authorities in the past have also lacked visibility. These are formidable handicaps in this period of NHS history.

REFERENCES

1. DEPARTMENT OF HEALTH AND SOCIAL SECURITY, and WELSH OFFICE, *Patients First. Consultative Paper on the Structure and Management of the National Health Service in England and Wales*, HMSO, London (1979)
2. DEPARTMENT OF HEALTH AND SOCIAL SECURITY, *Care in Action. A Handbook of Policies and Priorities for Health and Personal Social Services*, HMSO, London (1981)
3. BURNS, T. and STALKER, G.M., *The Management of Innovation*, Tavistock, London (1961)
4. KOGAN, M. *et al.*, *The Working of the National Health Service*,

Royal Commission on the NHS, Research Paper No. I, HMSO, London (1978)

5. BROWN, R. G. H., *Reorganising the Health Service*, Robertson, Oxford (1979)

6. For example, HAYWOOD, S. and ALASZEWSKI, A., *Crisis in the Health Service*, Croom Helm, London (1980)

7. OWEN, D., *In Sickness and in Health*, Quartet Books, London (1976), p. 113

8. DEPARTMENT OF HEALTH AND SOCIAL SECURITY, *Report of a Research Working Group on Inequalities in Health*, (Chairman: Sir D. Black) DHSS (1980)

9. HOUSE OF COMMONS, *Second Report from the Social Services Committee on Perinatal and Neonatal Mortality* (Chairman: Renee Short), HMSO, London (1980)

10. The problem of blocked beds is a recurring theme in the care of the very elderly. Elderly people may be unable to return home from a period in hospital without considerable nursing and or social work support, thus 'blocking' acute beds for other patients.

11. *Report of the Royal Commission on the National Health Service* (Chairman: Sir Alec Merrison) Cmnd 7615, HMSO, London (1979), Ch. 18

12. GOLDIE, N., 'Private Medicine – a logical development or an aberration? Report on a conference on National Health Care Systems in Non-growth Economies', *Scandinavian Journal of Social Medicine*, Supplementum 28, Stockholm (1981)

13. *Report of the Royal Commission on the National Health Service*, *op.cit.*, p. 289

14. SHEARER, A., 'The Health Care Market', *New Society*, 19 Feb 1981

15. GOLDIE, N., *op.cit.*

16. For example, THE POLITICS OF HEALTH GROUP, *Going Private. The Case Against Private Medicine*, available from 9 Poland Street, London W1 (1982)

17. KOGAN, M., *op.cit.*

18. PERRIN, J. *et al.*, *Management of Financial Resources in the National Health Service*, Research Paper, No. 2, Royal Commission on the National Health Service, HMSO (1979)

19. BROWN, R. G. S., *Reorganising the National Health Service*, *op. cit.*

20. HAYWOOD, S. and ELCOCK, H., *The Buck Stops Where? Accountability and Control in the National Health Service*, Institute of Health Studies, Hull (1980)

21. HAYWOOD, S. and ALASZEWSKI, A., *op. cit.*
22. Quoted by ALASZEWSKI, A., TETHER, P. and MCDONNELL, H., 'Another Dose of Managerialism?' Commentary on the Consultative Paper 'Patients First', *Social Science and Medicine*, Vol. 15A, No. 1, Jan. 1981
23. KLEIN, R., 'Normansfield: Vacuum of Management in the NHS', *British Medical Journal*, 23–30 Dec. 1978
24. DEPARTMENT OF HEALTH AND SOCIAL SECURITY and WELSH OFFICE, *Patients First: Consultative Paper, op. cit.*
25. *The Times Health Supplement*, 26 March 1982
26. HOUSE OF COMMONS, Social Services Committee, *The Government's White Papers on Public Expenditure in the Social Services. Third Report, Session 1979–80*, HC 702, HMSO, London (1980); HOUSE OF COMMONS, Social Services Committee, *Public Expenditure on the Social Services, Third Report, Session 1980–81*, HC 324, HMSO, London (1981)
27. HOUSE OF COMMONS, Public Accounts Committee, *Financial Control and Accountability in the NHS, 17th Report, Session 1980–81*, HC 255, HMSO, London (1981); HOUSE OF COMMONS, Public Accounts Committee, *Financial Control and Accountability in the NHS, 17th Report, Session 1981–82*, HC 375, HMSO, London (1982)
28. KLEIN, R., 'Auditing the NHS', *British Medical Journal*, Vol. 285, 11 Sept. 1982, pp. 672-3

Part three
CONTROVERSIES IN HEALTH POLICIES

This chapter aims to explore the trends in the major causes of illness and death in the UK and the way in which these have changed in the last century. These changing patterns in the leading causes of ill-health have provoked considerable discussion and controversy and present fundamental challenges for policy makers and to those concerned with providing health services.

In general terms the incidence of infectious diseases has declined in the UK as well as in other advanced industrial societies while diseases with a much more complex pattern of causality (aetiology) lying in the genetic, social and behavioural spheres, have tended to increase; such as diseases of the circulation, the cancers and accidents. Explanations of these changes are of vital importance to health policies for the population but our understanding of the biological and social processes at work, given the present state of knowledge, is limited. This is complicated by the fact that disciplines have tended to work within different explanatory frameworks to explain disease and ill-health. There is a contrast for example between the approach taken by the medical or biological sciences and the social sciences in explaining disease, health, illness and their incidence. There are, furthermore, differing theoretical approaches within the disciplines. This, and subsequent chapters, draw on recent work on the social bases of, and social production of, ill-health.

The changing pattern of ill-health, and the increased interest of social scientists in health and illness has been part of the process of shifting the paradigm of the way in which these phenomena are perceived and understood. These shifts are shown in diagrammatic form in document 31. There has tended to be greater questioning of the general applicability of the medical or disease model of illness. There has been a recognition that the concepts of disease, illness and health present problems of definition and themselves colour our view of the world. The first sections of this chapter therefore examine the concepts of disease, illness and health, and the measurement of mortality and morbidity.

CONCEPTS OF DISEASE, ILLNESS AND HEALTH

The concept of disease is rooted in the growth of scientific medicine which developed around the classification of disease entities in the nineteenth century. These disease entities were based on ideas of organic malfunctioning which in turn rested on a mechanistic view of normal bodily functioning. The diagnosis and treatment of such malfunctioning is the core of the medical task and it is around the identification, classification and treatment of diseases that the practice of medicine has grown in Western industrial societies. [Document 21 describes the 'medical model'.]

Illness is commonly distinguished from disease. Field, for example, comments that illness 'refers primarily to an individual's experience of ill-health and is indicated by a person's feelings of pain, discomfort and the like'. [1] It is thus possible to have an illness without disease and disease without illness. Disease is independent of social behaviour, while illness is culturally specific, dependent on folk definitions of normality which may or may not have a relationship to biomedical definitions. Illness has moral, psychological and social dimensions as well as physical, and therefore illness states or categories are as much a reflection of group definitions and responses as individual ones.

Health is an altogether more difficult concept and has been given a variety of interpretations. Within medical systems of thought, health has been seen as the absence of disease; to heal is essentially to make whole or restore to health. Healing by this definition becomes the preserve of the medical profession who have knowledge of disease processes. Health can also be considered as adequate functioning in a physical sense. The ability to perform certain tasks for example, can be taken as a measure of health. This can be extended to include mental and social functioning. The wider the definition the more subject to interpretation the notion of health becomes. Dubos sees health as adaptation to changes in nature and society. Health becomes 'freedom from pain, discomfort, stress and boredom . . . social, as well as biological, adaptation to environment and community'. [2] The World Health Organisation definition takes the concept of health a step further to describe it in positive terms as a 'state of complete, physical, mental and social well-being not merely the absence of disease and infirmity'.

Health seen as the converse of illness may vary according to different personal, social and cultural meanings given to it and there has been some exploration of the different meanings attached to health by anthropologists and sociologists. To give just two examples, certain middle-class Parisian women in a study by Herzlich[3] referred to health as a 'feeling of equilibrium', or well-being. However Blaxter and Patterson in a survey of attitudes to health among working-class women in Aberdeen found much lower expectations.[4] One respondent commented:

> After I was sterilised, I had a lot of cystitis, and backache because of the fibroids. Then when I had my hysterectomy I had bother with my waterworks because my bladder had a life of its own and I had to have a repair . . . Healthwise I would say I'm OK. I did hurt my shoulder – I mean, this is nothing to do with health but I actually now have a disability, I have a gratuity payment every six months . . . I wear a collar and take Valium then, just the headaches – but I'm not really off work a lot with it.

Despite the limitations of the 'disease model', the health status of nations and groups continues to be measured by the numbers of deaths and the amount of *medically* defined disease or sickness. This simply reflects the absence of more reliable measures. The measurement of health and the problems associated with it are discussed below followed by a discussion of the changing patterns of disease which is our main source of information on the causes of ill-health.

THE MEASUREMENT OF ILL-HEALTH

The health status of populations is measured by the use of data on mortality (deaths) and morbidity (disease and sickness). Mortality statistics are readily available and relatively reliable, but are only of limited value. They indicate what people die of, and at what age. They give a broad picture of the changing causes of death and can be used to measure changes in life expectancy. The mortality rate can be suggestive of the varying material circumstances of different groups because it is indicative of various 'at risk' factors in populations. However it is only a very crude indicator of the state of health of people who remain alive. A falling death rate may not mean an improvement in general basic health and many kinds of chronic ill-health, particularly among adults, which affect the quality of life, may not be reflected in mortality rates.

The Infant Mortality Rate (IMR), that is the number of deaths per 1,000 births during the first year of life, is generally acknowledged as being a more sensitive indicator of a society's general health status. This is because the number of infant deaths tends to be dependent on social and living conditions and the availability of health services which affect health status at all ages. Butler and Bonham also suggest that IMR is indicative of the number of near deaths which present with defects and deaths at a later stage. 'Like an iceberg we see only a proportion of the ill results, the deaths. But we must not forget the submerged and larger fraction, the near deaths and the harm they cause.'[5]

Data relating to morbidity, the amount of disease and sickness, are a more useful guide to health but the present range of morbidity statistics in the UK is limited. The main source of regular information is the General Household Survey of some 16,000 households which is carried out annually. The survey provides information on respondents' own recollections of episodes of ill-health making a distinction between acute illness and chronic illness (where there is long-standing sickness which affects activity). Questions have been changed periodically so that there are difficulties in making comparisons over time. This kind of information does rely on self-reporting and subjective definitions of illness. There are no large-scale regular health surveys of the population which offer *clinical* evidence about the distribution of disease and sickness although there have been one-off, small studies.

Information on morbidity can also be derived from data gathered for other purposes. Statistics on sickness absence, for example, are collected for the Department of Health and Social Security for the payment of sickness benefit. However they relate only to those who are employed and although they reflect professionally-determined clinical criteria of sickness and disability, disease categories can be very broadly framed. A 'respiratory tract infection', for example, can cover a multitude of symptoms, diseases and illnesses.

There is also data on the *use* of NHS services which can be taken as a measure of the amount of sickness for which there has been a consultation with a GP or which has led to the use of a hospital out-patient or in-patient facility. However these statistics too depend on the willingness to consult. Many studies have found a 'submerged iceberg of sickness' in the community which is never brought to the medical profession. This may be because conditions are defined as 'normal' due to age or occupation, because other remedies are being used or because there is little faith in the efficacy of medical intervention.[6]

Despite the limitations of the mortality and morbidity data, they are our main source of information on the changing patterns of death and disease. They are important not only for what they tell us about changes in the patterns but also because they have an important effect on how the problems of ill-health are understood. These understandings have in turn an effect on the policy-making environment and on demands for change in the provision of health services.

CHANGING PATTERNS OF MORTALITY

The most dramatic improvement in mortality rates has occurred among the very young and this has been progressive since the beginning of the nineteenth century. In Britain, at the beginning of the twentieth century 10 per cent of children born died within the first year. The present rate (at the end of the 1970s) is 1.3 per cent.[7] More than 98 per cent of babies now survive their first year of life. This is a pattern which is similar to that of other industrialised societies although the IMR in the United Kingdom has in recent years begun to lag behind that in other comparable countries. Figure 7 shows that

Fig. 7. Infant mortality; international comparisons

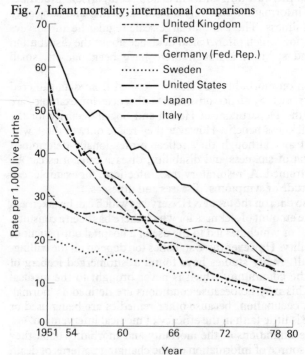

Source: *Social Trends*, No. 12, HMSO London (1982), p. 120

Sweden, Japan, Finland and France have better infant mortality rates though the rates of improvement for all has tended to flatten in recent years.

Mortality rates for other age groups vary according to sex and age but show a gradual improvement, particularly in the age groups under forty. Expectation of life at birth in the United Kingdom was 48.0 years for males and 51.6 for females at the turn of the century. By 1951 this had risen to 66.2 and 71.2 respectively and by 1978 there was a further increase to 70.0 years for males and 76.1 for females.[8] A recent study by WHO has suggested that there has been a general slowing down in the improvement in life expectancy. 'For males as well as females there is a noticeable, almost universal, reduction in the rate of decline of mortality with a virtual standstill or even setback for males.'[9] Table 9 shows the life expectancy at various ages for males and females in England and Wales. Life expectancy is shorter in

Table 9. Life expectancy – England and Wales

Age	1948–50		1958–60		1973–75	
	M	F	M	F	M	F
0	66.3	71.0	68.1	73.9	69.5	75.7
1	67.7	72.0	68.8	74.3	69.8	75.8
25	45.3	49.4	45.9	51.0	46.6	52.4
45	27.0	30.9	27.1	32.0	27.7	33.2
65	12.2	14.6	12.1	15.2	12.4	16.4

Source: DHSS, *Health and Personal Social Service Statistics for England and Wales*, HMSO, London, various years.

Northern Ireland and Scotland which accounts for differences between these and figures for the UK as a whole.

Changes in the leading causes of mortality and morbidity

Two factors stand out in any examination of major causes of death and disease in this century in the UK and indeed in most industrialised societies. The first is the *decline* in the incidence of infectious diseases and the second is the *increase* in diseases of the circulation (this includes heart attacks and strokes), cancer and respiratory diseases as the major causes of death in adults both male and female. The table in the document section [doc 23] shows the trends for Great Britain. The increase in deaths from lung cancer and myocardial infarction has

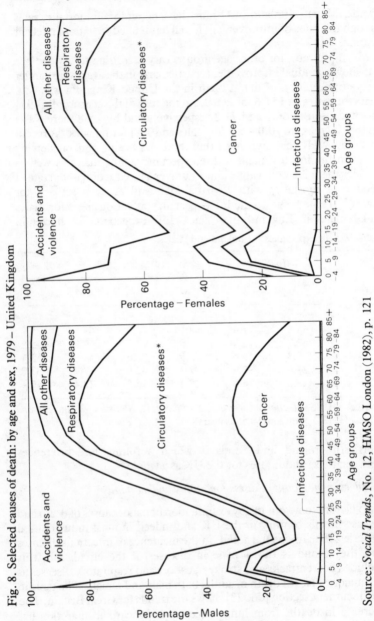

Fig. 8. Selected causes of death: by age and sex, 1979 – United Kingdom

Source: *Social Trends*, No. 12, HMSO London (1982), p. 121
*Includes heart attacks and strokes.

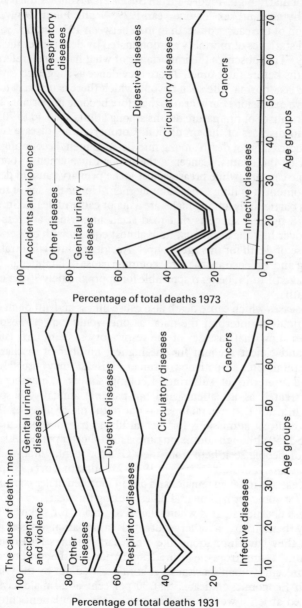

Fig. 9. Selected causes of death in men: a comparison between 1931 and 1973

The cause of death: men

Percentage of total deaths 1973

Percentage of total deaths 1931

Age groups

Age groups

Respiratory diseases

Accidents and violence

Other diseases

Genital urinary diseases

Digestive diseases

Circulatory diseases

Cancers

Infective diseases

Genital urinary diseases

Accidents and violence

Other diseases

Digestive diseases

Respiratory diseases

Circulatory diseases

Cancers

Infective diseases

Source: *Social Trends*, No. 9, HMSO London (1977)

been particularly high. Figure 8 from *Social Trends* shows the causes of death by age and sex for one year 1979. While Figure 9 gives a comparison of the causes of death in men between 1931 and 1973.

Overall statistics of mortality are dominated by deaths over the age of seventy. This obscures the importance of what have been referred to as 'deaths before their time'. There is evidence as suggested earlier that there is a 'normal' life span beyond which there is unlikely to be progressive extension. Early deaths therefore become important. The two major causes of premature deaths among adults aged 40 to 70 are cancer and diseases of the circulation. Coronary heart disease is the largest single cause of death among middle-aged men, accounting for one-third of the deaths. Cancer is the major cause among women. Among the cancers, while breast cancer is the primary cause of death among women, it is lung cancer among men. Under the age of forty accidents particularly among males are a major cause of death. Smith, using 1978 figures, suggests that road accidents, which are responsible for over half the accidents, rank almost equally with cancer as a chief cause of death for this age group.[10] Accidents, involving traffic, poisoning and violence are the most common cause of fatalities among children aged 1 to 14, being responsible for approximately 30 per cent of the deaths.[11]

The diseases which cause death also cause illness and although it is more difficult to interpret the data, as one would expect, hospital discharges show that diseases of the respiratory system, circulatory diseases and cancer account for the highest number of discharges from hospital after in-patient treatment. Disease may also take a heavy toll in terms of suffering. Looking simply at numbers of patients treated as in-patients and out-patients annually, hospital statistics indicate that mental illness is one of the major illnesses. The number of direct admissions for mental illness has increased three-fold since 1950 although admission time is for a shorter period. A large number of people seek help from their GPs for mental illness. The second national morbidity survey in 1970–71 found that over a sample of practices, one in seven females and one in fourteen males consulted their GP for some form of mental illness during this year.[12]

Sickness absence figures where claims are made for sickness and invalidity benefit are another source of information on sickness although they have limitations like other data. Figures for example concern only claims from the insured population and therefore tend to underrepresent women's sickness. A study carried out by the Office of Health Economics indicates that 30 per cent of all male days of certificated absence were due to diseases of the circulation, chronic bronchitis and arthritis and rheumatism for the year 1978–79. [13]

Among children, as with mortality, accidents are a frequent cause of sickness and injury. At the more severe end of the spectrum the Hospital In-patient Inquiry in 1977 estimated that accidents caused nearly 128,000 children aged 1 to 14 to be admitted to hospital as in-patients in England and Wales. [14] This again was a fraction of the accidents treated but not admitted by Accident and Emergency Departments. The numbers involved in childhood accidents and estimated costs involved are shown in Table 10.

Table 10. The number and cost of childhood accidents

	Number	Cost (£m) (Dec 1980)
Deaths (1979)	925	–
Hospital inpatients (1977)	128,000	31.1
New A & E cases (1979)	2,000,000	31.4
GP consultations (1979)	1,334,000	5.5
		68.0

Source: Office of Health Economics, *Accidents in Childhood*, OHE Briefing No. 17, Sept. 1981

In summary, the pattern of death and disease in the UK, in line with patterns in other industrialised societies, has changed during the century. The decline in infectious disease has led to increasing numbers surviving into middle and old age of each cohort of births. The largest single factor has been the greater survival rate of infants in the first year of life. The age structure of the population has changed so that there are large numbers of old and very elderly people, bringing a greater demand for medical and social services [doc 16]. Demand has increased not only for acute medical services but for care and support since old age brings an increase in chronic illness, disability and dependency.

While the incidence of infectious diseases had declined, the emergent pattern of disease, diseases of the circulation, cancer, respiratory disease, of accidents, mental illness and other behaviour-related conditions has added to the amount of chronic illness and disability in the community. There has been considerable speculation and argument as to the causes of the change, the reasons why infectious diseases have declined and the so-called diseases of affluence increased. We now turn to this issue.

SOCIAL FACTORS AND THE CHANGING PATTERN OF MORTALITY
AND MORBIDITY

The debate about the causes of the changing pattern of disease and
illness has generated a number of theories which draw on different
frameworks or paradigms of explanation. Any brief account is bound
to oversimplify the complexity of the issues involved but this section
will attempt to identify the main explanatory approaches and examine
the relationship between disease and social class, an area of investi-
gation which generated intense interest and activity among medical
and social researchers in the latter half of the 1970s.

Social factors and disease: explanations

Recent explanations of the changing patterns of illness and disease
have stressed the importance of social and economic factors in causation. This marks a break from the past. The theory of disease which
lay at the heart of the growth of nineteenth century scientific medicine
and the medical or curative model has already been described. The
germ theory of disease rested on the assumption that single diseases
had single causes and this seemed to be a convincing explanation in
the context of a prevalence of infectious disease. Vaccination, immunisation and drugs therapies appeared to be effective in combating
disease. However, germ theory had serious weaknesses and one of the
most important was the fact that only some people exposed to pathogens contracted diseases. Why should certain people be more susceptible than others? In the attempt to explain this there has been a return
to the even earlier nineteenth century tradition which was concerned
to demonstrate that disease was linked to the environment in which
people live and the way they live. The two extracts in the document
section given an example taken from Engels describing factory work
in the nineteenth century and a recent study of women production-
line workers by Ruth Cavendish [doc 25]. Both relate illness to
production processes and ways of working.

Blume suggests that there have been two major disciplinary
approaches in attempting to understand the relationship between
social factors and disease or illness. One is the epidemiological
approach, the second the sociological.[15] Epidemiology is a study of the
distributions and states of health in human populations. It is concerned therefore with the effects of combinations of factors, social and
environmental, as well as biological, which affect the incidence of
specific diseases in individuals. It suggests the multi-causality of
illness and disease rather than the mono-causality of germ theory.

Sociological explanations on the other hand are primarily concerned with demonstrating a link between modes of social organisation and social structure on disease and illness in societies and groups. The focus is on susceptibility to disease or illness in general rather than with specific disease categories and the susceptibility of particular groups or classes with similar social characteristics rather than individuals. They could be called 'general susceptibility theories'.

Multi-causal explanations of changes in patterns of disease   In a major contribution in the epidemiological tradition stressing multi-causality, McKeown in *The Role of Medicine*,[16] argues that the decline in mortality from infectious diseases has been the consequence of improvements in nutrition and standards of living from the early nineteenth century onwards. These improvements led to changes in reproductive behaviour which further strengthened resistance to infection while interventions in public health through environmental improvements of water supply and sanitation lessened the likelihood of the spread of pathogens. Thus medical intervention through vaccination and immunisation, with the possible exception of diphtheria and poliomyelitis, has had a minimal effect on mortality rates.

Implicit in McKeown's account is a notion that human health rests on the capacity of the individual to resist disease. People are well but become ill for a variety of reasons. In turning to contemporary disease patterns where non-infective diseases predominate McKeown suggests that part of the explanation lies in the higher survival rates among infants and increased longevity. People who live longer are more exposed to a range of diseases which have a complex of causes. Causes may be sought in a range of genetic, behavioural and environmental factors and in the present state of knowledge there can only be alternative hypotheses about the hazards of particular diseases in specific individuals. Thus there is a strong behavioural association between smoking and lung cancer. People who smoke have a high incidence of lung cancer. But genetic and environmental factors may also be involved. Environmental pollution at home or at work may increase risk and so may genetic factors. In the case of other diseases environmental pollution is more directly involved. Working with asbestos brings a very high risk of mesothelioma. Silicosis is an occupational hazard of miners, byssinosis of cotton workers, but there may also be factors which predispose families or individuals within these occupations to the disease. It is unusual to be able to identify a disease with a single clear-cut identifiable causal link. Huntington's Chorea, for example, is believed to be of wholly genetic origin. Other diseases tend to have a complex aetiology depending on a variety of factors; life style, behaviour, work, as well as inherited susceptibility.

The 'general susceptibility' of groups and societies to disease. Socio-logical explanations of the changing disease pattern take a number of different forms as there are a variety of theoretical approaches within sociology. In general however sociological theories all emphasise the importance of social structure and institutions on patterns of health and disease. Dubos and Powles represent a form of Social Darwinism. Both describe modern disease patterns as evidence of maladaptation to industrialisation. Dubos argues:

> It is a dangerous error to believe that diseases and suffering can be wiped out altogether by raising still further standards of living, increasing our mastery of the environment and developing new therapeutic procedures. The less pleasant reality is that, since the world is ever changing, each period and each type of civilisation will continue to have its burden of disease created by the unavoidable failure of biological and social adapta-tion to counter new environmental threats.[17]

Powles presents evidence to suggest that certain diseases occur particularly in advanced industrial societies, for example, arterio-sclerosis, diabetes, diverticulitis. Ways of living and particularly diet are involved.[18] Other sociological approaches suggest that the capi-talist mode of production is implicated in the creation of disease. Production for profit ignores the risks to workers of the production process and despite overwhelming evidence of risks to health, govern-ments are slow to intervene. It is also argued more generally that patterns of living in advanced industrial societies create hazards. Cassel, for example, suggests that changing social conditions lead to stress and stress increases susceptibility to disease in general. A variety of social circumstances have been investigated along these lines. For example widowers are shown to have a death rate three to five times higher than married men of the same age for every cause of death.[19] In all these situations, however, although there appears to be 'an association' between social factors and illness it is difficult to establish a precise linkage. The term cause is used in a very general rather than a specific way.

Research has also been stimulated into the relationship between rising levels of unemployment and ill-health. Brenner in a well-known study has attempted to establish a link between levels of production, and unemployment and ill-health. He suggests that recessions, and wide-scale economic distress exert an impact on health status indi-cators – IMR, maternal mortality and national mortality rates, especially deaths ascribed to cardiovascular disease, cirrhosis of the liver, suicide and homicide rates and rates of first admission to mental hospital.[20]

The high rates of unemployment in the UK have led to more research on this topic. In an attempt to link macro- and micro-social variables, Colledge in a small-scale study of unemployment in Newcastle argues that a reduction in the general level of economic activity triggers off a sequence of events which ultimately is shown up in increased levels of ill-health and death rates. This is because of the increased level of stress in individuals. The stress is caused by social pressures, financial difficulties, family and marital relationships, a disruption of daily living patterns, a challenge to the ingrained work ethic.[21] The response to this stress varies with personality and socio-economic position, but there is a significant number of cases where the result is ill-health of one sort or another. This is supported by Fagin's research on health and unemployment, the conclusions of which are reproduced in the document section [doc 26]. Social factors are shown therefore 'to produce' or increase susceptibility to disease.

SOCIAL CLASS AND ILL-HEALTH

Both the epidemiological and sociological approaches are attempts to explain the changing patterns of disease from different perspectives. Both approaches have been drawn towards using social class as an analytical tool to explore the patterns of incidence of particular diseases; in this they have been stimulated by the concern of politicians and the public. A Conservative Minister, Sir Keith Joseph, set up the Court Committee to examine Child Health Services following his interest in the 'cycle of deprivation'. The conclusion of the report in 1976 was that 'in many crucial respects our findings have given us profound anxiety about the state of child health in this country, about the shortcomings of services and those working in them, and about the prospects for new generations if they are to grow up in the same deprived physical and emotional circumstances as many children today have to contend with'[22] [doc 22]. David Ennals, a Labour Minister, set up the Black Committee to pursue further the relationship between health and social class and this provides a rich source of information on inequalities in health.[23] The decision by the Select Committee of Health and Social Services to investigate the trends in neonatal and perinatal mortality reflected the continuing concern for the lack of further improvement in infant mortality. Its findings were published in the Short Report in 1981.[24]

Most studies of the relationship between social class and ill-health use the Registrar General's classification of occupations on which to base a division of the population into five broad social classes. These groupings encapsulate a number of variables such as income, property, occupation and education which are highly correlated with each other. Broadly speaking most investigations into disease and illness have revealed a higher incidence of illness in the lower social classes.

The Black Report states that class differences in morbidity and mortality are a constant feature of the entire human life time:

> They were also found at birth, during the first year of life, in childhood, adolescence and in adult life. In general they are more marked at the start of life and in early adulthood. Average life expectancy provides a useful summary of the cumulative impact of these advantages and disadvantages throughout life. A child born to professional parents, if he or she is not socially mobile, can expect to spend over 5 years more as a living person than a child born to an unskilled manual household.[25]

Figure 10 below shows the persistent class inequalities at different stages of life.

In relation to infant mortality, although this continues to improve the class gradient has persisted. Figure 11 below illustrates the trends.

Social progress, whilst reflected in an overall decline in various rates of mortality has not given rise to any significant improvement in the health experience of the manual classes relative to the professional and managerial classes and this is particularly the case with infant mortality. Children born into unskilled manual workers' families are four times more likely to die in their first year of life than those born into professional families.

There is also a class gradient in the main causes of mortality in childhood accidents and respiratory diseases. The same is true of morbidity, growth and cognitive development as well, although the available data here are rather thin. The Court Report commented, 'We have already had occasion to refer repeatedly to the correlation between social class and the prevalence of ill-health and disability in children . . . There is now extensive evidence that an adverse family and social environment can retard physical, emotional and intellectual growth, lead to more frequent and more serious illness and adversely affect educational achievement and personal behaviour.'[26]

In relation to adult health the Black Report suggests that out of eighty-two disease categories listed in mortality statistics to constitute the Standardised Mortality Rate (SMR) there is a class gradient in sixty-eight of the categories. These cover chronic diseases, motor

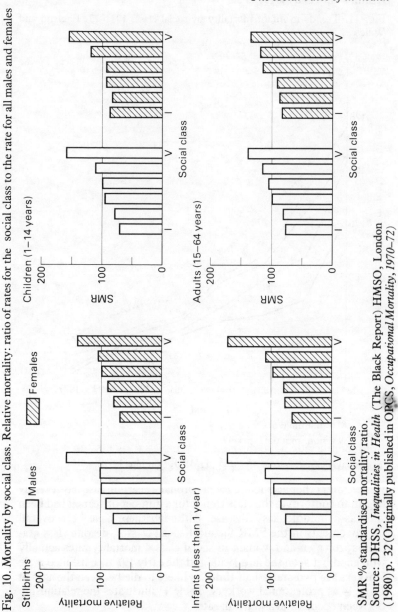

Fig. 10. Mortality by social class. Relative mortality: ratio of rates for the social class to the rate for all males and females

SMR % standardised mortality ratio.
Source: DHSS, *Inequalities in Health* (The Black Report) HMSO, London (1980) p. 32 (Originally published in OPCS, *Occupational Mortality, 1970–72*)

159

Fig. 11. Trends in infant mortality by social class, 1911–77, England and Wales

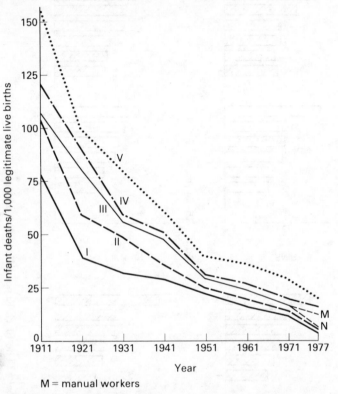

M = manual workers
N = non-manual workers

Source: OPCS, *Trends in Mortality*, HMSO, London (1978)

vehicle and other accidents. Even coronary heart disease has recently begun to conform to the class trend; for a number of years it had been seen as a 'middle-class' disease. Although there have been overall improvements in the SMR for most social classes, despite class gradients, for men and women in social class 4 mortality rates actually worsened between the late 1950s and the early 1970s. Unskilled male workers are two-and-a-half times as likely to die between the ages of 15 to 44 as professional workers. Table 11 illustrates the relationship between occupation and death rates.

These figures tend to make nonsense of the comment that contem-

Table 11. Mortality by occupation unit: Men 15–64 (Selected examples)

Occupation units	Direct age-standardized death rate (per 100,000)	SMR⋆
Relatively low death-rate		
University teachers	287	49
Physiotherapists	297	55
Paper products makers	302	50
Managers in building and contracting	319	54
Local authority senior officers	342	57
Company secretaries and registrars	362	60
Ministers of the Crown, MPs, senior government officials	371	61
Office managers	377	64
Primary and secondary school teachers	396	66
Sales managers	421	70
Architects, town planners	443	74
Civil service executive officers	467	78
Postmen	484	81
Medical practitioners	494	81
Relatively high death-rate		
Coal miners (underground)	822	141
Shoemakers, and shoe repairers	898	156
Leather products makers	895	147
Machine-tool operators	934	156
Watch repairers	946	154
Coal miners (above ground)	972	160
Steel erectors, riggers	992	164
Fishermen	1028	171
Deck, engineering officers and pilots	1040	175
Labourers and unskilled workers, all industries	1247	201
Policemen	1270	109
Deck and engine room ratings	1385	233
Bricklayers' labourers	1644	274
Electrical engineers (so described)	1904	317

Source: Adapted from OPCS, *Occupational Mortality*, Decennial Supplement 1970–72, England and Wales, HMSO, London (1978)
⋆ Standardized Mortality Rate (SMR) is an index for mortality which is adjusted for the age distribution of the group being studied.

porary disease patterns reflect the 'diseases of affluence'. It is the poor who experience greater ill-health in industrial societies and if the mortality rates were as good in social class 4 and 5 as in social class 1, Britain would be in line with the 'healthiest' countries in the world league, Sweden and Finland. In many respects, however, data on class and mortality and morbidity present problems; first, problems of interpretation and second, problems for policy.

THE INTERPRETATION OF DATA ON CLASS, MORTALITY AND MORBIDITY

The major difficulty of much information on the relationship between class and illness is that of itself, it explains very little. Social class does not *cause* ill-health but it is associated with it. Low social class brings a general susceptibility as a consequence of the higher incidence of other variables associated with class, low incomes, occupation, diet, etc. Both the epidemiological and sociological explanations referred to earlier have attempted to explain the linkages but both have weaknesses. The former, because they are based on illness in individuals fail to explain the context in which health and illness behaviour occurs in different classes. For example they may explain that more men in social class 5 smoke but not why they do or why social class 5 women tend to be late attenders at antenatal clinics. There is also difficulty in explaining the causes of ill-health which are not based on disease as in the case of accidents or mental illness. On the other hand sociological explanations may suggest factors which create vulnerability to disease in general but are less effective in explaining the incidence of particular diseases in particular individuals and frequently weak on what action to take, short of radical social change.

It may be that the way forward lies in continuing to identify groups which are very susceptible to ill-health and explore the circumstances which make them more vulnerable to particular diseases and threats to health. Brown and Harris's work on depression in women using various psychosocial variables has suggested that particular groups of working-class women are vulnerable to a specific illness, depression.[27] This study combines both the epidemiological and sociological perspectives.

In other areas there is simply too little information to resolve conflicts over the 'causes' of ill-health. Take accidents to children where children of parents in social class 5 are five times as likely to have an accident in childhood than those in social class 1. Accidents have been linked to the lack of safe play space. The Black Report argued that 'apart from the specific danger from road traffic, it is likely that the working class child lives in a more dangerous physical environment than middle class children. Derelict slum housing about to be cleared, deserted canals, mineshafts and factories, railway lines and rubbish tips; all these present dangers to the child in the urban industrial area.' Susceptibility is therefore linked to social/environmental factors. Brown and Harris on the other hand found that the mother's psychiatric state and the presence of a serious long-term difficulty or threatening life event was related to increased accident risk in children and in another study Brown and Davidson found that maternal psychiatric disturbance led to increased irritability and loss of interest in the children. This, they suggested, gave rise to new behaviour patterns in children and a greater risk of accidents. Susceptibility here is linked to psychosocial factors.[28] It seems that illness, disease or accidents can be explained in different ways depending on the perspective of the researcher.

If certain groups are susceptible to accident, disability and ill-health, there is also evidence to indicate that disadvantage is cumulative. In a detailed study, *The Health of Children*, Blaxter suggests that there is an inherited element.[29] Children of professional and managerial class parents tend to be taller than those with parents in social class 5. (A difference of 3.3 cms at seven years old.) There is strong evidence relating the birth weight of the child to the height of the mother. Low birth weight itself is linked to high infant mortality and morbidity. Disadvantage may thus be passed on through generations. Although a good environment can compensate for low birth weight, one which is not satisfactory can represent a cumulative hazard. Poor nutrition and child care can reinforce disadvantage.

Blaxter has drawn a profile of the adult at greatest disadvantage. This is broadly speaking a person who has carried through life 'at risk' factors from conception through birth, and childhood, with particularly disadvantageous social and environmental conditions which are part of the living and working environment (for example working in an asbestos factory or in a polluted northern city). This may be exacerbated by having inadequate access to health services and by behaviour characteristics such as smoking, drinking and a tendency not to use available preventive and curative services [doc 33]. Poor health, as Rainwater comments, may be reinforced by culture 'just as lower class people become resigned to a conception of themselves as persons who do not function very well socially or psychologically, they become resigned to bodies which function less well physically'.[30]

It is quite clear that the social production of disease is complex and that if health status is to be improved then a range of social and environmental factors need to be taken into account as well as factors relating to the individual and individual behaviour. This is implicit in the above quotation. One necessary step is a much finer social occupational class breakdown linked with parallel studies of small populations who are particularly susceptible.

STRATEGIES FOR CHANGE IN HEALTH POLICY

The state of knowledge and the conflicting paradigms of explanation of ill-health present difficulties for policy-making as well as research. There are difficulties in establishing where to break the cycle of ill-health and in determining who or what is primarily to blame for that ill-health. As in the case of poverty, explanations of the cause of ill-health tend to make *a priori* assumptions about where the problem lies and use this as a guide to policy. Hirsch puts it like this: 'the conservative viewpoint sees the problem as residing in the individual and tries to change him, and the reformist viewpoint sees the problem as residing in the environment and tries to change it. The reform viewpoint sees troubled individuals and blames that on the environment.'[31]

It is possible however to identify *three* main approaches to health policy. The first focuses on the individual and aims to change individual behaviour as a way of improving health. The second concentrates on achieving a more equal distribution of health services according to need as a way of improving health and the third, or structuralist approach, seeks broader changes in areas of social life well beyond conventional health services. The third approach may incorporate the second, as does the Black Report, but there are advantages in discussing them separately.

Individualist strategies

Much of the work carried out within the epidemiological tradition does suggest that individual behaviour and family behaviour may be the most appropriate point at which to intervene as a step towards improving health. Comment has already been made on the well-established link between smoking and lung cancer, and the high rate of accidents, particularly car accidents, in men aged between 15 to 40. There is also an established relationship between alcoholism and cirrhosis of the liver and considerable controversy about the association between high levels of cholesterol and/or sugar on the incidence of coronary heart disease. As a general strategy it has been suggested by McKeown and others that the best hope for improving health lies in changing individual behaviour. Many of the policies for prevention discussed in Chapter 10 rest on this premise and are discussed further in that context.

In the same tradition, although more positively, Belloc and Breslow in a study in the United States attempted to relate personal behaviour more generally to physical status.[32] They assessed the effects on health of following seven rules: (a) no smoking of cigarettes; (b) sleeping for seven hours a night; (c) eating breakfast; (d) keeping weight down; (e) drinking moderately; (f) exercising daily and (g) not eating between meals. It was concluded that health and longevity increased with the number of rules followed. For people over seventy-five following all the rules, health was said to be as good as for those aged 35 to 44 who followed less than three; and life expectation at age forty-five was eleven years longer for people following six or seven rules than for those following less than four. Strategies to improve health by changing individual behaviour rest on the assumption that information and education on health services will encourage individuals to effectively optimise their own health.

The distribution of health services

The second approach to the problem of improving the health of the population has concentrated on ensuring that health services are more readily available. There is strong evidence to suggest that the distribution of health services is unequal, particularly if the level of provision is related to need. There has already been some discussion of this issue in Chapter 5 in relation to geographical maldistribution of services regionally. The point to be made here is that there is also evidence that health services are least adequate for those who suffer the greatest ill-health, social classes 4 and 5: that there is what Julian Tudor-Hart calls 'an inverse care law'.[33] This argument has three aspects. First, it is suggested that in areas of the country where there are greater numbers in the lower social classes, who have greater health needs, there are fewer health services and second, that this is exacerbated by unequal *use* of services by those who most need them, third there is less expenditure overall on the health care of the lower social classes.

Class and the availability of health services   It is of course a complex matter to determine whether services are distributed or used in exact ratio to need. Conclusions of research on this question are indicative of the general trends rather than definitive statements of statistical accuracy. Furthermore the picture is complicated by the variety of health services where it is possible to assess distribution according to class: hospital services, in-patients, out-patients, dental services, preventative services, GP services, etc.

It is proposed here only to look at the distribution of GPs as the inequitable distribution of hospital facilities and hospital manpower has been discussed already. Furthermore, the GP service as the source of primary care acts as the point of referral, so the distribution in a sense matters more.

A study by Political and Economic Planning in 1944 pointed to the relationship between the affluence of areas and the distribution of GPs.

> In Hastings before the war there was one GP for every 1,178 persons, while in South Shields there was one for every 4,105 . . . Thus the number of residents per GP was twice as great in Kensington as in Hampstead, thrice as great in Harrow; four times as great in Bradford, five times in Wakefield, six times in West Bromwich and seven times in South Shields. This disparity in distribution is even more serious than it appears from these figures because 'under-doctored' districts are usually also poor districts with high rates of sickness and mortality and in special need of a good medical service.[34]

Butler in 1976 concluded that with regard to GPs the NHS

> has not brought about any dramatic shift in their location. The broad pattern of staffing needs have not changed dramatically over the last 20 or 30 years. Areas which are currently facing the most serious shortages seem to have a fairly long history of manpower difficulties, whilst those which are today relatively well supplied with family doctors have generally had no difficulties in past years in attracting and keeping an adequate number of practitioners . . . Certain areas of the country are medically deprived in the sense that existing services are unable to cope with the demands placed upon them, while others have a relative abundance of medical resources in relation to their needs.[35]

The same tends to be the case with other NHS personnel and facilities.

The distribution of facilities however does not necessarily say anything about the use of services and the share of public expenditure going to particular social classes. It may be that social classes 4 and 5 use health services more than professional or managerial classes.

The use of health services by social class There has been a lively debate on this issue. The flames have partly been fanned by American academics who deplore the inequities in their own market-oriented medical systems and see the NHS as an achievement in collective intervention. Martin Rein, has argued that the 'lowest social classes make greater use of hospital in-patient services . . . and . . . they receive what appears to be of as good quality as that secured by other social classes'.[36] Rein's examples are drawn however from the south of England where in any case the availability and quality of services tends to be higher than in other parts of the country, and most critics suggest that he made insufficient allowance for greater needs. There is clearly controversy in relation to use of hospital and GP services but after a detailed survey of the available evidence the Black Committee concluded that class differences in need were not fully reflected in health service use.[37] The results of two studies on the use of health services are reproduced in the document section [doc 24].

Cartwright and O'Brien comment that the 'quality' of care received by higher social classes may be superior to that received by lower social classes. 'There appears to us to be fairly conclusive evidence that the middle class made more use of preventive services, and to suggest that the middle class may in relation to a number of services, receive better care.'[38] 'Better care' is difficult to pinpoint precisely but the Black Report cites studies which suggest that women from social class 5 not only experienced the lowest degree of intensive care during their pregnancies, but were very much more likely to have their babies induced in hospital. Consultation times tended to be longer with higher social classes and there was evidence to show that home visits by consultants to patients in terminal care favoured these groups also.

Health service expenditure by social class The third aspect of class inequalities relates to health service expenditure and logically, if there are inequalities in the two areas already discussed, less is likely to be spent on the lower social class. Two examples may be given of studies which relate expenditure to social class. Noyce, Snaith and Trickey analysed the expenditure by local authorities in the three branches of the health service in 1971/72. They found a significant positive correlation between the percentage of the population in professional and managerial socioeconomic groups in both community health expenditure and hospital revenue expenditure. They conclude 'evidently as late as 1971/72 no effort was achieving success in directing new capital to deprived regions'.[39]

More recently Le Grand in *Strategy of Equality* has examined the distribution of expenditure per head in the NHS and found that higher social groups incurred higher levels of expenditure.[40] As the basis of calculation he used data on current costs to the NHS of units of utilisation and numbers of people by social class reporting illness. Table 12 below shows the findings.

Table 12. Public expenditure on health care by socio-economic group – All persons – England and Wales 1972

Socio-economic group	Expenditure per person: percentage of mean	Expenditure per person reporting illness: percentage of mean
Professionals, employers and managers	94	120
Intermediate and junior non-manual	104	114
Skilled manual	92	97
Semi- and unskilled manual	114	
Mean (£)= 100	18.1	103.2

Source: Calculated as in Le Grand, *Strategy of Equality*, George Allen & Unwin (1982) p. 26

These inequalities in distribution and access to health services have led to a pressure for policies to increase equality of provision. RAWP policies have been described in the previous section. The Short Committee too put a good deal of emphasis on the importance of improving antenatal facilities and care. There are criticisms of this approach as more services do not *necessarily* correlate with better health care and improved mortality rates. However among service providers there is a belief that it can. Baird, has shown in Aberdeen that despite a situation in which the environmental and social characteristics of the population are by no means ideal (for example the social class distribution and the physique of mothers was considerably less advantageous to good results than those in the south of England) improvements have been achieved in terms of indices such as the perinatal mortality rate which compare with the best in the UK.[41]

Structuralist strategies

The third broad approach to policies in relation to a reduction of ill-health places an emphasis on the need to change social conditions and social inequalities in general as a precondition to the reduction of illness and disease. Such policies, of which the recommendations of the Black Report on Inequalities in Health is a prime example, emphasise the link between poverty and ill-health and inequalities in the work place and the environment. Townsend, drawing on information from the Royal Commission on Income and Wealth and on his own study of poverty, argues that 'the conditions under which men and women make their livelihood, the degree of insecurity and stability, the scope for self-fulfilment and job-satisfaction and the physical and mental character of the task itself are all important determinants of health status'.[42] So the Black Report is concerned to alleviate the wider causes of inequality, in family income, in housing, in environmental improvements as well as in improved access to health services. The recommendations of the Report for changes outside the health service are reproduced in the document section [doc 27].

Structuralist strategies have a wide agenda of social reform covering a range of approaches and activities. Health issues have become in recent years a rallying point for a number of pressure groups, campaigning for example for the abolition of lead in petrol, or concerned with drawing attention to the high level of risk in exposure to asbestos.

FINAL COMMENT

This chapter has attempted to review the evidence in relation to the major causes of ill-health, and to account for the different approaches to explaining them. It has been suggested that different modes of explanation may partly account for different approaches to policy questions as they do in relation to poverty. Governments in Britain have so far failed to act positively upon the overwhelming evidence that there are strong relationships between social conditions and ill-health. The major response has been to attempt to improve access to NHS services although the difficulties of achieving this in view of the politics of the NHS was pointed out in Chapter 7. Moreover, simply providing services does not necessarily improve health status.

In contrast to the Lalonde Report on the Health of Canadians which defines health as a major policy issue, health policies in Britain have tended to be fragmented and piecemeal with increasing health services.[43] Recently preventive health policies have focused on changing individual behaviour but this focus must broaden if it is to ameliorate the consequences of avoidable risks to health.

REFERENCES

1. FIELD, D., 'The Social Definition of Illness', in TUCKETT, D. (ed.) *An Introduction to Medical Sociology*, Tavistock, London (1976)
2. DUBOS, R., *The Mirage of Health*, Allen & Unwin, London (1960)
3. HERZLICH, C., *Health and Illness: A Social Psychological Analysis*, Academic Press, London (1976)
4. BLAXTER, M. and PATTERSON, E., *Mothers and Daughters. A Three-generational study of Health Attitudes and Behaviour*, Heinemann Educational, London (1982)
5. BUTLER, M. R., and BONHAM, D. E., *Perinatal Mortality: The first report of the 1958 British Perinatal Mortality Survey*, E. & S. Livingston, Edinburgh (1963)
6. WADSWORTH, M. E. J., BUTTERFIELD, W. J. H. and BLANEY, R., *Health and Sickness: The Choice of Treatment*, Tavistock, London (1971)
7. BLAXTER, M., *The Health of Children. A Review of Research on the Place of Health in Cycles of Disadvantage*, Heinemann Educational, London (1981), p. 35
8. *Social Trends*, No. 12, Table 7.1, p. 119. HMSO, London (1981)
9. OFFICE OF HEALTH ECONOMICS, *Medicines and the Quality of Life*, Briefing No. 19, Sept. 1982, OHE, London
10. SMITH, T., 'Cause of Death: Attitude of Mind', *The Times Health Supplement*, 11 Dec. 1981
11. OFFICE OF HEALTH ECONOMICS, *Accidents in Childhood*. OHE Briefing No. 17, Sept. 1981
12. OPCS, *Morbidity Statistics from General Practice: Second National Study 1970–1971*, HMSO, London (1976)
13. OFFICE OF HEALTH ECONOMICS, *Sickness Absence – a Review*, OHE Briefing No. 16, Aug 1981
14. OHE, *Accidents in Childhood, op. cit.*
15. BLUME, S., 'Explanation and Social Policy: "The" problem of social inequalities in health', *Journal of Social Policy*, Vol. 11, Pt. 1, Jan. 1982
16. MCKEOWN, T., *The Role of Medicine. Dream, Mirage or Nemesis?*, Blackwell, Oxford (1979)
17. DUBOS, R., *Man, Medicine and Environment*, Pall Mall Press, London (1968), p. 75
18. POWLES, J., 'On the Limitations of Modern Medicine', *Science*,

Medicine and Man, **1** (1973), 1–30

19. CASSEL, J., 'Psychological processes and "stress": theoretical formulations', *International Journal of Health Services,* 4 (1974), 471

20. BRENNER, H. M., 'Health costs and benefits of economic policy', *International Journal of Health Services,* 7 (1977), 581–623

21. COLLEDGE, M., *Unemployment and Health,* North Tyneside Community Health Council (1981)

22. DEPARTMENT OF HEALTH AND SOCIAL SECURITY and DEPARTMENT OF EDUCATION AND SCIENCE, *Fit for the Future. Report of the Committee on Child Health Services* (Court Report) (Chairman: Sir Donald Court), Cmnd 6684, HMSO, London (1976)

23. DEPARTMENT OF HEALTH AND SOCIAL SECURITY, *Report of a Research Working Group on Inequalities in Health* (Black Report) (Chairman: Sir Douglas Black), DHSS, London (1980), Ch. 2

24. HOUSE OF COMMONS, *2nd Report from the Social Services Committee on Perinatal and Neonatal Mortality* (Chairman: Renee Short), HMSO, London (1980)

25. DEPARTMENT OF HEALTH AND SOCIAL SECURITY, Black Report, *op. cit.,* Ch. 3 and 4

26. DEPARTMENT OF HEALTH AND SOCIAL SECURITY, Court Report, *op. cit.,* Ch. 1 and 2

27. BROWN, G. and HARRIS, T., The Social Origins of Depression, Tavistock, London (1978)

28. OHE, *Accidents in Childhood, op. cit.*

29. BLAXTER, M., *Health of Children, op. cit.*

30. RAINWATER, L., 'The Lower-class: health, illness and medical institutions' in DEUTSCHER, I. and THOMPSON, E. J. (eds), *Among the People: encounters with the poor,* Basic Books, New York

31. HIRSCH, C., quoted in WILDAVSKY, A., *The Art and Craft of Policy Analysis,* Macmillan (1979), Ch. 2

32. BELLOC, N. B. and BRESLOW, L., 'Relationship of Physical Health Status and Health Practices', *Preventive Medicine,* 1 (1972), 409–21

33. TUDOR-HART, J., 'The Inverse Care Law', in COX, C. and MEAD, A. (eds), *A Sociology of Medical Practice,* Collier-Macmillan, London (1968)

34. POLITICAL AND ECONOMIC PLANNING, 'Medical Care for Citizens,' *Planning,* No. 222, 1944

35. BUTLER, J., *Family Doctors and Public Policy,* Routledge & Kegan Paul, London (1973)

36. REIN, M., 'Social Class and the Health Service', *New Society,*

14 (1969), 807
37. DEPARTMENT OF HEALTH AND SOCIAL SECURITY, Black Report, *op. cit.*
38. CARTWRIGHT, A. and O'BRIEN, M., 'Social Class Variations in Health Care and the Nature of GP Consultations' in STACEY, M. (ed.), *The Sociology of the NHS*, Sociological Review Monograph, No. 22, Keele University (1976)
-39. NOYCE, SNAITH, A. and TRICKEY, J., 'Regional Variations in the Allocation of Financial Resources to Community Health Services', *The Lancet*, 1 (1974), 554
40. LE GRAND, J., *Strategy of Equality. Redistribution and the Social Services*, George Allen & Unwin, London (1982) Ch. 3
41. Quoted in BLAXTER, M., *op. cit.*, Ch. 11
42. TOWNSEND, P., 'Toward Equality in Health Through Social Policy', *International Journal of Health Services*, 11 (1), 1981
43. MINISTRY OF NATIONAL HEALTH AND WELFARE (CANADA), *A New Perspective on the Health of Canadians* (Chairman: M. Lalonde), Ottawa (1974)

vention are then examined and assessed. The final section suggests that these reflect a particular set of assumptions and that the issue of prevention is essentially political; the present structure of services, however, inhibits the development of policies for prevention.

THE DIMENSIONS OF PREVENTION

Within medical and epidemiological work a distinction is usually made between primary, secondary and tertiary prevention. The full definition of these terms from the White Paper Prevention and Health, 1977, is reproduced in the document section [doc 28]. Primary prevention refers to attempts to prevent ill-health arising in the first place and is concerned with the promotion of appropriate attitudes to health, secondary prevention refers to the procedures used to identify disease at a very early pre-symptomatic stage, before an individual is aware of being ill. Treatment can then be given to prevent the disease from developing into something more serious and life-threatening. Finally tertiary prevention has been used to describe the process of rehabilitation and returning a patient to adequate or normal functioning after a period of illness or treatment to minimise disability for individuals and families and the community, or more positively, to restore effective function and preserve social roles. In this chapter the focus is on primary prevention.

Billis, in an attempt to clarify the concept of prevention, has argued that when used in relation to the physical world the most straight-forward meaning of prevention is 'to stop'.[2] Prevention is concerned with intervening in the interaction between two factors which create a result which is considered undesirable: thus mosquito bites human which causes malaria or more problematically human eats sweets which causes tooth decay or smokes cigarettes which 'cause' illness. Prevention is generally about action taken to avoid the occurrence of a particular anticipated consequence. Causal relationships may however vary considerably in complexity. It was pointed out in Chapter 8 for example that the causal factors in many contemporary illnesses were complex and frequently disputed. However irrespective of the complexity of the problem there can be intervention at a number of points in the chain of events:

1. The causal factor can be eliminated. Mosquitoes can be eliminated by spraying. Cigarettes or sweets may be banned entirely.
2. A barrier can be erected between the causal factor and the human being. Mosquito nets may be used, 'harmful' substances removed from cigarettes. Teeth may be coated with fluoride.

Chapter nine

POLICIES FOR PREVENTION

Over recent years, a series of government reports, consultative documents, white papers and pamphlets have heralded a major change in government policy in the field of health.[1] There is a new emphasis in these publications on the importance of prevention, and attention is drawn to the role that the individual and the community can play in promoting and safeguarding the nation's health. The concept of prevention has far-reaching implications for responsibilities within the health service and for health in the community.

The increasing popularity of prevention and the government's response reflects a number of factors which have been discussed in previous chapters. First, the pattern of disease and illness has changed and it has been argued that much ill-health is avoidable particularly through a change in individual behaviour. Second, there has been an increasing disillusionment with the benefits of curative medicine. Paradoxically advances in medicine have been paralleled by an awareness that no intervention is wholly safe and that much chronic illness is not amenable to treatment. Third, there has been the consistent concern with the cost of the NHS. This was a dominant theme in the first section of this book and prevention is seen as providing a cheaper alternative to the continued expansion of curative medicine.

Prevention is thus an attractive proposition, furthermore, it has a breadth of appeal. To the left it is part of the progress towards a better society where the social ills of capitalism will be diminished, to the right prevention holds out the hope of reduced government intervention of concrete and effective policies. This breadth of appeal conceals the very real difficulties which surround the concept of prevention and its realisation in concrete and effective policies. This chapter begins by examining the dimensions of 'prevention', then looks at three areas where prevention has been proposed as a major strategy for improving health. Recent government policies in relation to pre-

improving the conditions that produce good health . . . the task is to reinforce and build on changes (in public attitudes and awareness) that task will fall to commercial and voluntary organisations as well as to the Government, the NHS and public bodies . . . much of the work has to be undertaken locally.[15]

Care in Action also stresses the importance of health care professionals in the dissemination of information. GPs are expected to play a preventive role in primary health care, dentists the main source of information on oral hygiene. The booklets published by governments are designed for health care professions so that, in effect, the information from governments is to be filtered through a variety of professionals. In the case of GPs and dentists, who are independent contractors, there is no way of ensuring that preventive work is carried out.

Smoking and health: government policy

The main thrust of government activity in the area of prevention has been through health promotion and education as a strategy for changing the behaviour of individuals and activity has been greatest in relation to smoking. There is a stronger association between smoking and ill-health than any other single variable and the least disagreement about that association. Lung cancer, coronary heart disease and a range of respiratory diseases have all been linked with smoking. There is also evidence to suggest that to give up smoking significantly reduces the risk. This makes smoking an ideal target for prevention.

There has been some preventive action through regulation by governments. Advertising has been limited, packages carry health warnings, taxes have been increased on tobacco. However advertising has not been banned completely and an annual increase in taxes has been rejected. Governments have been unwilling to take stronger regulatory action 'because cigarette smoking is a long standing habit practised by nearly half the population, it would be totally unrealistic to expect smokers to give up the habit . . . '[16] It is also argued in Prevention and Health, 1977 that tax increases raise the cost of smoking for those least able to afford it and, given their dependence on tobacco, some smokers may forego necessities. Governments have ostensibly eschewed regulation on the grounds of individual liberty, although there are those who argue that they have equally feared the cost of the loss of tax revenues. The main strategy has therefore been education and persuasion, a reliance on the provision of information to raise awareness and a sense of individual responsibility, such a response is expected from those who on another level are viewed as

whole field of health care from the prevention of disease and disability in the new-born to the maintenance of health in old-age'.[9]

The striking factor in all the publications on prevention and health has been the emphasis on individual responsibility. 'Much ill-health in Britain today arises from overindulgence and unwise behaviour . . . the greatest potential and perhaps the greatest problems for preventive medicine now lies in changing behaviour and attitudes to health. The individual can do much to help himself, his family and the community by accepting more direct responsibility for his own health and well-being.'[10] The intellectual origins of this emphasis on individual responsibility follow from an emphasis on illness in the individual and the medical model and have been referred to in Chapter 8. 'Personal behaviour, what people do or not do to themselves,' says McKeown, 'is now relatively more significant (in determining health) than food deficiency and environmental hazards'.[11] Illich who has attacked modern medicine still characterises health in terms of the work ethic. He sees health as a 'personal task' in which successes depend upon 'self-awareness, self-discipline and the inner resources by which each person regulates his own daily rhythm and actions, his diet and his sex'.[12] Prevention and Health (the 1977 White Paper) suggests that early diagnostic and screening facilities as well as being of unproven efficacy may detract from individuals' sense of responsibilities for themselves. This too is very much in tune with the approach of Illich [see also doc 32].

The main role of government is then seen to lie in making information available.

> The primary responsibility for his own health falls on the individual, the role of the health profession and of the government is limited to ensuring that the public have access to such knowledge as is available about the importance of personal habits on health and at the very least no obstacles are placed in the way of those who decide to act on that knowledge.[13]

A series of booklets designed 'particularly for those working in the health, social and education services as health educators' have been produced in recent years. 'Eating and Health' and 'Avoiding Heart Attacks' are recent examples.[14]

Clearly the diffusion of health education responsibilities to a wide variety of bodies is the extent of government's commitment to this issue. Care in Action, the 1981 handbook on priorities, explicitly suggests a mixed economy in relation to prevention.

> The preventive role of NHS services is to give information available about the risk to health and to minimise such risks by developing the services and

for prevention identify changing individual behaviour and government regulation as possible bases for action.

GOVERNMENT POLICY ON PREVENTION: THE GENERAL APPROACH

There is no doubt that the changing pattern of major disease categories has influenced government thinking about prevention in the 1970s and we now look at government statements. Two themes are evident in a number of recent publications. The first is the concern for rising costs of health care and the second for the continuing high rates of mortality and morbidity in particular diseases such as heart disease and cancer. Prevention and Health: Everybody's Business, in 1976, the reports of the Public Expenditure Committee on Preventive Medicine, during 1976/77 and the White Paper Prevention and Health published in 1977 outline both the government's analysis and response to these problems.[7] The response is summed up in the last of these documents as, 'an unequivocal change in policy'; a clear emphasis on prevention as a strategy for change, and a strategy aimed at changing behaviour. These documents highlight the importance of individual behaviour, lifestyle and risk-taking in contemporary illness and disease. The role of government is seen to be primarily concerned with encouraging healthier lifestyles through providing information, and in funding health education and health promotion. Implicit in this is the allocation of responsibility, and blame, for ill-health to the individual and a diffusion of blame and responsibility from governments to a variety of bodies. There is thus perceived to be a limited role for government and an increased task for other statutory bodies, quangos or voluntary bodies in health education.

The objective of Prevention and Health (the 1977 White Paper) is spelt out:

the first (aim) is to secure that greater emphasis is placed in the Health and Personal Social Services on prevention . . . particular priority should be given to the care of the young and to concentrating on groups and people most at risk. Secondly . . . to ensure that people are encouraged to take more responsibility for their own health . . . to enable them to do so, there should be a greater flow of reliable information and advice.[8]

The Priorities documents in 1976 had earmarked an extra £2 m. increase in 1979/80 for preventive medicine and health education, particularly fluoridation, family planning and antenatal care. Although the impact was diffused by an extremely wide definition of prevention, 'the ideas behind preventive medicine permeate the

Table 13. Reliably established (as of 1981), practicable* ways of avoiding the onset of life-threatening cancer

	Percent of all US cancer deaths known to be thus avoidable
Avoidance of tobacco smoke	30
Avoidance of alcoholic drinks or mouthwashes	3
Avoidance of obesity	2
Regular cervical screening and genital hygiene	1
Avoidance of inessential medical use of hormones or radiology	<1
Avoidance of unusual exposure to sunlight	<1
Avoidance of current levels of exposure to currently known carcinogens (for which there is good epidemiological evidence of human hazard) in (i) occupational (ii) food, water or urban air	

Excluding ways such as prophylactic prostatectomy, mastectomy, hysterectomy, oophorectomy, artificial menopause or pregnancy.

Source: Peto, R., 'Why Cancer?' *The Times Health Supplement*, 6 Nov. 1981, p. 14

Better Dental Health concluded that there is now the knowledge and capability to prevent most dental disease.[6] The report indeed widens the definition of prevention in relation to dental health to include every item of dental treatment.

The report suggests that good oral hygiene, particularly the regular brushing of teeth, would prevent the onset of gingival disease while an overall reduction in the consumption of sugar would have a profound effect on the incidence of dental decay. However, the fluoridation of water is the 'single measure available to the community that if implemented would have the most dramatic effect on the level of dental decay in the UK'. In the case of dental disease, therefore, strategies have been followed through health education and health promotion the reduction of risks can lead to improvements in mortality rates.

Although the relationship between risk factors and the incidence of coronary disease are not well understood – any preventive strategy could, in theory, attempt to affect smoking, or cholesterol levels or levels of blood pressure or all three. The two latter are believed to be related to diet and exercise. There is however some disagreement on which factor or factors in diet are primarily to blame. Unsaturated fats, or sugar or lack of dietary fibre, all have been implicated. However the relationship between smoking and heart disease has been most clearly established. It remains the most obvious contender on which to base a preventive policy.

Cancer

Our second example of a disease where a policy for prevention has been suggested is cancer. Doll and Peto have recently argued that a large proportion, 80–90 per cent of cancers, are theoretically avoidable.[4] Cancer of course is in many respects a term covering a whole spectrum of diseases, each of which has a particular set of causative factors. In relation to lung cancer, the major cause of cancer deaths among men, an important causal relationship has been identified with smoking. Up to one-third of cancer deaths are attributable to smoking. Other factors such as alcohol consumption, occupational cancers, environmental pollutants, sexual activity, nutritional and other dietary factors are implicated with particular kinds of cancer but their overall effect is either smaller, or less well established than the link between smoking and lung cancer. Table 13, constructed by Peto, reproduces the practicable ways of avoiding the onset of life-threatening cancer. On this sort of evidence those concerned with health may point to the curtailment of smoking as the obvious contender for a preventive stategy.

Dental caries and periodontal disease

Our third example of the scope for prevention is from the area of dental health. The Royal Commission on the NHS commented in 1979 that by any standard 'the dental health of the nation is poor'. In 1968, 37 per cent of the population of England and Wales over the age of sixteen had no natural teeth. Periodontal disease was present in 73 per cent of the 16 to 34 age group and in 90 per cent of those over thirty-five in the same year.[5] In 1981 a DHSS working party, *Towards*

3. Or the human being can take action or be treated in various ways to avoid hazards. They may avoid areas with mosquitoes, give up smoking and sweet eating.

It is clear that preventive action involves a series of judgements about the causal chains in operation, about the most effective strategies for intervention and about the key actors in the process. Governments may have an important role in advising and giving information to change behaviour or in restricting behaviour through regulation. In practical terms the key actors in the process of intervention have been governments through regulation, and historically, particularly in the nineteenth century, governments have stopped the spread of disease through regulating the supply of water and the collection of refuse. Recently in government policy there has been *less* emphasis on regulation and *more* on persuasion through changing individual behaviour. We turn now to three areas of current concern, coronary heart disease, cancer and dental caries and periodontal disease, to look at present thinking about the causal chains leading to these conditions to explain the shift from regulation to personal responsibility. In each of the areas the costs of treatment and care are high and claims have been made that risks are largely avoidable through changing individual behaviour.

Avoiding coronary heart disease

There has been considerable effort put into investigating the causes of coronary heart disease internationally. This is because the incidence is very high and so are the costs. In a study of coronary heart disease an Office of Health Economics publication (OHE) estimates that the cost to the NHS of the treatment of those suffering from coronary heart disease in 1981 was approximately £255 m. per year and this is something of an underestimate.[3] 60 per cent of this sum is attributable to hospital in-patient care. In addition, in terms of sickness absence 26 million working days were lost in the same year, costing the National Insurance Fund £115 m. in payments. The social burden of the disease is of course also considerable both to the individual sufferers and their families.

In order to prevent coronary heart disease, the risk factors have to be identified. There is a broad consensus that the disease is strongly linked with cigarette smoking, high serum cholesterol levels and raised blood pressure. Together they can increase by eight-fold the chances of a coronary event. There is also evidence from the United States and Australia to suggest that where active prevention policies

THE LIMITS OF PREVENTION: CHANGING INDIVIDUAL BEHAVIOUR

If the campaign to reduce smoking has had a limited effect this is even more so with other areas of health education and promotion. There are difficulties in providing clear-cut, unambiguous advice and this may be because causative factors are disputed. For example, this has tended to be the case with dietary factors and coronary heart disease. Health education moreover needs to be adequately funded, linked to an appropriate administrative structure, targeted towards particular groups and straightforward, acceptable and practical without being alarmist in its approach, to be effective.

Graham, in a critique of the effects of preventive work with mothers and young children which attempts to improve child care and child health, has suggested that a strategy which seeks to underline individual responsibility is misguided.[20] She argues that mothers already do take their responsibilities for their children seriously and that health promotion and health education may increase uncertainty. The problem for many parents and particularly women as they still do most of the mothering, is the network of conflicting roles in which they find themselves. Admonitions to do this, or that, may be irreconcilable with demands already being placed on the mother. As family patterns become more complicated with more single parent families and serial marriages this may be even more the case. Graham suggests that health education can only really become effective if it is more holistic in its approach. It must include an understanding of vulnerability to health risks due to social and emotional circumstances and an awareness on the part of health educators of the culture and the home circumstances of families they are attempting to reach.

On a broader platform there are those who have rejected the individualistic basis of much recent government policy in the area of prevention on the grounds that this ignores the social and environmental determinants of ill-health. Crawford argues that self-responsibility, self-reliance and self-discipline reflect the capitalist ethic of bourgeois individualism. It rests on a victim-blaming ideology. 'It instructs people to be individually responsible at a time when they are becoming less capable as individuals of controlling their health environment, the ideology tends to obscure the reality of class and the impact of social inequality on health.'[21]

The emphasis on individual responsibility thus plays down the wider economic and environmental influences on health, and assumes that the individual has the power and autonomy to carry out decisions which affect lifestyle. It also tends to draw attention away from inequalities in access to life chances, goods and services and the way in which they contribute to health. Cancer rates, coronary heart disease and dental disease are in general higher in lower social classes. In contrast to Doll and Peto whose research on cancer was referred to earlier in the chapter, Epstein in *The Politics of Cancer*, argues that all cancer rates are rising and stresses the importance of the place of work in determining cancer rates, smoking and other behavioural characteristics are taken as residual rather than as determining factors. On this basis Epstein suggests that 20 — 40 per cent of cancers are work-related.[22]

It is clear that the controversies over the 'causes' of ill-health and where to break into the cycle lie at the heart of any discussion of prevention. Changing individual lifestyle is one approach but it has also been argued that there should be greater government regulation in the interests of health. Such strategies, it is suggested, are both more effective and appropriate.

REGULATORY STRATEGIES

Warner has suggested that a classification can be made of different kinds of preventive health measures along a continuum which distinguishes between different kinds of strategy by the extent to which they depend upon active, passive or no involvement of the target individual or population.[23] He comments that the greater degree of dependency on activity by the recipient the less likely the success of the programme. General environmental programmes which need little or no effort on the part of the individual such as clean air measures, or the addition of vitamin D to milk, the removal of sugar from paediatric medicines, the marking of the sugar content on all foodstuffs, the addition of fluoride to water supplies can be extremely effective. These are regulatory activities and must be carried out by governments. As programmes demand more active involvement so they become less effective and have an increasing class bias in their take up. Vaccination and immunisation programmes need some participation. Rates of vaccination and immunisation have been falling over the years and this may be due to different degrees of awareness of health in the population and what Rose called the paradox of prevention.[24] Rose has commented that individuals are unlikely to be greatly motivated to subscribe to measures which offer substantial benefits to the community but may carry fewer advantages and greater risks to each individual participant. Concern over vaccine damage is a case in point. Individuals may prefer to take the risk of damage from whooping cough and the like, than accept the very small risk of damage from vaccination although this has had undoubted benefits to the community. More information and other incentives may thus have to be introduced to make programmes effective.

The kinds of programmes where prevention is likely to be least effective are those which involve the individual in taking the initiative, particularly where there has to be an element of repetition, for example not smoking or taking fluoride pills. Legislation may of course help to change habitual behaviour; the compulsory wearing of seat belts is an important step towards reducing mortality and morbidity in road accidents.

Difficulties however arise in the case of regulatory policies at a general policy-making level. Legislation which seeks to 'interfere with the liberty of the individual' frequently raises opposition at a Parliamentary level and in local government. There is a dislike of and antagonism to what is seen as paternalism. In a study of the reasons for the failure to implement fluoridation programmes in a number of Scottish authorities[25] Brand found that there were two major reasons for the failure to implement this cheap and effective way of preventing tooth decay, one related to administrative structure, the second to politics. Administrative arrangements in relation to water are complex as the agreement of a number of local authorities which share a common water supply under a particular Water Board is needed. This created difficulties. Second, the fluoridation of water was frequently left to a free vote in local councils rather than being a party issue. Councillors were thus often without leadership or sufficient information on which to make a judgement. In the absence of clear guidance they fell back on 'folk' knowledge and resisted attempts to interfere with the 'purity' of the water supply.

This case study may have a wider applicability to health issues as these have not on the whole been seen as major party issues. The politics of health are not clearly developed and this may reflect the existence of a national health service and the consensus which has surrounded it. Governments, irrespective of party, have found regulation in health matters, in times of peace at least, politically unacceptable. This is despite the fact that there may be clear benefits to the collectivity in promoting or preventing certain kinds of behaviour through regulation.

Mill, the nineteenth-century liberal political philosopher, suggested that the avoidance of harm to others was the only legitimate reason for legally compelling someone to do something they would not otherwise do, self-regarding actions properly falling outside the law. This was based on the conviction that each individual was the best judge of his/her own welfare. In practice, however, it is very difficult to separate self-regarding from other-regarding activities. Pregnant mothers who smoke put the foetus at greater risk as they tend to have lower birth weight babies, who in turn are more vulnerable. Smokers pollute the environment for others as there is an element of 'secondary' smoking. With a national health service the costs of treating those whose illness is associated with smoking fall on the community as a whole, to which all citizens have contributed. There seems little justification therefore in terms of libertarian arguments for not increasing the extent of regulation in relation to health.

It is unlikely that the debate over increasing the amount of regulation or concentrating on health education to change lifestyle will be readily resolved. And in a sense the argument is an academic one. There is overwhelming evidence that both the workplace and general environment are major arenas in which the production of ill-health occurs and that there are relatively simple regulatory measures which could be introduced, some involving compulsory health measures such as fluoridation, others concerned with prohibiting actions or activities, such as the addition of lead to petrol. There needs to be a greater willingness to investigate and regulate and fundamental to this is greater visibility for public health issues. Interestingly it has been suggested that the British population as a whole tends to be more fatalistic and apathetic towards health issues than North Americans.[26] Political awareness is necessary whether the approach to prevention focuses on changing society or the individual. However, one factor which inhibits the development of a politics of health care is the present structure and provision of preventive health services to which we now turn.

ADMINISTRATIVE CONSTRAINTS TO PREVENTION

There is an extraordinarily complicated network of services providing primary, secondary and tertiary prevention which are the consequences of a highly fragmented system of provision of health services and the division of labour within it. To give just two examples, J. N. Morris comments that twelve central government departments and agencies are concerned with the control of pesticides, although this is hardly a priority area.[27] At a local level there are a large number of individual health workers with responsibilities for promoting better health; health visitors, for example, have a statutory responsibility for health education and the prevention of ill-health through visiting mothers with new babies and in relation to young children. District nurses have an important role in educating informal carers to share part of the caring task. GPs are implicitly and occasionally explicitly involved in health education and prevention particularly in relation to babies, children, family planning, the old and the chronically ill. Health education officers are employed by local authorities or health authorities to promote health education. District Community Physicians (DCPs) have a role in monitoring ill-health and preventive health services in their areas. Clinical medical officers look after the health of school children. All these workers are likely to use different information systems and ways of operating. The reason for the fragmentation is that health services have been organised around institutions and agencies concerned with treatment rather than prevention.

The 1974 reorganisation of the health service did nothing to simplify this situation. Before 1974, Medical Officers of Health had a responsibility for personal health services in the community within local government, the authority which provided environmental health services, and therefore had control over the selling of food, safety of public housing and environmental pollution. The Medical Officer of Health had a clearly defined responsibility for the health of a defined community and co-ordination with the environmental health services was relatively easy as they were within the same authority. In 1974, however, responsibility for environmental health remained with local government, while District Community Physicians became integrated with the structure of management of curative services in the health districts, under the general administration of the Area Medical Officer. DCPs could be used in a consultative capacity by local authorities on environmental health matters. In its evidence to the Merrison Commission the Society of Community Medicine felt that this change had brought disadvantages. 'Despite many advances and improvements in environmental control, especially in the more traditional sectors of water and air, there is little evidence that the physical environment continues to improve; rather the reverse, with the environment being continually and subtly degraded.' [23] They go on to argue that the community physician is now less in the public eye since the change in structure in 1974 and that some of the impetus for the development of services has, as a consequence, been lost.

This lack of clear responsibility for community and environmental health at local level is mirrored by the lack of a single departmental responsibility at central government level. Occupational health, for example, is the responsibility of the Health and Safety Executive of the Health and Safety Commission. Its remit is 'the reactions of workpeople to their working environment and the prevention of ill-health arising from working conditions'. The Department of the Environment is responsible for the aspects of environmental health which come under local government while the DHSS is concerned with community health services. Unless there are clear responsibilities for health at both central and local level, then it is too easy for professional commitment or political lobbying to be diffused among the plethora of agencies involved and prevention remains piecemeal and largely ineffective. Administrative fragmentation means lack of linkages into the main decision-making structure which can generate commitment to particular preventive policies and commit resources to seeing them through.

FINAL COMMENT

It is clear that there are many difficulties in the way of developing sound preventive policies. These are inextricably related to what are identified as the major causes of illness and death. The search for these causes is complex and difficult because deciding where to look or at which groups in the population, involves judgements of value. Furthermore there are deficiencies in knowledge and disputes about the relative weight to be given to particular causative factors. Preventive strategies to date have tended to take a predominantly individualist perspective and this has been influenced by the dominance of the disease or medical model which concentrates on illness in the individual. Preventive strategies have also been influenced by the way health services are at present provided and the particular division of labour between professionals. Just as the individualist strategy blames individuals, so structures based on treatment fragment responsibility for prevention. Both underestimate the relationship between poverty and ill-health, and the effect of the workplace on ill-health. Strategies to prevent ill-health in the future, if they are to be effective, will inevitably involve attempting to decrease the extent of deprivation and also to increase the amount of regulation over health matters. The former can only be achieved by concentrating more resources where there are the greatest health problems. As Tawney comments, 'public health is purchasable; within natural limitations a community can determine its own death rate'.[29]

REFERENCES

1. DEPARTMENT OF HEALTH AND SOCIAL SECURITY, *Priorities for*

Health and Personal Social Services, HMSO, London (1976); *Prevention and Health: Everybody's Business*, HMSO, London (1977); *First Report from the Expenditure Committee*, Session 1976/77; *Preventive Medicine*, Vol. 1, Report, HMSO, London (1977); *Occupational Health Services: The Way Ahead*, HMSO, London (1977); *Eating for Health*, HMSO, London (1978); *Avoiding Heart Attacks*, HMSO, London (1981); DEPARTMENT OF HEALTH AND SOCIAL SECURITY, SCOTTISH OFFICE and WELSH OFFICE, *Prevention and Health*, Cmnd 7047, HMSO, London (1977)

2. BILLIS, D., 'At Risk of Prevention', *Journal of Social Policy*, Vol. 10, Pt. 3, July 1981

3. OFFICE OF HEALTH ECONOMICS, *Coronary Heart Disease. The Scope for Prevention*, Paper 73, Office of Health Economics, London (1982)

4. PETO, R., 'Why Cancer? The causes of cancer in developed countries', *The Times Health Supplement*, 6 Nov. 1981, reporting on work for United States Congress by DOLL, R., and PETO, R.

5. *Report of the Royal Commission on the National Health Service* (Chairman: Sir Alec Merrison), Cmnd 7615, HMSO, London (1979), Ch. 9

6. DEPARTMENT OF HEALTH AND SOCIAL SECURITY, Report of the Dental Strategy Review Group. *Towards Better Dental Health*, HMSO, London (1981)

7. *op. cit.*, reference 1

8. DEPARTMENT OF HEALTH AND SOCIAL SECURITY, *Prevention and Health*, 1977, *op. cit.*, p. 1

9. DEPARTMENT OF HEALTH AND SOCIAL SECURITY, *Priorities for Health and Social Services*, 1976, *op. cit.*

10. DEPARTMENT OF HEALTH AND SOCIAL SECURITY, *Prevention and Health*, 1977, *op. cit.*, p. 39

11. MCKEOWN, T., *The Role of Medicine. Dream, Mirage or Nemesis?*, Blackwell, Oxford (1979), p. 90

12. ILLICH, I., *Limits to Medicine: Medical Nemesis. The Expropriation of Health*, Marion Boyars, London (1976)

13. DEPARTMENT OF HEALTH AND SOCIAL SECURITY, *Prevention and Health*, 1977, *op. cit.*

14. See reference 1

15. DEPARTMENT OF HEALTH AND SOCIAL SECURITY, *Care in Action. A Handbook of Policies and Priorities of the Health and Personal Social Services in England*, HMSO, London (1981)

16. DEPARTMENT OF HEALTH AND SOCIAL SECURITY, *Prevention and Health*, 1977, *op. cit.*, Ch. VI

17. CENTRAL STATISTICAL OFFICE, *Social Trends*, No. 12, HMSO, London (1981), Table 7. 17
18. DEPARTMENT OF HEALTH AND SOCIAL SECURITY, *Prevention and Health*, 1977, *op. cit.*
19. OFFICE OF HEALTH ECONOMICS, No. 73, *op. cit.*, p. 50
20. GRAHAM, H., 'Prevention and Health: every mother's business, a comment on child health policies in the 1970s' in *The Sociology of the Family: New Directions for Britain*, Sociological Review Monograph 28, University of Keele (1979)
21. CRAWFORD, R., 'You are Dangerous to Your Health: the ideology and politics of victim blaming', *International Journal of Health Services*, 7 (4), 1977
22. EPSTEIN, S., *The Politics of Cancer*, Doubleday, New York (1979)
23. WARNER, K. E., 'The Economic Implications of Preventive Health Care', *Social Science and Medicine*, Vol. 13c, 1979, 227–37
24. ROSE, G., 'Strategy of Prevention: lessons from cardio-vascular disease', *British Medical Journal*, Vol. 282, 1847–51, 6 June 1981
25. BRAND, J. A., 'The Politics of Fluoridation: A community conflict', *Political Studies*, Vol. XIX, No. 4, 430–9
26. OHE, *The Prevention of Coronary Heart Disease*, *op. cit.*
27. MORRIS, J. N., 'Epidemiology and Prevention', Milbank Memorial Fund *Quarterly, Health and Society*, Vol. 60, No. 1, 1982
28. *Report of the Royal Commission on the National Health Service*, 1979, *op. cit.*, Ch. 5
29. TAWNEY, R. H., *Equality*, Allen & Unwin (1938), p. 168

Chapter ten
THE NHS AND ITS USERS

Almost everyone in Britain is affected by the NHS. Most people (99 per cent) are registered with GPs as NHS patients and the proportion of the population wholly covered by private insurance remains small. The large majority or their relatives therefore, will use the NHS, for care or treatment, during the course of their lives. Even if they do not use the service they are likely to contribute to it as taxpayers or as payers of national insurance. In the rather disparate literature on the relationship between the NHS and the public there have been three broad perspectives which have been taken, to examine that relationship; the political, the economic and the social. These are essentially different ways of approaching the study of the individual in relation to social institutions.

This chapter aims to look at these disparate ways of conceptualising the relationship between users and potential users of health services and the NHS; that large, professionally-dominated and bureaucratically-provided service. The first section looks briefly at political relationships and the attempts to increase democracy in the NHS, the second examines health service users as 'consumers' of health care, both passive and active. The third section takes a social perspective to look at the part individuals play in the process of health care as health workers themselves. The assumption there is that illness and its management constitutes a problem for all individuals and social groups. Everyone is therefore involved in health work although roles may be distributed differently. The role distribution in health work in Western industrial societies tends to demean health work other than that professionally provided and this is seen to pose a particular problem when the divisions between the content of professional and non-professional tasks becomes blurred as in the case of community care. The problem here lies in reducing the distance between the professional and lay-user or healer and increasing co-operation in the management of illness.

It is suggested in conclusion that an analysis of these different dimensions of the relationship between the NHS and its users may help to clarify policy objectives.

DEMOCRACY AND PARTICIPATION IN THE NHS: THE POLITICAL DIMENSION

The NHS compared to other institutional structures providing social services lacks democratic controls. There is no elected tier and therefore, theoretically, the Secretary of State for Health and Social Services is accountable to Parliament for money spent in the NHS, for policies pursued and for mistakes made. The very scope of this task and the unwieldy nature of parliamentary scrutiny weakens accountability and sensitivity to democratic pressures. Accountability and democracy are slippery concepts and cannot be fully developed here. Mackenzie in *Power and Responsibility in the NHS*[1] does take a broad approach to these issues. It is sufficient for our purposes to describe briefly the mechanisms which exist to call health ministers and their civil servants to account for their actions in the NHS, in addition to the mechanisms described in Part two.

Health Ministers deal with many thousands of issues through written and verbal questions both in the House of Commons and outside it, every year. Complaints are investigated by the Health Service Commissioner, by internal hospital inquiries, and by the service committees of the FPCs in relation to GPs, dentists, opticians and pharmacists. There are *ad hoc* committees and commissions of inquiry into a variety of specific issues, many of which have been referred to in earlier chapters in this book. Standing Advisory Committees to the DHSS have a general brief to keep a constant review of particular aspects of the NHS. At the House of Commons, the Public Accounts Committee on Expenditure and the Select Committee on the Social Services have taken up particular issues of their choice to investigate more fully and have been particularly active in recent years. Infant mortality, expenditure on the health services and medical careers have been topics investigated by the Social Services Committee while the Public Accounts Committee has concerned itself with accountability. The details of the most relevant reports are given in the list of statutes and committees at the end of this book.

Despite these mechanisms for ensuring accountability at a national level the lack of an elected tier at a local level does lead to the absence of an overt focal point for local issues and local policies to be formulated around elected representatives. Health policy has largely been the concern of a few interested and involved national politicians, higher civil servants at the DHSS, the representatives and advisers of professional bodies and on occasions the unions representing workers in health care. Although there is little doubt that chairmen, members and officers of health authorities lobby the DHSS, the political process of decision-making is largely hidden from public view. The public have therefore had little chance to participate in the formulation of health policy at a local or national level and although there has been considerable pressure group activity at a national level, at local level the community interest is particularly weakly represented.

The decision was made in 1946 to make the NHS a centralised service. The reasons for this were largely political; the medical profession and the voluntary movement were diametrically opposed to local government control. However, in addition to this central government and the Ministry of Health did not wish to lose control of such an expensive service or their ability to achieve a more even distribution of resources. A nod to democracy was made through ministerial appointments of local people to the management committees of the hospitals and the Regional Hospital Boards. This was however not the kind of system of representative democracy on which local government in Britain rests. The actions of the local authorities gain legitimacy through the election of representatives who claim to pursue the interests of the local community and those who elected them. The importance of local government is its potential to respond to local needs within the limits of national policies and local resources.

The substitute for locally elected health authorities was the representation of interest groups, particularly those involved in producing the service. Thus Bevan appointed lay people to represent the community interest and health professionals, mainly doctors, to his new health service bodies, the HMCs and RHBs. Doctors were in this way given 'full participation in the administration' of the service. This was participative rather than representative democracy. However time was to show that local lay interests were weakly reflected in the activities of the boards and committees. Crossman later called these 'self-perpetuating oligarchies' in his impatience at the failures of field authorities in the NHS to respond to inadequacies and weaknesses of the service.[3] The phrase may owe more to political rhetoric than analysis although research studies had shown that members of health authorities were predominantly middle class, elderly and male.[4]

Bevan's solution to managing the health services was based on the assumption that running them was uncontroversial. There was an implicit acceptance that health care was about providing professionally-determined, predominantly medical services, and that the professionals could be left to determine needs and the level of services for the community. As it became increasingly apparent during the late 1960s and early 1970s that the health service was failing to adapt itself to changing needs and priorities, changes were sought. Part of the aims of the 1974 reorganisation was to increase democratic participation. The assumption was that this would facilitate the implementation of national priorities and make the service more sensitive to local needs. Greater democracy was to be introduced in two ways, though both were within the tradition of participative rather than representative democracy. The first aimed to increase lay and professional representation within the health authorities, the second to create a new institution, the Community Health Council, to represent the public.

The health authorities, region and area, were to contain members representing the professions, including nursing. Local interests were to be represented through appointing nominees from local authorities although other members were chosen for the personal contribution they could make to the service. Their role was to make major policy and strategic planning decisions and meetings were to be public, with no subcommittee structure.

From the evidence of research studies it seems that these devices have not achieved a lively and informed involvement of appointed members. Haywood and Alaszewski, on the basis of their research on a number of areas and regions, suggest that the impact of members on the running of the authorities has been small.[5] They argue that this is essentially due, not to members' lack of experience and expertise, but to their lack of power. In contrast to local government where political groups gain legitimacy in relation to the officers of the council, by being elected to carry out a particular programme, there is no such group cohesion or party programme among local health authority members. Thus, they have no coherent approach to policy. Nor do they have a power base. They tend to act as individuals. This suggests that the attempt at democratisation of health authorities, particularly the increase of local authority members by Barbara Castle, has not brought an increased control over decision-making at a local level by the appointed bodies. Power has tended to remain with the professional service-providers over whom management controls, as suggested in Chapter 7, are also weak.

Patients First aimed to increase the receptivity of the health authorities to local needs. The new districts will be concerned with the provision of services at a more local level and there is intended to be a much closer relationship between those planning and those managing services. The membership of the authorities is smaller and there are fewer conflicting pressures as there were for example between the interests of different districts in multi-district areas. Problems remain however. There has been no change in the distribution of power and members of the districts are likely to suffer from the same weaknesses as their predecessors.

Community health councils

The second aspect of the attempt to increase the democratic element in health service provision was through the establishing of the Community Health Councils (CHCs), an entirely new institution in 1974. CHCs were also intended to increase the amount of participation in the health service through the 'representation of interests'. This notion was however, ambiguous and was interpreted in different ways. It was suggested on the one hand that CHCs should consist of local people knowledgeable about the health services and representing the interest of particular groups in need. These, by definition, would *not* be representatives of the public at large. On the other hand CHCs were said to exist to represent the interests of the public, a different matter entirely. This ambiguity has never been satisfactorily resolved.

In 1974 CHCs were established in each health district, 229 in all, in England and Wales. They were funded by the regions and one-third of the membership was drawn from voluntary organisations, one-half appointed by local authorities, and one-sixth by the Regional Health Authority. This composition was influenced by the desire to achieve a structure which reflected expertise in the health services as they affected minority groups, those interested in the handicapped and disabled, for example. The Council was serviced by a small secretariat and was to work from a local office in each district. The functions and powers of the CHCs were broadly two-fold. They were to comment upon local services, and be consulted on the future plans and intentions of the health authorities. CHCs were given a special role in relation to hospital closures. An Area Health Authority could not close a hospital without CHC approval and if this was not forthcoming, the matter was to be referred to the Secretary of State for a final decision. To enable them to perform these functions CHCs were given a right of access to information and the right to visit health service premises. The second main function of the CHC was to be a source of information and advice to the public, particularly in helping them to channel their complaints in the appropriate direction.

Ham suggests that the efficacy of CHCs, despite their theoretically wide powers, has been affected by the dominant political culture of representative democracy.[6] Members of health authorities (whose own legitimacy is in any case weak because they are not elected) and their officers have tended to see CHCs as speaking only for themselves or narrow sectional interests. They may see *themselves* as representing the true public interest and see little payoff in the time spent in their dealings with CHCs. These factors may explain the hostility to the Councils from many quarters in the health service, particularly for example from Family Practitioner Committees most of which have not allowed CHC representatives into the non-confidential part of their meetings. The role of CHCs is also limited by their resources. Information, knowledge and expertise are important if groups are going to influence decision-making and with the limited budgets they possess, the influence of CHCs on decision-making is inevitably limited.

In its consideration of the role of CHCs, the Royal Commission on the NHS argued that CHCs should primarily be seen as consumer bodies and not part of the management of the NHS. There is however confusion over this issue. The DHSS has stated that the CHCs have been given a special role in relation to the planning process, that they should be consulted and help to determine the setting of priorities and in helping to encourage the better use of resources. On the other hand the Association of Community Health Councils in their evidence to the Royal Commission argued that their ability to represent the consumer was strongest when they were not seen as part of the process of management.[7] Part of the problem certainly lies in the lack of precision with which the terms 'participation' and 'consultation' have been used. Ham quotes a national survey in which 68 per cent of Community Health Councils were shown to have had disputes with the Area Health Authorities on the meaning of participation and consultation.[8]

In an illuminating article attempting to show the gradations of meaning involved in the notion of participation, Sheree Arnstein, an American academic, has constructed a ladder of participation to describe the different degrees of power.[9] This ranges from what Arnstein calls manipulation and therapy, through informing, consultation and placation, to partnership, delegated power to citizen control, where power is held by citizens rather than governments or service providers. The powers of Community Health Councils are limited to the lower rungs of the ladder of participation, which amounts to 'tokenism'. They are given information, they are consulted, there may be some room for negotiation although this depends on the stage at which they are consulted. If it is at a late stage in the planning process, for example, it adds up to little more than tokenism.

CHCs may make their greatest impact in providing information which gives new perspectives to problems. The survey carried out by Kensington and Chelsea CHC on access to primary health care in the inner city revealed a paucity of NHS general practitioners in this particular area and a high proportion of people not registered with GPs either because they could not find a GP to take them or because they had not bothered to register.[10] The Royal Commission on the NHS was also concerned about health care in inner cities and in 1981 the Acheson Committee produced a highly critical report on primary health care in Inner London.[11] The work of Kensington and Chelsea CHC could thus be seen as part of the process of recognition and identification of the problem of inner city care. Community Health Councils in London were also able to collect information on the cumulative effect of the bed closures in the London area in the latter part of the 1970s. There is no official overall London Health Authority, so here again they played a useful role in collecting and pooling information. The production of such information could secure a minimal power base for Community Health Councils and it will be interesting to see how their role develops in relation to the new District Health Authorities during the 1980s.

In summary, the various innovations in democratic practice introduced in 1974 have been unable to change the basic distribution of power in the NHS. Perhaps the greatest contribution of CHCs has been in providing a source of information, advice for the public, and as a potential focal point for expressing the views of those concerned with health care. Perhaps their greatest weakness is that they have, on the whole, lacked the capacity to challenge the dominant values in health care based on the medical or disease model of health.

HEALTH SERVICE USERS AS CONSUMERS: THE ECONOMIC DIMENSION

To describe the health service users as consumers is to use the language of the economic market. The assumption is that there is a product 'health services' which are produced and available on demand or need, in the case of the NHS without price, to be consumed by health service users. Some versions of the argument suggest a passive, others an active consumer.

Passive consumers

Abel-Smith suggests that the idea of a passive consumer is a more accurate description.[12] Once a person has presented himself for treatment, then the use of resources is determined by the professional. Professionals may use a number of devices to ration the use of resources such as queueing or 'cooling out' to cope with the absence of price and there is little, within the NHS, that the consumer can do to affect resource use. Furthermore, patients are unable to easily question the strategies or choices involved in diagnosis and treatment. The consumer is most helpless when most in need and, typically, unable to judge the quality of the treatment or its technical appropriateness. This is the case whether the consumer pays for the treatment or not. Neither are consumers able to judge the cost of health care and Abel-Smith comments, 'there are few fields of consumer expenditure where the consumer is as ill-equipped to exercise this theoretical sovereignty as in the health services'.

This may also be because few episodes of ill-health are similar. Patients are unable to build up expertise in dealing with these and it is difficult to form a judgement about treatments and disposals because failure to achieve results may be due to the peculiarities of the particular patient. The product is in other words infinitely varied. It is difficult to judge who is or is not a technically good doctor or what constitutes the good hospital. This view of the essentially helpless health service user is well represented in the sociological literature discussed in the next chapter. However these observations may be much less applicable to chronic illness or where the education and social class of the 'consumer' brings greater equality of knowledge. Davis and Horobin have collected a fascinating series of personal accounts of coping with illness in *Medical Encounters*.[13]

To a certain extent this passive acceptance of health care is borne out by consumer-satisfaction surveys of the NHS. The Royal Commission on the NHS specially commissioned two surveys of users and patients. Both surveys found the level of general consumer satisfaction with health services was high. In the study on patients' attitudes to the hospital service over 80 per cent of in-patients thought that the service they received was good or very good.[14] Simpson's study of primary care services for old people and children in a rural and an inner city area, concluded that 'on the whole, while always capable of improvement, the NHS did provide an accessible primary care service which was generally appreciated by its users'.[15] Although the *general* level of professed satisfaction was high, there were in fact a large number of specific complaints. Among out-patients, for example, over 25 per cent complained about difficulties in getting information about their progress. This rose to 31 per cent for in-patients. One in four adult in-patients complained that doctors had discussed their condition as if they were not there. Waiting times also caused complaints. 16 per cent of patients at out-patient clinics waited an hour after their appointment time and another 8 per cent for forty-five minutes. There were also complaints about lack of privacy and early waking times in hospitals. Nearly half of the patients surveyed complained of being woken too early. In fact 44 per cent were being woken before 6.00 a.m. and 76 per cent before 6.30 a.m. The Royal Commission comments 'This seems to us a prime example of the hospital being run for the convenience of its staff rather than the patient. We do not believe that the in-patients' day cannot be so organised so that the majority of patients are able to wake up at roughly their usual time.'[16]

What is surprising is that such a high level of grumbles and grievances should be seen as compatible with a very high level of reported satisfaction. As far as the NHS is concerned consumers do appear to be passive. Perhaps Cartwright is right when she suggests in her study of patients and their GPs that 'behind the satisfaction of most patients there lies an uncritical acceptance and lack of discrimination which is conducive to stagnation and apathy'.[17] This brings us full circle to Abel-Smith's point that over much medical practice users lack the knowledge and will to critically assess the treatment they receive. They are patients rather than consumers, they complain about the 'hotel' aspects of care rather than treatment, the quality of which they cannot judge. To look at the question another way around, there seems to be a high capacity for health systems to generate loyalty among their recipients.

The term consumer has in fact been deliberately injected into discussions about health services by some writers in an attempt to place the users of services within the debate about health service provision. Too often the patient's views receive little attention. The Royal Commission on the NHS was practically unique in looking at services from the user's perspective. The Commission did attempt to take a slightly wider look at the objectives of health services [doc 8] and to examine aspects of health care which are weakly developed often because they are peripheral to curative medicine and to the interests of the 'professional monopolisers'. Blaxter in a study of the rehabilitation services carried out for the Commission, looked at the network of referrals between health workers and agencies. This was intended as a measure of the relative weight of use by 200 physically impaired people of different services but it also shows how the Health and Personal Social Services appear to the consumer, a bewildering network of agencies and individuals.[18] A chart from the study is reproduced in document 29. Such a state of affairs may encourage passivity.

Active consumers

Health service users and patients may be passive in relation to the NHS but studies of illness behaviour have indicated the model of illness behaviour based on the passive consumer or patient and active doctor is an over-simplification and may be a reflection of the kinds of surveys carried out. People may be very active in relation to their health. Those with symptoms do not automatically declare themselves ill and take to their beds, nor do they necessarily consult a doctor. As David Robinson showed in his study of families in South Wales decision-making in the process of becoming ill is determined by a wide range of perceptions and evaluations which are influenced by social structure, by class, by family roles and work demands.[19]

The first line of defence in illness is often self-medication. Cartwright and Dunnel in *Medicine Takers, Prescribers and Hoarders* found that 41 per cent of their national sample had taken painkillers during the previous fortnight, 14 per cent indigestion remedies, 14 per cent skin ointments and antiseptics, 13 per cent throat and cough remedies.[20] People also consult others within their social network about signs and symptoms and choose to consult practitioners other than those provided through the NHS. This may be as a substitute for, or complementary to the NHS; it may be a precursor to conventional treatment or used when this has failed.

Hard evidence on the extent of alternative medicine is difficult to come by. Hewitt and Wood recorded the numbers of acupuncturists, naturopaths, chiropractors and osteopaths registered by their organisations in 1975 and estimated that there were 200,000 people consulting during the year.[21] Inglis's study, *Fringe Medicine*, suggests that there is a substantial field of healing activity outside orthodox allopathic medicine.[22] Groups who feel they are not well catered for by orthodox medicine have turned to alternative medicine. The women's health movement for example has spread information about self-care and 'holistic medicine'. There have been attempts to develop a more social model of illness as an alternative to the disease model and Roberts's *Women, Health and Reproduction* is a collection of essays in which the general argument is that the disease model of illness is inappropriate to the handling of many aspects of women's health care.[23] Bart, in an account of a self-help abortion clinic, demands the handing over of 'medical technologies' arguing that these should not remain the property of the medical profession in a hospital setting. The working of a Well Woman Clinic is also described in the book. This is concerned with counselling and support, the sharing of health problems and treatments to develop ways of coping among women.

Small scale studies of Asian Communities also indicate the continued use of alternative health care. Hakim doctors trained in one or both systems of Indian medicine continue to practise in this country. For both women and particular ethnic groups there has sometimes been a failure of the NHS to understand sufficiently the cultural and emotional dimensions of illness which may make the NHS unacceptable. Brent Community Health Council explores these issues in its booklet, *Black People and the Health Service*.[24]

Further signs of active consumerism can be found in the growth and development of organised self-care around particular illnesses and disabilities. Mutual self-care groups exist for many specific conditions and Henry and Robinson's study has provided an account of the mutual support derived from the experience of sharing and learning among those with similar difficulties. Self-help groups may offer an understanding of pain, disability and dying in a supportive and non-stigmatising environment.[25]

The growth of private medicine must also be seen as the result of active consumerism, although this formally embraces the medical model. The reasons behind the growth, already referred to in Chapter 8, are complex. It may reflect the level of income, the desire to guarantee speedy treatment and better standards of the 'hotel' aspects of patient care or simply the increase in the numbers of groups (companies and trade unions) taking out subscriptions to private medical insurance as a benefit for their members. Goldie has calculated that of the 1.6 million subscribers in 1980, one million were members through group schemes.[26] This growth suggests a demand for acute medical care at a time when the NHS is attempting as a matter of policy to switch resources to care in the community and is indicative of the existence of the tension between the demand as expressed by the individuals and the needs of the collectivity expressed by governments. Those who opt for private medicine however do accept the medical model of illness and become 'passive consumers' subject to professional decisions. They are in no better position to judge the 'quality' of medical care they are receiving and do so in a context where their rights are less guaranteed.

HEALTH SERVICE USERS AS HEALTH WORKERS: THE SOCIAL DIMENSION

There are those who totally reject the use of the term consumer as being inappropriate to what can generally be called the 'human service industries'.[27] Hughes, for example, argues that the patient is part of the process of health care.[28] The patient brings conditions to the doctor in the first place and is actively involved in the process of 'producing' effective treatment. The patient does not consume a product but *is* part of the production of recovery or health. Treatment is interactive and negotiated. There have been a number of studies of health care from this perspective: Roth's account of long-stay hospitals[29] and Stimson and Webb's study of the patient's view of general practice, *Going to see Doctor*.[30] These emphasise the on-going drama of an illness episode of which the consultation is a small part of a longer process of managing illness. The consultation is anticipated and made sense of by the patient afterwards, and may or may not result in the patient following advice given. These studies and others suggest that the patient is very much part of the production of health care. Analyses which exclude the patient from the consideration of issues in health care encourage the objectification of the patient and bring a rigid distinction between work *to* people and work *for* people. Human service industries which are only concerned with doing work *to* people simply fail to achieve the services *for* them. If patients are considered part of the process of health work then they are more likely to co-operate in their own treatment. Illich argues that 'medical procedures often turn into a kind of black magic, when instead of mobilising his healing powers, they transform the sick man into a limp and mystified voyeur of his own treatment'.[31] The rejection of the term 'consumer' can thus be seen as part of the process of attempting to reconceptualise roles in health care so that the role of medical expert is only one part. This is particularly important in understanding those areas of health and medical care which do not fit the acute illness, passive patient/authoriative doctor model. Much health care is concerned with the management of chronic illness, with the discomforts of disability and old age, with the management of self-limiting and trivial illness, where a variety of people may be involved in health care work.

Celia Davies has argued that health care can be seen as a field of work in which there are participants of various kinds providing health care within or outside the institutional setting. It is an arena in which occupational identities are forged and status is established; where some work is paid and similar work unpaid. Health policies and organisational structures aid or discourage a particular division of labour as they establish boundaries between different health care roles. Health workers and the organisational arrangements for the delivery of care may serve to socialise individuals into health roles thus reinforcing them. Davies, herself, found that in a study of new mothers and health workers, the latter sought to socialise the mother into appropriate behaviour in the division of labour, for example about which issues help should be sought and which health problems could be considered as trivial.[32]

Individuals could be said to be health workers therefore, in two dimensions. They perceive, define, make choices and cope with all stages of illness in themselves and they perform a similar role in the health care of others. Changes in the pattern of disease which have brought more long-term illness and disability and the attempts to come to terms with these in policy terms through the development of community care for dependent groups have underlined the fact that there is no simple divide between health on the one side and professionally-defined illness on the other. Neither is there a clear distinction between lay people on the one hand and professionals on the other. Attempts to break down barriers organisationally are occurring as there is greater recognition of the social aspects of illness. Parents may stay in hospital with their children, there have been experiments with patients-groups in primary care,[33] community health workers have been employed to encourage particular ethnic groups, such as pregnant Asian women, to use health services. The redefinition of health service users as health workers may aid the reconceptualisation of health roles.

SUMMARY

This chapter has attempted to examine the relationship of the individual to health care in a number of different ways. First, by using the political model of wo/man to look at the limited extent of account-ability and participation of the public in the health system. Second, by examining the concept of the health care 'consumer' which rests on an economic model of wo/man and third by exploring the role of the individual as health worker in the social management of illness. Each model of wo/man tends to yield a different policy prescription and all, singly, have limitations. They do collectively reveal some of the complexities of the relationship between health care users and providers in contemporary health care.

REFERENCES

1. MACKENZIE, W. J. M., *Power and Responsibility in Health Care. The National Health Service as a Political Institution*, Oxford University Press, Oxford (1979)
2. PATEMAN, C., *Participation and Democratic Theory*, Cambridge University Press, Cambridge (1970)
3. CROSSMAN, R., *A Politicians View of Health Service Planning*, University of Glasgow (1972) p. 23
4. ROYAL COMMISSION ON LOCAL GOVERNMENT, *Representation and Community*, Appendix 7, Vol. III, Research Appendices, Cmnd 4040 II, HMSO (1969)
5. For example, BROWN, R. G. S., *Reorganising the NHS*, Robertson, Oxford (1979) and HAYWOOD, S. and ALASZEWSKI, A., *Crisis in the Health Service*, Croom Helm, (1980)
6. HAM, C., 'Community Health Council Participation in the NHS Planning System', *Social Policy and Administration*, **14** (3), Autumn 1980
7. *Report of the Royal Commission on the National Health Service* (Chairman: Sir Alec Merrison), Cmnd 7615, HMSO, London (1979), Ch. 11
8. HAM, C., *op. cit.*
9. ARNSTEIN, S. R., 'A Ladder of Citizen Participation', *American Institute of Planners Journal*, July 1966
10. KENSINGTON, CHELSEA, WESTMINSTER, SOUTH DISTRICT, *The Family Doctor in Central London. A survey of general practitioner services* (1977), 89 Sydney St, London SW3
11. LONDON HEALTH PLANNING CONSORTIUM, *Primary Health Care in Inner London* (Chairman: Donald Acheson), May 1981
12. ABEL-SMITH, B., *Value for Money in Health Services*, Heinemann, London (1976), Ch. 4
13. DAVIS, A. and HOROBIN, G., *Medical Encounters, the Experience of Illness and Treatment*, Croom Helm, London (1977)
14. GREGORY, J., *Patients' Attitudes to the Hospital Service*, Royal Commission on the National Health Service Research Paper No. 5, HMSO, London (1978)

15. SIMPSON, R., *Access to Primary Health Care*, Royal Commission on the National Health Service Research Paper No. 6, HMSO, London (1979)

16. *Report of the Royal Commission on the NHS*, *op. cit.*, Ch. 10

17. CARTWRIGHT, A., *Patients and their Doctors*, Routledge & Kegan Paul, London (1967), p. 216

18. BLAXTER, M., *Principles and Practice in Rehabilitation*, Appendix G, Royal Commission on the NHS, *op. cit.*

19. ROBINSON, D., *The Process of Becoming Ill*, Routledge & Kegan Paul, London (1971)

20. DUNNELL, K. and CARTWRIGHT, A., *Medicine Takers, Prescribers and Hoarders*, Routledge & Kegan Paul, London (1972)

21. HEWITT, D. and WOOD, P. H. N., 'Heterodox Practitioners and the Availability of Specialist Advice', *Rheumatology and Rehabilitation*, **14** (1975), 191

22. INGLIS, B. *Fringe Medicine*, Faber, London (1964)

23. ROBERTS, H. (ed.), *Women, Health and Reproduction*, Routledge & Kegan Paul, London (1981)

24. BRENT COMMUNITY HEALTH COUNCIL, *Black People and the Health Service*, (1981)

25. HENRY, S. and ROBINSON, D., 'The Self Help Way to Health' in ATKINSON, P., DINGWALL, R. and MURCOTT, A. (eds), *Prospects for the National Health Service*, Croom Helm, London (1979)

26. GOLDIE, N., 'Private Medicine: a logical development or an aberration?' Report from a conference on National Health Care Systems in Non-growth Economies. *Scandinavian Journal of Social Medicine*, Supplementum 28, Stockholm 1981

27. STACEY, M., 'The Health Service Consumer: A Sociological Misconception' in STACEY, M. (ed.), *The Sociology of the National Health Service*, Sociological Review Monograph 22, University of Keele (1976)

28. HUGHES, E. C., *Men and their Work*, Free Press, Glencoe, Illinois (1958)

29. ROTH, J., *Timetables, Structuring the Passage of Time in Hospital and other Careers*, Bobbs Merrill, Indianapolis (1963)

30. STIMSON, G. and WEBB, B., *Going to see Doctor. The consultation process in general practice*, Routledge & Kegan Paul (1975)

31. ILLICH, I., *Limits to Medicine: Medical Nemesis. The Expropriation of Health*, Marion Boyars, London (1976), p. 121

32. DAVIES, C., 'Comparative Occupational Roles in Health Care', *Social Science and Medicine*, Vol. 13a, No. 19

33. For example, PRITCHARD, P., 'The People's Practice', *The Health Service*, 11 June 1982; RAKUSEN, J., 'Patient Power', *The Times Health Supplement*, 5 March 1982

Chapter eleven

DOING BETTER AND FEELING WORSE: CRITIQUES OF HEALTH CARE

By the mid-twentieth century most advanced industrial societies developed state financed health systems and health expenditures were rising along with growth rates. There was an expansion of investment and spending on health care facilities and an increase of professionals and others involved in health work. The belief was that medicine had made and was making a significant contribution to the health and happiness of individuals. Dollery, writing in the late 1970s, sums up the mood:

> Some of the early achievements in the treatment of infectious disease were so miraculous as almost to surpass belief. They literally changed the world. The watch and wait while the pneumonia of the young adult progressed through crisis to lysis or death. Ths agony of a child with otitis media or worse still osteomyelitis, the long-drawn-out vigil of the patient with pulmonary TB coughing away his life. Anti-bacterial chemotherapy made the cure of such scourges almost a matter of routine. It was a time of optimism. Science appeared to have the salvation of the world in its hand and mankind could look forward to an era of healthy ease and modest luxury. The budgets of the Medical Research Council and the National Institutes of Health increased exponentially and journalistic comment about medical research was almost always eulogistic.'[1]

A greater scepticism has developed during the 1970s and 1980s which is not simply about less lusty growth rates but also awareness that in most western industrial societies increased spending has not necessarily brought improvements in health. Despite state financed health services problems have persisted. Research has shown that there have been continuing inequalities in the distribution of health services and therefore inequalities in access. The burden of ill-health, furthermore, has been greatest among groups living in certain regions and among members of particular groups such as ethnic minorities, the lower social classes, or those working in hazardous occupations.

Lifestyle has been shown to have a profound effect on health status.

Health care systems have appeared to be resistant to change and have frequently failed to adapt to meet new demands created by the increased burden of dependency characteristic of advanced industrial societies. It has been suggested that they have been more concerned with the curing of illness rather than the provision of care or the prevention of ill-health. Health care has been criticised for being bureaucratically organised and alienating for the individual.

These doubts, many of which have been referred to in previous chapters, have been brought into focus in a number of critical attacks on health care by a variety of academics and polemicists. The criticisms have in turn brought a mood of greater pessimism about contemporary health care. There has been a sense of, in Wildavsky's phrase, 'doing better and feeling worse'[2] in relation to health services. The criticisms have taken different starting points from which to pinpoint the inadequacies of health care and have drawn on different frameworks of analysis, on this basis they have been grouped into 'critiques' in this chapter. This tends to oversimplify and perhaps distort the work of particular writers, and to exaggerate the differences of approach. However, it does serve to clarify the sets of assumptions on which 'critiques' rest.

THE PROFESSIONAL DOMINANCE CRITIQUE

This approach suggests that the dominance of the medical profession legally, politically, administratively and morally is the analytical key to understanding the distribution of resources and power in health care, and the shortcomings of health services. Eliot Freidson whose books *Professional Dominance* and *The Profession of Medicine* laid down the bones of the argument in 1970,[3] has been particularly influential in generating further work. His criticisms were not new. G. B. Shaw, for example, developed a scathing attack on the medical profession in the Preface to *The Doctor's Dilemma* in 1911[4] [doc 30]. Freidson however did take a more critical stance to the role of the profession than had prevailed during the age of optimism in the 1950s and 1960s.

As a sociologist, he stressed the autonomy of the medical profession in the political organisation of health care, in the division of labour in medical care and in relation to the treatment of illness. He argued that the status of the profession is derived from political activity which is legitimated by political and social elites through a system of state licensing. Medical practitioners, organised around their particular discipline, he suggested, give Western systems of medical care their basic and characteristic structure.

Parry, in a discussion of the rise of the medical profession in England, draws on the work of Freidson to argue that the process of professionalisation itself is a strategy for achieving a monopoly position in the delivery of health care and that since the foundation of the General Medical Council in 1858, which gave the profession the right to establish qualifications and debar individuals without them from calling themselves a medical doctor, the profession has increased its area of influence.[5] Although this role is mediated by the state in Britain the control of a basic core of skills, an increasing division of labour in medicine and health care, and a structure of institutional contacts has enabled doctors to consult and be consulted about a wide range of health policies. Furthermore they have a key position in the delivery of health services in the National Health Service. Through the exercise of clinical autonomy, the right to decide what is best for the patient, they in fact act as gatekeepers in the distribution of material goods and resources in health care.

Those who have looked at the role of the medical profession from this perspective argue that the profession can, with its autonomy over technique and control of its own work, dominate the practice of health care. In Freidson's words they can

> drive a wedge into other zones of practice to maintain control over facilities, the organisation of service delivery and training . . . All the work done by other occupations and related to the service of the patient is subject to the order of the physician. The profession alone is held competent to diagnose illness, treat or direct the treatment of illness and evaluate the service. Without medical authorisation little can be done for the patient by para-professional workers. The client's medication, diet, excretion and recreation are all subject to medical orders. So is the information given to the patient. By and large, without medical authorisation, paramedical workers are not supposed to communicate anything of significance to the patient about what his illness is, how it will be treated, and what are the chances of improvement.[6]

This dominance does not stop at the boundaries of the health system but may extend to other personal service workers outside the health system, to teachers, social workers and the like.

Medical dominance has a further dimension. Its influence and power is strongest at the level of the doctor-patient relationship. Freidson again suggests 'the medical profession had the first claim to jurisdiction over the label illness, and anything to which it might be attached, irrespective of its ability to deal with it effectively'.[7] It is this control over an area of knowledge and set of ideas which has been the source of much analysis and criticism around what has been referred to as the 'medicalisation thesis'. This has been developed to argue that medicine has sought to 'take over' increasing areas of social life. 'All kinds of problems', says Zola, 'roll to the doctor's door . . . from sagging anatomies, to unwanted pregnancy, childlessness to genetic counselling, from laziness to crime'. Medicine has become a form of social control, 'by naming the spirit that underlines the deviance, authority places the deviant under control of language and customs and turns him from a threat to a support of the social system'.[8] So it is argued, medicine has the tendency to 'make' diseases, such as child-battering, alcoholism, schizophrenia, as well as to dominate the institutional mechanisms which have been developed to cope with them.[9]

Certainly the practice of medicine is a moral exercise as well as a technical one. Kennedy in *The Unmasking of Medicine* in 1981 argued that the medical profession's jurisdiction in the giving and with-holding of treatment, in relation to abortion, mental handicap, as well as in the designation of diagnostic categories such as alcoholism, or depression conceals judgements about the person and the person's status. Thus choices are made which should rightly be left to the individual.[10] Oakley's study of childbirth, *Women Confined*, is an account of the medicalisation of childbirth, where technical expertise and medical criteria take precedence over other forms of knowledge and therefore medical choices overtake personal ones. The study was based on interviews with women at different stages of pregnancy and post-partum and gives a graphic picture of doctors' and mothers' views of pregnancy, and the fundamental difference in their pers-pectives on the meaning of childbirth.

Doctors

(a) define reproduction as a specialist subject in which only doctors are experts in the entire symptomatology of childbearing.

(b) the associated definition of reproduction as a medical subject, as exactly analogous to other pathological processes as topics of medical knowledge and intervention.

(c) the selection of limited criteria of reproductive success, i.e. peri-natal and maternal mortality rates.

(d) the divorce of reproduction from its social context, pregnant patienthood being seen as a woman's only relevant status.

(e) the restriction of women to maternity . . . their derived typifica-tion as 'by nature' maternal, domesticated, family-oriented people.[11]

This failure of the medical profession and the medical model of illness to recognise patients as persons in scientifically-based medical systems has been underlined by the work of some anthropologists and other social scientists who have examined the handling of illness in cultures different from our own.[12] These studies have shown that other health systems may be more successful in handling the social dimensions of illness which involve readjustment, pain and suffering, despite the undoubted successes of scientific medicine in the biological sphere. Thus in less industrialised societies, physical and behavioural changes in individuals' illness may be coped with through particular rituals which are meaningful in terms of the culture and help to reintegrate the individual within it.

Young, an anthropologist who worked with the Amhara describes the process through which the group deals with an illness episode.

> A sickness episode begins when the principal (actor) and or his relative decide the range of symptoms into which his signs could be translated. Next they must obtain the services of someone, whose medical powers are appropriate to this range of symptoms: under certain circumstances, they may have power enough themselves to translate the signs. Their choices of diagnostician decides what set of rules will be played, what individuals (including therapists and pathogenic agents) and audiences can be mobilised, and what sort of social states will be involved. The therapist's task is to communicate and legitimize the episode's outcome, and this too, takes place according to rules shared by sick persons, healers, and audiences.

These rituals and rules can help to provide an answer to the fundamental questions raised by all illness . . . why is this happening to me and how do I cope with this? It also involves the group in an episode which is potentially threatening to its stability.[13]

The medical or disease model represented by the medical profession with its concentration on the individual, acted on by biological forces, underestimates the importance of the circumstances leading to illness, the social relations of illness and the importance of other health workers in the handling of illness states.

Perhaps the best known polemic on the medicalisation thesis is Illich's *The Limits to Medicine* where the author argues that institutionalised medicine has become a threat to health through social, clinical and structural 'iatrogenesis', or damage done by the provider.[14] These terms are described and illustrated in document 32. As a Christian Socialist Illich has mounted a moral crusade against many aspects of modern industrial and professional society which he sees as attacking the autonomy and sense of responsibility of the individual.

His critique has been directed mainly at curative medicine and its limitations. Although few would fully endorse his emphasis on the destructive power of modern medicine, he has helped to encourage a greater scepticism about its benefits.

The professional dominance critique can account for the political influence and power of the medical profession in terms of its control over an area of knowledge. It is less able to explain why that knowledge has been and is so highly valued. After all Cochrane in *Efficiency and Effectiveness*, McKeown in *The Role of Medicine* and a number of other medical and sociological studies have shown how the 'scientific' bases of medical practice have been exaggerated and pointed to the fashionable nature of many therapies.[15] Why is it then that medical knowledge continues to hold such sway? The link with science and high technology may be important in mystifying the public. It may also be that the public has a vested interest in attributing the power to care and heal to the profession. After all, those who mediate in the process of illness and death in any society have had a position of power. Moreoever it may be that the critics of medicine have underestimated its achievements in alleviating suffering and disability. This ambivalence to the medical profession is illustrated by the extracts in document 30. A further criticism of the professional dominance approach is that it has failed to relate medical power to the wider distribution of power in society and to the reasons why political and social elites should support medicine's claims. Before turning to this issue however we will examine the political economy critique which is rather briefly discussed as many of the issues were dealt with in greater detail in Chapters 8 and 9.

THE POLITICAL ECONOMY CRITIQUE

The focus of the political-economy critique is on the political and economic circumstances which create particular patterns of illness and disease and secondarily on the lack of appropriateness of societal responses to these. McKeown argued in 1974 that significant improvements in health had occurred during the nineteenth and early twentieth centuries due to improvements in the standard of living and not due primarily to medical intervention.

> It (the modern improvement in health) began in the eighteenth century and was reflected in a decline in mortality which has continued, with interruptions, until the present time. The improvement was initiated by an increase in food supplies which resulted from the Agricultural Revolution

that spread throughout Europe after 1700. From about 1870 this influence was powerfully supported by improved hygiene, particularly in respect of water supplies and sewage disposal. In the twentieth century, further advance followed the introduction of effective preventative and therapeutic measures (immunisation and drugs). The contribution of the last influence to the total decline in mortality was relatively small and the improvement in human health was therefore due predominantly to a change in reproductive behaviour and to modification of the environment by provision of food and protection from physical hazards.[16]

Thus, the improvement of health was primarily due to economic factors and social changes, secondarily to political factors, through social intervention, and thirdly to medical intervention.

Work carried out on the social bases of ill-health during the 1970s referred to in Chapter 8, sought to demonstrate the relationship between disease, ill-health and specific social and economic factors. The Centre for Studies in Health Policy has argued for example that we live in an 'ill-health promoting economy' and has commented on the values which support the pursuit of ill-health.

> The pinnacle of achievement in health has come to be equated with the spectacle of men and women becoming overstressed and under-exercised, indulging in excessive consumption of food, cigarettes and alcohol for a number of years before being rushed to an intensive care unit and submerged in expensive technology only when acute symptoms have prevented them from indulging in further consumption.[17]

Those who explain health and ill-health in terms of the political economy emphasise the importance of, and the need for, a collective response to such factors. McKeown has for example suggested that social action and inaction in the societal arrangements for the provision of food, shelter, transport and work bear the responsibility for certain classes of causes of ill-health. 'The physical environment which we have constructed, high rise housing, the extensive use of petrol-driven vehicles, the change in eating habits, methods of processing, manufacturing and distributing food, the manufacture and production of new products, all have brought new and unanticipated hazards.'[18] The social organisation of providing for the necessities of life whether in the public or private sector, plays a part in the aetiology of physical illnesses as well as being a factor contributing to stress related illnesses, depression and neuroses.

Furthermore, as the Black Report on Inequalities in Health demonstrated so effectively, the impact of hazardous social and environmental factors falls heavily on particular groups.[19] Social deprivation, measured by occupational class is associated with ill-health, and the

Health Policy and the NHS

use of and availability of health services tends to reinforce inequalities through lack of adequate services. There is also evidence to suggest particular occupations and lifestyles increase exposure to health hazards. The social causes of ill-health have been shown to be complex and varied. They remain embedded in the socioeconomic structure but affect smaller groups than was the case with the nineteenth century infectious diseases, along the lines of gender, ethnic group, occupation, geographical area, as well as class. Effects of deprivation and hazard are cumulative, poor growth, and physical development in adolescence and childhood are likely to influence susceptibility to disease throughout life and these in turn are affected by the social position, circumstances, health and habits of parents.

A political-economy critique has often, both now and in the nineteenth century, been effective in explaining the inequalities in health care and social conditions associated with ill-health. It has generated many policy proposals and strategies for the amelioration of conditions, the Beveridge proposals and the post-war welfare legislation among them. This approach has been less enlightening about the underlying power relationships which inhibit change. The Marxist critique attempts to tackle these questions arguing that both the patterns of illness and disease and the arrangements for health care, with its division of labour, professional and bureaucratic dominance, is a characteristic of the mode of production and the relationships of production in advanced capitalist society.

THE MARXIST CRITIQUE

According to the Marxist critique, the organisation and practice of medicine and the provision of health services supports capitalist organisation and the interests of the modern state. This accounts for inequalities, medical dominance and the ill-health promoting economy. As Marx and Engels put it, 'the ruling ideas of each age have ever been the ideas of its ruling class'. Navarro, for example, in *Class Struggle, the State and Medicine*,[20] explicitly rejects the view that the structure of medical services and its inequalities in the use of health services can be explained in terms of forces within the medical profession or result from lack of societal responsiveness to change. He seeks to show that class relations, and the class structure of British society, determines all the significant aspects of health policy and health care. Thus more is spent on the health care of the middle class, wealthier regions attract a greater share of health resources. The provision of a National Health Service with its concentration on curative medicine rather than on the need for care of dependent groups and prevention is also seen to reflect bourgeois ideology. Curative medicine and the medical establishment serves the interests of capital by concentrating attention on individual ill-health; a concentration on the individual depoliticises health issues and the major causes of ill-health. It diverts attention from the illness-generating conditions in the social structure, from polluted and polluting environments, from dangerous working conditions and the like.

The Marxist critique also emphasises the social control functions of medicine. It sees the recent emphasis on the responsibility of the individuals for their health and stress on behavioural factors in ill-health, smoking, excessive alcohol consumption, as diverting attention away from structural factors and the importance of social and political action in changing the structure of power. This approach embraces the medicalisation thesis arguing that medical knowledge is ideological. Susser comments that 'Starting with a relatively simple set of possibly effective procedures fulfilling some uncontrived human needs, medical care under capitalism has become transformed into an increasingly sophisticated, yet ineffective body of unnecessary values with increasing bio-technology, ancillary testing, ritualistic surgery, over-utilisation of hospital and superfluous appointments.'[21] This is reminiscent of Marcuse's arguments on the state's role in the creation of false needs in industrial societies.[22]

McKinley links these arguments to the analysis of the health care system as a large and profitable enterprise which is part of, and linked to, the business sector. This, he and others demonstrate in relation to the medical care systems in the USA.[23] The analysis has been less fully and rigorously developed in relation to Britain with its National Health Service except perhaps in relation to the drug industry. The industry is clearly part of an international network of capitalist enterprise. However what is interesting is how the relationship between the private sector and the NHS is managed. This is very complex as in some respects the NHS is a 'monopoly' buyer.[24]

The Marxist critique has been used in two further dimensions to analyse and explain the division of labour and hierarchy of power in the NHS itself. Both Doyal in *The Political Economy of Health*,[25] and Navarro explain the rigid division of roles in health care, between different health workers and the reduction of the patient to the object of the labour process in terms of the class structure and relations of production. Medical care, they suggest, develops as a product rather than a personal service under capitalism.

A socialist-feminist critique of health care is also partially developed by Doyal in highlighting the role of women in the division of labour in health care. It is pointed out that their position in the health system reflects their place in the social structure, the caring and less powerful role of nurses compared to the curing and leadership role of doctors; the hierarchy in medicine itself between male-dominated surgery and the more female-dominated specialisms such as community and child health. Oakley[26] and Ehrenreich and English[27] in different contexts argue that contemporary health care demotes women's expertise as healers as well as medicalising many areas of women's experience in the interests of male careers. Women play a large role in the health care of their families, they assume and are expected to assume prime responsibility for well and sick children and for dependent relatives, they are involved in pregnancy and child birth, they take the main responsibility for contraception, women are more subject to certain health problems, particularly depressive illness, probably because their greater role ambiguity leads to greater stress. Both their contribution as health workers and their particular needs in health care, it is suggested, are neglected or distorted in contemporary health care. These authors conclude that a capitalist and patriarchal social structure and the consequent social status and relationships are the explanation for the inadequacies of contemporary health care.

The foregoing critiques explain the shortcomings of health care and the limitations of health policy according to different frameworks of explanation. They share a scepticism about the benefits of the scientific advances in medicine. The final critique to be examined, that of the radical right while agreeing with many of the criticisms of modern health care, rests on embracing what modern medical care has to offer, and concentrates on enhancing the ability of the consumer to buy medical care in the market.

THE RADICAL RIGHT CRITIQUE

Unlike the professional dominance and Marxist critiques which are relatively weak on strategies for change the arguments of the radical right are extended into recommending changes in the mode of health care organisation. The aim is to reduce the role of government intervention in health care on the basis that health care is a good like any other and as such should be part of provision in the private, rather than the public sector. In Britain the critique has been promoted by the Institute of Economic Affairs and *The Litmuss Papers* represent a recent statement.[28] However, the arguments for privatisation are also implicit in some of the recent policy statements of the 1979 Conservative government referred to in Chapter 7 of this book.

The main criticism of the NHS by the radical right is that it is seriously underfunded. It is argued that facilities are inadequate, both in terms of the availability of up-to-date technology, equipment, trained manpower and on the 'hotel' side of health care. Hospital buildings are frequently old and ill-equipped. Waiting lists for relatively simple but not critical operations such as hernias, varicose veins or hip-replacements are long and although these are not life-threatening conditions they cause considerable discomfort and impair the quality of life. It is argued, and here they join forces with other critiques, that health institutions and procedures are bureacratic, alienating, time-consuming and the patient becomes an object rather than being treated as a patient. Moreover, freely available health care under the NHS does not encourage an individual sense of responsibility for health, nor regular surveillance and preventive measures. *The Litmuss Papers* comment that in the United States there has been a growth of health maintenance programmes as part of health insurance and there is generally a more positive attitude to health and more knowledge of aspects of personal lifestyles which are a threat to health. It has been suggested, for example, that the level of knowledge of the association between diet, exercise and smoking is much greater in the US than in Britain where it is believed that 'stress' causes heart disease. It may be that these factors explain the reduced rates of coronary heart disease in the US referred to in Chapter 9.

The Litmuss Papers also draw attention to professional frustration in the NHS. Covert rationing, queueing, inertia, resistance to change and appalling industrial relations are, according to the radical right, the result of public sector management. Professionals are being prevented from providing the service they wish to offer. 'The NHS must fail, because it does not supply the British people with the best medical care they want because it prevents them as individual consumers from paying for the services that suit their personal family circumstances, requirements and preferences', says Sheldon.[29]

The radical right seek to remedy the faults of the NHS through a system of health care funding which rests on a combination of private and state insurance linked to other measures which encourage the private sector to provide health care facilities. Their arguments rest on the idea of the rational sovereign consumer and a belief in a remedy to the ills of the NHS on the demand, rather than the supply side. There is however a secondary reason for promoting private health care. The private market is an export earner. It can attract foreign capital, and therefore take its place as part of the business revival promised to follow from the 1979 Conservative government's economic strategy. As part of that economic policy is to cut public expenditure, it is easy to see the attractions from an economic point of view of encouraging the development of private medicine and pursuing the feasibility of a major change in the funding of the NHS. The critique of the radical right is of course based on the assumption of a group of well-endowed, intelligent, healthy and rational consumers with an ability to protect their health and avoid illness through their individual action. Social and economic factors in the causation of disease are ignored and so are the collective benefits of a healthier population. Moreover it is assumed that individuals are able to evaluate the health care they are receiving and affect the standard and efficiency of care they receive. Neither argument is valid. The problem of evaluation of technical and professional activities remains despite 'consumer choice'.

FINAL COMMENT

There is no doubt that all the critiques mentioned above have presented a challenge to the NHS and to government policy in health care. Each contains a partially valid analysis of the shortcomings of the NHS. Their major contribution has been that they have shown that existing health policy and health care rests on a particular set of assumptions, on a predominantly medical model of illness and that this has limitations. A diagram constructed by Illsley and reproduced in the document section [doc 31] suggests the dimensions of change to accommodate criticisms through a new policy paradigm. Health care has become, as a result, a disputed area of policy and provision and is therefore an important political issue, even in Britain which has had a national health service since the 1940s. Criticisms have, however, occurred at a period when low growth rates and high unemployment, together with Conservative economic policies, are posing a threat to the maintenance and continuation of the NHS? If so many procedures are ineffective, if medicalisation is a form of social control, if medical intervention can be so damaging to the patient, if changes in lifestyle, modes of production, the distribution of income are more important than health and medical care then what is the justification for devoting such a large proportion of GNP to the NHS? Klein comments, 'Ideology and the politics of Utopia are in fashion: the conventional wisdom is that radical solutions, based on a new vision of society are required.'[30] In fact critiques of health have been more effective in analysing the deficiencies of health care and the NHS than in describing its achievements or in recommending feasible changes in policy.

REFERENCES

1. DOLLERY, C., *The End of an Age of Optimism*, London: The Nuffield Provincial Hospitals Trust, Oxford (1978)
2. WILDAVSKY, A., *The Art and Craft of Policy Analysis*, Macmillan (1980)
3. FREIDSON, E., *Professional Dominance: The Social Structure of Medical Care*, Atherton Press, New York (1970)
4. SHAW, G. B. S., *The Doctors Dilemma* (originally published 1911), Penguin, London (1956)
5. PARRY, N. and PARRY, J., *The Rise of the Medical Profession: a study of collective social mobility*, Croom Helm, London (1977)
6. FREIDSON, E., *Professional Dominance, op. cit.*
7. *Ibid.*
8. ZOLA, I. K., 'Medicine as an Institution of Social Control', *Sociological Review*, **20** (3) Nov. 1972
9. For example, SZAZ, T., *The Myth of Mental Illness*, Harper and Row, New York (1961)
10. KENNEDY, I., *The Unmasking of Medicine*, Allen & Unwin, London (1981)
11. OAKLEY, A., *Women Confined: Towards a Sociology of Childbirth*, Robertson, Oxford (1980)
12. For example: LOUDON, J. B. (ed.), *Anthropology in Medicine*, Academic Press, London (1976); MACLEAN, U., *Magical Medicine*, Penguin, London (1971)
13. YOUNG, A., 'Some Implications of Medical Beliefs and Practices for Social Anthropology', *American Anthropology*, **78** (5) 1976
14. ILLICH, I., *Limits to Medicine. Medical Nemesis. The Expropriation of Health*, Marion Boyars, London (1976)
15. For example: COCHRANE, A. L., *Effectiveness and Efficiency. Random Reflections on Health Services*, Nuffield Provincial Hospitals Trust (1971); STACEY, M. *et al.* (ed.), *Health Care and Health Knowledge*, Croom Helm, London (1977); BLAXTER, M., 'Diagnosis as Category or Process. The Case of Alcoholism', *Social Science and Medicine*, No. 12, 1978
16. MCKEOWN, T. and LOWE, *An Introduction to Social Medicine*, Blackwell, Oxford (1974), p. 20
17. DRAPER, P., BEST, G. and DENNIS, J., *Health, Money and the*

National Health Service, Unit for the Study of Health Policy, London (1976), p. 28

18. MCKEOWN, T., *The Role of Medicine. Dream, Mirage or Nemesis?*, Blackwell, Oxford (1979)

19. DEPARTMENT OF HEALTH AND SOCIAL SECURITY, *Report of a Research Working Group on Inequalities in Health* (Chairman: Sir Douglas Black), DHSS (1979)

20. NAVARRO, V., *Class Struggle, The State and Medicine: an historical and contemporary analysis of the medical sector in Great Britain*, Robertson, Oxford (1978)

21. MCKINLEY, J., 'The Business of Good Doctoring or Doctoring as Good Business: reflections of Freidson's view of the medical system', *International Journal of Health Services*, 7 (3), 1977

22. MARCUSE, H., *One Dimensional Man*, Abacus (1972)

23. MCKINLEY, J., 'A Case for Refocussing Upstream: the political economy of illness' in JACO, E. G. (ed.), *Patients, Physicians and Illness*, Free Press (3rd edn) (1979)

24. ABEL-SMITH, B., *Value for Money in Health Services*, Heinemann, London (1976), Ch. 6

25. DOYAL, L., *The Political Economy of Health*, Pluto Press, London (1979)

26. OAKLEY, A., *Subject Woman*, Penguin, London (1982)

27. EHRENREICH, B. and ENGLISH, D., *For Her Own Good. 150 Years of the Experts' Advice to Women*, Pluto Press, (1979)

28. SHELDON, A. (ed.), *The Litmuss Papers*, Centre for Policy Studies, London (1980)

29. SHELDON, A., *The Lessons of Centralised Medicine*, in *ibid*.

30. KLEIN, R., 'Ideologies, Utopias, and the Debate about Health Care', *British Medical Journal*, Vol. 282, 24 Jan. 1981

Part four
ASSESSMENT

Chapter twelve
CHALLENGES FOR THE FUTURE

The system of health care as it has developed through the NHS and the Welfare State is, in the 1980s, confronting its successes and its failures. The provision of medical and health care has been built mainly around the disease model of illness and curative medicine. It has been fostered by the rapid growth of medical technologies and the continuing development of drug therapies, cushioned by economic growth and the broad consensus on economic and social policy; the Butskellism of the 1950s and 1960s. These factors have helped to provide the means of reducing the threat to survival of severe illness. Their very success has (1) obscured the social bases of illness, and collective responsibilities for the maintenance of health; (2) has drawn attention away from the importance of creating a personal awareness of the foundations of wellness and (3) has released and created new needs for care, counselling, rehabilitation. Although attempts have been made by governments to develop policies which move towards meeting new needs through attempting to achieve a more equal distribution of resources throughout the country, by promoting services which meet the needs of dependent groups, and by raising the level of consciousness of illness-producing behaviour, the results in terms of outcome appear to have been small.

There has been a persistent gap between the rhetoric and the reality, between the policy intent and policy implementation at different levels of the health system. The 1970s have brought critiques of health care which have re-emphasised the importance of the relatively neglected paradigms of health policy, based on the maintenance of health and the relief and management of pain and suffering. These rested on alternative ways of seeing and interpreting health and ill-health and in many respects their re-emergence has created a new rhetoric, and a reinterpretation of the role of governments in health policy. They have pointed out that matters of health frequently take second place to the realisation of economic and political interests. In capitalist societies profits are put before health, and that therefore the costs and hazards of manufacturing processes and of pollution are insufficiently taken into account by modern governments. The interests of users of health care it is suggested have been hidden and invisible under the screen of professionally-dominated bureaucratic medicine.

A debt is owed to those who have helped to raise the level of consciousness about health and have brought health issues nearer the centre of political debate. Health care and health policy can no longer be seen to be solely as technical or professional matters but are part of a broader discussion of social inequalities and social policies. However the new rhetoric must not be allowed to obscure the benefits of the NHS in the cure of illness and the relief of suffering. These benefits may not be readily measurable but this does not mean that there has been no progress. The cure of illness remains centrally important to any health policy and the NHS remains a civilised way of fulfilling this role. Although more effort must be devoted to developing preventive policies in parallel with those for cure, it must be recognised that prevention is inherently difficult. For example, it is one thing to say that in theory all road accidents are preventable and quite another to have no road accidents or deaths. There are problems in developing effective procedures due to gaps in existing knowledge. There are also conflicts of interest and value involved. In other words strategies for prevention, as well as the problem of reaching the right balance between cure, prevention and care are essentially political as they are areas of dispute. The NHS because of its structure and the distribution of power within it, is ill-equipped to resolve these conflicts in an open and democratic manner. The remainder of this conclusion will elaborate on the issues raised here; the relationship between health and social policy, the intrinsic conflicts which face any health system and the imperviousness of the NHS to outside influences.

HEALTH IS PART OF THE WELFARE STATE

Recent work on the social bases of ill-health, its relationship to poverty and deprivation, conditions of work, and particular kinds of environment have been discussed at various points in this book. The findings are clear, the poor are sicker and the effects of ill-health are cumulative. Poor growth and development, in adolescence and child-hood, will influence susceptibility to disease throughout life. Services for the maintenance of income, the provision of adequate housing,

education and improved social services, the availability of employment, leisure and recreation are therefore essential to maintaining and
improving health and preventing illness. Health policies are affected
by the presence or absence of collective intervention in other areas of
social policy and it is the interaction of services in the different areas of
provision which is crucial. The lack of effectiveness of policies to
alleviate poverty has been one factor leading to the inequalities in
health status between different social classes. The existence of the
NHS and the apparent solving of the 'Giant' of illness has tended to
obscure the relationship between standards of living and ill-health.
Governments and the informed public were more concerned with the
interaction of social, economic conditions and their effects on health
in the 1860s and 1930s than today. The Black Report on Inequalities
in Health is in this sense a restatement of the collectivist tradition of
the Beveridge Report and the role of the state in providing a range of
social services. Its recommendations are concerned with the relief of
poverty and deprivation as much as with the improvement of health
services.

CONFLICTS IN HEALTH CARE

A restatement of the importance of health services as part of a wider
programme of social intervention must not be allowed to obscure
certain fundamental problems and conflicts of value in the provision
of health services. One basic problem facing health care providers,
irrespective of the type of social and political organisation, is the
difficulty of relating the input of resources into health services, (or
other social services for that matter) to improvements in health or
health outputs. There is all too little monitoring of treatments or
disposals in health care whether this is in the sphere of curing,
prevention or caring. Questions of effectiveness can be particularly
important when arguments are being made to develop new services, as
opposed to maintaining expenditure on existing ones. When the
expenditure of public money is involved, there is a need to know that
this is being spent effectively, yet the measuring of effectiveness is
essentially difficult and raises questions of choice and, therefore, of
value.

Questions of value are also involved in the collection and use of
information and data in health care. Statistics about health and illness
are frequently inadequate. Mortality statistics are available but are of
little use of their own, while measures of morbidity depend upon the
adequacy of surveillance of illness and sickness. The most useful

statistics are often those kept on individuals over a period of time as they can relate lifestyles and experience to ill-health and trace relationships. There is a need for better information systems on the incidence of illness in the population so that evaluative work can be carried out. This may involve the keeping of much more detailed information on individuals and populations and their histories so that epidemiological work can be done and it raises a host of ethical questions about individual rights and professional freedom and the confidentiality of data. Jean Robinson, for example, discusses some of these issues in an article on the incidence of cervical cancer.[1] She suggests that collection of data on the relationship between promiscuity and cervical cancer has acted as a smoke screen and drawn attention away from pollutants at the work place, dirt, dust and so forth, on women and their husbands, and *its* association with cancer.

There is a further set of moral and ethical problems raised by attempts to use health resources more effectively and efficiently in relation to who decides and whose interest is involved. Underlying these issues there is a fundamental dilemma which presents itself in relation to all health care, the claims of the individual and the interests of the collectivity. There is for example the conflict of interest between the professional who is committed to curing and caring for a particular individual patient, and the necessity for resources to be used in the national interest. MacKenzie puts it in the following way:

> on the one hand, there are the traditions and the organisation of caring and curing. The guiding maxim and myth is that of personalised individual relations. The professional owes to the client (or patient) services without limit or qualification. The person whose need is in question is entitled to everything, to absolute finality. He or she may in his or her own interest be deceived; but must not be betrayed. There are many patients, their needs may conflict and compete, but each relationship is unique and demands infinite respect. We are in the presence of pain and death. On the other hand the intervention of public management, the exclusion of bargaining in the market, implies that every one is to count for one and no more than one . . . once it is realised that resources are not infinite, there must be a rule of allocation; and it must be a rule of equality, subject only to some informed, independent and unbiased adjudication of need.[2]

This kind of conflict can rarely be resolved, but must be managed at various levels in ways which are acceptable and visible. Emphasis on individual cure and care is the source of the immense strength, benefit and popularity of modern medical care. It poses great problems for governments who are charged with the allocation of resources, particularly when these are not increasing. It is one of the reasons for the difficulties of making RAWP reallocations effective and also developing policies for prevention and for the care of dependent groups.

Preventive policies are intrinsically about protecting populations, to ensure the maintenance of health and the prevention of disease, and the responsibility for carrying out this function falls on governments and a range of health workers acting on behalf of the community. One weakness of recent government policy has been to underestimate the role and obligation of governments to protect health. Reliance on changing individual behaviour to improve health is no substitute for collective action.

Not that the arguments for and against collective intervention are as simple as those taking the Marxist critique sometimes imply. Public health involves weighing up risks and benefits to the individuals as against risks and benefits to the collectivity. The campaign to increase the rate of whooping cough vaccination is a case in point. The vaccination rate for whooping cough had fallen in 1982 to 30–40 per cent of the child population of one year olds, partly as a consequence of media coverage of the small risk of brain damage to children after vaccination. The incidence of whooping cough has increased in the early 1980s, bringing increased disability and deaths to a proportion of children. There is now a campaign to vaccinate 4 to 5 year olds as well as younger children but controversy over the issue continues.[3] Interventions of governments in many areas of public health involve a weighing of costs and benefits. The process is essentially political and the function of those representing the 'community' pressure groups, the media and critics of contemporary health care should be to reveal and make public whose interests and benefits are involved in the practice and provision of health care. Unfortunately, health issues because they are about suffering, lend themselves to over simplification and sensationalism.

THE RESISTANCE OF THE NHS TO CHANGE

There are, however, structural factors which hinder the operation of the democratic process in health care in Britain, making the NHS resistant to change. The two major factors responsible are the power of the medical profession as decision-takers in the service, and the organisation of the NHS itself. It has been argued in the course of this book that despite, and probably because of, the centralised nature of the NHS, the effective decision-makers in health care are the clinicians. They affect policy outcomes despite the policy intentions of governments.

Haywood and Alaszewski in their recent book *Crisis in the Health Service*[4] draw on Lukes's theory of power to analyse the three dimensions in which medical dominance operates in the NHS and this is illuminating. Lukes's first dimension of power is the 'capacity of an individual or group to modify the conduct of other individuals or groups in observable conflicts'.[5] The medical profession, although they have not won *all* observable conflicts, have considerable power particularly in areas relating to their pay and conditions of service. The original structure of the NHS reflected this, and so have the later reorganisations of the NHS. The 1982 decision to restore the autonomous status to Family Practitioner Committees, rather than include them in the administrative structure of the District Health Authorities, is a case in point. The Merrison Commission strongly recommended an integration of these functions with those of the main health authorities as a way of improving the general coverage of primary health care services. Organisations representing GPs have always been hostile to any changes which inhibit their freedom to adopt their own pattern of practice. Generally speaking, the ability of the medical profession to modify the conduct of other groups has only been weakened when they are divisions of interest between groups *within* medicine.

Lukes's second dimension of power is concerned with the 'ability of groups or individuals to control the issues on the agenda for discussion, and the rules of the game, in relation to the way in which the issues on the agenda are handled'. There are clearly areas of medical activity which have been ruled off the political agenda or which have not progressed beyond preliminary skirmishing. These relate to the accepted autonomy of the doctor to diagnose and treat the patient in whatever way is deemed to be most appropriate. Despite the rising drug bill, there are no 'controls' on the GP's freedom to prescribe. There can be suggestions made by FPCs that GPs should change their methods of prescribing and these are monitored by the Prescription Prescribing Authority, but very little is known about these 'investigations' and how pressure is brought to bear. There has been a general resistance on the part of the profession to attempts to pursue methods of controlling clinical decisions and their financial implications, just as there has been resistance to monitoring the efficiency and effectiveness of medical regimes. Complaints systems for patients along the lines recommended by the Davies Committee[6] have been another casualty, kept off the political agenda like the attempts to extend the remit of the Parliamentary Commissioner for the NHS to cover complaints about clinical judgement.

Lukes draws attention to these areas of non-decision:

> Decisions which result in the suppression or thwarting of a latent or
> manifest challenge to the values and interests of the decision-maker . . . a
> means by which demands for change in the existing allocation of benefits
> and privileges in the community can be suffocated before they gain access
> to the relevant decision-making arena – or, failing all these things, are
> maimed or destroyed in the decision-making stage of the policy process.[5]

At a local level in the health service, perhaps to an even greater extent
than at national level, policies have been kept off the agenda. The
development of facilities in the community has given way to on-going
hospital based expenditure. Accountability to the health authorities is
also weak. Consultants and GPs although not budget holders themselves, make demands for services. In the hospital, for example,
demands are made for nurses, special diets, beds, pathology, x-rays,
in general practice, for drugs or referrals to hospital. These demands
rest on clinical decisions and controls over the process are few. There
is little incentive to review existing practices and find cheaper ways of
doing things. There may be systems of medical audit within
specialisms, and the 'Cogwheel' changes have improved medical
management, but ultimately spending decisions are determined by
the criteria of clinical judgement. There is little organisational space
for the administrators and managers in the hospital to suggest changes
across specialisms, neither is there the power to do so. It was pointed
out in Chapter 7 that these grass-roots decisions, which may be
perfectly reasonable and justifiable in their own terms, may also affect
the allocation of development monies, where choices can be pre-
empted by the revenue consequences of earlier clinical decisions.

The third dimension in Lukes's analyses of power is the ability 'to
prevent people, to whatever degree, from having grievances by
shaping their perceptions, cognitions and preferences in such a way
that they accept their role in the existing order of things, either
because they see it as natural or unchangeable, or because they value it
as divinely ordained and beneficial'. It is here that the basis of the
influence and power of the curative/disease model of health lies.
Despite the alternative paradigm of the maintenance of health suggested in the introduction this has barely broken the surface of public
debate, particularly at a local level in the health authorities. Questions
of priorities in terms of the broad spectrum health needs of the
community scarcely arise. This is of course because illness *now* always
appears more pressing than the maintenance of health at some later

date; and because the funding of existing services appears more pressing than an assessment of priorities. This reflects the view of the lay public as much as health providers. There is a general disinterest in public health, while the closure of a hospital generates intense hostility. Possibly because there is a loss of employment and the loss of a facility involved, there is a visible focus for opposition. Furthermore, the structure of the health services increases the power of the curative/disease model and the professional providers and reduces the influence of countervailing interests, where these exist among the corporate rationalisers and the community interest.

THE CONSEQUENCES OF NHS STRUCTURE ON THE DISTRIBUTION OF POWER

McLachan has suggested 'The NHS is the first public institution of any size concerned with a welfare service universally available in which a different kind of democracy from that traditionally understood was introduced.'[7] In other words the NHS has a centralised structure with no elected tier at a local level. The groups which represent the interests of the collectivity, the corporate rationalisers, and the community interest are weakly reflected in the NHS for a number of reasons. Despite a high degreee of centralisation at a national level, in fact effective accountability in the health service has remained a problem. The DHSS, because it is responsible for such a large and complex service, becomes concerned with an enormous amount of detailed decision-making which detracts from its ability to look at broader issues. Furthermore, at the level where policy is implemented, at the local level in the health authorities, members and chairman appear from the research studies to be relatively impotent in making policy decisions which go against the interests of service providers, professionals *or* administrators, even if they wish to do so. Unlike local authorities, health authorities lack legitimacy. They have not been elected and evidence suggests there is uncertainty about whom or what they represent.

Certainly as far as the public is concerned health authority members, unlike councillors, lack visibility. They lack the authority and the ability to mobilise the 'community interest'. This can and does occur in relation to issues under the jurisdiction of local authorities. Furthermore, health authority members do not have the same relationship with professional and administrative staffs as their counterparts in local government. In the local authorities chief officers are accountable to the council and its committees which are controlled by the majority party and have been elected to follow through a particular programme of policies. Health authorities are apolitical in this sense and there are disadvantages to this lack of democratic accountability. Local authorities can and do lobby central government in the interests of their authority. Health authorities and their members tend to lack political clout in this respect, and are largely irrelevant to the actual running of the service. Members tend to have little effect on the internal decision-making of the hospital or community health services. There is no necessity for members of a health authority to sharpen their minds in preparing a local health policy for their areas as they do not have to face an electorate. This means that knowledge of health services and issues in health are in general low, even among the politically aware. Health issues simply tend not to be on the agenda. In the absence of extra resources to promote particular health policies at central government level or new initiatives by administrators at local level, professionals continue to dominate both conceptions of health and resource allocation within the service.

Health authorities at the local level as a consequence of their relationship to the professional health care providers, to the DHSS and their lack of relationship to the particular populations and communities, have tended to maintain a narrow focus on what constitutes health care and policy. They have not been concerned to understand the forces which influence health and ill-health in their areas. The local authorities which provide housing, transport, education, personal social services and planning, environmental health, leisure and recreation, have been impelled, to some extent to face the consequences of the interaction of their separate services upon each other and the trade-offs to be made between different policies within their remit, particularly in inner city areas. Health authorities have not, and this is a structural weakness in the NHS.

A further weakness of structure is the fragmentation of the community health services between local government, general practice and the health authorities. At central level there is also a division of responsibility for preventive health, this time between different departments and *ad hoc* agencies. This fragmentation diffuses responsibility and makes choices of the proper balance between cure, care and preventive policies more difficult.

If political issues in health services are to find expression then the more locally based District Health Authorities could be an appropriate focus for such activity. Where DHAs are coterminous with local authorities there is a good basis for officer/administrator collaboration and also at member level. This could provide a possible basis for the development of a broad concept of health care. However at present, the two factors which brought improvements in health in the nineteenth century are lacking. The sanitary authorities in the Victorian towns had a combination of elected councils and medical officers of health with a reforming zeal. They had both the power and the authority over issues relating to public health in their areas of jurisdiction. In the absence of such factors, the political impetus for change may have to come from what Alford refers to as the 'repressed' community interest,[8] pressure groups, the media, political groupings, trade unions, etc. It is remarkable how in recent years there has been increased activity and the growth of groups concerned with issues in health. These groups may provide the activists with sufficient reforming zeal to bring improvements in public health. Their activities may also serve to raise the level of consciousness in what people may do for themselves, and for each other in maintaining and promoting their health, and in seeking out and developing alternative forms of health care, where those which are available are either ineffective or inappropriate.

REFERENCES

1. ROBINSON, J., 'Cervical Cancer, a Feminist Critique', *The Times Health Supplement*, 27 Nov. 1981
2. MACKENZIE, W. J. M., *Power and Responsibility in Health Care. The National Health Service as a Political Institution*, Oxford University Press, Oxford (1979), Ch. 10
3. Letter from the Chief Medical Officer to GPs and District Medical and Nursing Officers, 6 Sept. 1982, and also PRESTON, N. W., 'Whooping Cough Immunisation: Fact and Fiction', *Public Health* (London) **94** (1980), 350–5
4. HAYWOOD, S., and ALASZEWSKI, A., *Crisis in the Health Service*, Croom Helm, London (1980), Ch. 7
5. LUKES, S., *Power: a radical view*, Macmillan, London (1974)
6. DEPARTMENT OF HEALTH AND SOCIAL SECURITY, *Report of the Committee on Hospital Complaints Procedure*, HMSO, London (1973)
7. Quoted by MACKENZIE, W. J. M., *op. cit.*, Preface
8. ALFORD, R., *Health Care Politics*, University of Chicago Press (1975)

Part five
DOCUMENTS

LABOUR (ANEURIN BEVAN) AND CONSERVATIVES (RICHARD LAW) DEBATE THE INTRODUCTION OF THE NATIONAL HEALTH SERVICE

MR BEVAN: The first reason why a health scheme of this sort is necessary at all is because it has been the firm conclusion of all parties that money ought not to be permitted to stand in the way of obtaining an efficient health service. Although it is true that the national health insurance system provides a general practitioner service and caters for something like 21 million of the population, the rest of the population have to pay whenever they desire the services of a doctor. It is cardinal to a proper health organisation that a person ought not to be financially deterred from seeking medical assistance at the earliest possible stage. It is one of the evils of having to buy medical advice that in addition to the natural anxiety that may arise because people do not like to hear unpleasant things about themselves, and therefore tend to postpone consultation as long as possible, there is the financial anxiety caused by having to pay doctors' bills. Therefore, the first evil that we must deal with is that which exists as a consequence of the fact that the whole thing is the wrong way round. A person ought to be able to receive medical and hospital help without being involved in financial anxiety.

In the second place, the national health insurance scheme does not provide for the self-employed, nor, of course, for the families of dependants. It depends on insurance qualification, and no matter how ill you are; if you cease to be insured you cease to have free doctoring. Furthermore, it gives no backing to the doctor in the form of specialist services. The doctor has to provide himself, he has to use his own discretion and his own personal connections, in order to obtain hospital treatment for his patients and in order to get them specialists, and in very many cases, of course – in an overwhelming number of cases – the services of a specialist are not available to poor people.

Not only is this the case, but our hospital organisation has grown up with no plan, with no system; it is unevenly distributed over the country and indeed it is one of the tragedies of the situation, that very often the best hospital facilities are available where they are least needed. In the older industrial districts of Great Britain hospital facilities are inadequate. Many of the hospitals are too small – very much too small.

Furthermore – I want to be quite frank with the House – I believe it is repugnant to a civilised community for hospitals to have to rely upon private charity. I believe we ought to have left hospital flag days behind. I have always felt a shudder of repulsion when I have seen nurses and sisters who ought to be at their work, and students who ought to be at their work, going about the streets collecting money for the hospitals. I do not believe there is an hon. Member of this House who approves that system. It is repugnant, and we must leave it behind – entirely. But the implications of doing this are very considerable.

I have been forming some estimates of what might happen to voluntary hospital finance when the all-in insurance contributions fail to be paid by the people of Great Britain, when the Bill is passed and becomes an Act and they are entitled to free hospital services. The estimates I have go to show that between 80 per cent and 90 per cent of the revenues of the voluntary hospitals in these circumstances will be provided by public funds, by national or rate funds. [An HON. MEMBER: 'By workers' contributions.'] And, of course, as the hon. Member reminds me, in very many parts of the country it is a travesty to call them voluntary hospitals. In the mining districts, in the textile districts, in the districts where there are heavy industries it is the industrial population who pay the weekly contributions for the maintenance of the hospitals. When I was a miner I used to find that situation, when I was on the hospital committee. We had an annual meeting and a cordial vote of thanks was moved and passed with great enthusiasm to the managing director of the colliery company for his generosity towards the hospital; and when I looked at the balance sheet, I saw that 97½ per cent of the revenues were provided by the miners' own contributions; but nobody passed a vote of thanks to the miners . . .

MR LAW: . . . We accept the principle, and we accept the consequences that flow from it. We understand, for example, that once we are committed, as we are gladly committed, to the principle of a 100 per cent, service, we require an enormous expansion and development in the health services as a whole. We understand, once we accept the principle, that we are committed to a far greater degree of coordination, or planning as it is usually called, than we have ever known before . . . if my right hon. and learned Friend the Member for North Croydon (Mr Willink) had still been Minister of Health, had the General Election result gone another way, I do not doubt that he would have introduced, before this, a Bill which would have differed from this Bill only in that my right hon. and learned Friend would not have attempted to control, own and direct the hospital services of this country or to interfere with that age-old relationship which exists, always has existed, and in our view ought to continue to exist, between a doctor and his patient. Therefore, the right hon. Gentleman is not entitled to say – he has not said it, but he might – that we will the end without the means. We will both the end and the means. We will this end, a comprehensive and efficient health service. We are willing to support any practicable means that will give us that end.

But we differ from the right hon. Gentleman on this issue. We believe that the right hon. Gentleman could have reached his end, and a better end, by other means, and by better means. We believe that he could have established a health service, equally comprehensive, better coordinated and far more efficient, if he had not been determined to sweep away the voluntary hospitals; if he had not been determined to weaken the whole structure of English local government by removing from the field of local government one of the most important and vital responsibilities of local authorities; and if he had not sought to impose upon the medical profession a form of discipline which, in our view and in theirs, is totally unsuited to the practice of medicine, an art, a vocation, however you like to call it, which depends above all else upon individual responsibility, individual devotion and individual sympathy.

From: *Hansard*, 30 April 1946

Document two
THE SCOPE OF THE HEALTH SERVICE IN 1948

NATIONAL HEALTH SERVICE BILL, 1946
Introductory

1. The Bill provides for the establishment of a comprehensive health service in England and Wales. A further Bill to provide for Scotland will be introduced later.
2. The Bill does not deal in detail with everything involved in the service. It deals with the main structure. Within that structure, further provision will be made by statutory regulations – on lines which the Bill lays down and subject always to the control of Parliament.

Scope of the service

3. The Bill provides for the following kinds of health services:

　　(i)　Hospital and specialist services – i.e. all forms of general and special hospital provision, including mental hospitals, together with sanatoria, maternity accommodation, treatment during convalescence, medical rehabilitation and other institutional treatment. These cover in-patient and out-patient services, the latter including clinics and dispensaries operated as part of any specialist service. The advice and services of specialists of all kinds are also to be made available, where necessary, at Health Centres and in the patient's home.

　　(ii)　Health Centres and general practitioner services – i.e. general personal health care by doctors and dentists whom the patient chooses. These personal practitioner services are to be available both from new publicly equipped Health Centres and also from the practitioners' own surgeries.

　　(iii)　Various supplementary services – including midwifery, maternity and child welfare, health visiting, home-nursing, a priority dental service for children and expectant and nursing mothers, domestic help where needed on health grounds, vaccination and immunisation against infectious diseases, additional special care and after-care in cases of illness, ambulance services, blood transfusion and laboratory services. (Special school health services are already provided for in the Education Act of 1944.)

(iv)   The provision of spectacles, dentures and other appliances, together with drugs and medicines – at hospitals, Health Centres, clinics, pharmacists' shops and elsewhere, as may be appropriate.

Availability of the service

4.   All the service, or any part of it, is to be available to everyone in England and Wales. The Bill imposes no limitations on availability – e.g. limitations based on financial means, age, sex, employment or vocation, area of residence, or insurance qualification.

5.   The last is important. If the National Insurance Bill now before Parliament is passed into law, almost everyone will become compulsorily insurable, and after payment of the appropriate contributions will become entitled to the various cash benefits – including sickness and maternity benefits – for which that Bill provides. A proportion of their contributions will be used to help to finance the health services under the present Bill, but the various health service benefits under the present Bill are not made conditional upon any insurance qualification or the proof of having paid contributions. There are no waiting or qualifying periods.

6.   The service is to be available from a date to be declared by Order in Council under the Bill, and it is hoped that this will be at the beginning of the year 1948.

The service to be free of fees or charges

7.   The health service is to be financed partly from the exchequer, partly from local rates, partly from the help (mentioned above) which part of the National Insurance contributions will give. There are to be no fees or charges to the patient, with the following exceptions:

(i)   There will be some charges (to be prescribed later by regulations) for the renewal or repair of spectacles, dentures and other appliances, where this is made necessary through negligence in the care of the articles provided.

(ii)   There will be charges (taking into account ability to pay) for the provision of domestic help under the Bill and for certain goods or articles (e.g. supplementary foods, blankets, etc) which may be provided in connection with maternity and child welfare or the special care or after-care of the sick.

(iii)   It will be open to people if they wish, in certain cases, to pay for additional amenities within the arrangements of the service – e.g. to pay extra for articles or appliances of higher cost than those normally made available, or to pay charges for private rooms in hospitals (which they will nevertheless be able to obtain free where privacy is medically necessary).

General organisation of the service

8.   The Bill places a general duty upon the Minister of Health to promote a

comprehensive health service for the improvement of the physical and mental health of the people of England and Wales, and for the prevention, diagnosis and treatment of illness. To bring physical and mental health closer together in a single service, it transfers to the Minister the present administrative functions of the Board of Control in regard to mental health (the Board retaining only its quasi-judicial functions connected with the liberty of the subject).

9. The Bill proposes that the Minister shall discharge his general responsibility through three main channels:

(a) For parts of the service to be organised on a new national or regional basis – i.e. hospital and specialist services, blood transfusion and bacteriological laboratories for the control of epidemics – the Minister is to assume direct responsibility, but he is to entrust the actual administration of the hospital and specialist services to new regional and local bodies under the Bill. These bodies are to act on his behalf in suitable areas to be prescribed by him, and they are to include people of practical experience and local knowledge and some with professional qualifications. Special provision is made for hospitals which are the centres of medical and dental teaching.

(b) For parts of the service to be organised as a function of local government – i.e. the provision of new Health Centre premises and a variety of local domiciliary and clinic services – direct responsibility is put upon the major local authorities, the county and county borough councils. They will stand in their ordinary constitutional relationship with the central Ministry, but their general arrangements for these local services are made subject to the Minister's approval.

(c) For the personal practitioner services both in the Health Centres and outside – i.e. the family doctor and dentist and the pharmacist – new local executive machinery is created, in the form of local Executive Councils. One half of the members of each of these Councils will consist of people nominated by the major local authorities and by the Minister, and the other half of people nominated by the local professional practitioners concerned. There will normally be an Executive Council for each of the major local authorities' areas, and they will work within national regulations made by the Minister.

10. By the Minister's side, to provide him with professional and technical guidance, there is to be set up a Central Health Service Council. This will include people chosen from all the main fields of experience within the service – with various standing committees of experts on particular subjects, medical, dental, nursing and others.

From: *The National Health Service Bill*, Cmd 6761, HMSO (1946)

THE 1944 WHITE PAPER: AN ACCOUNT OF THE INADEQUACIES OF EXISTING HEALTH SERVICES

The record of this country in its health and medical services is a good one. The resistance of people to the wear and tear of four years of a second world war bears testimony to it. Achievements before the war – in lower mortality rates, in the gradual decline of many of the more serious diseases, in safer motherhood and healthier childhood, and generally in the prospect of a longer and healthier life – all substantiate it. There is no question of having to abandon bad services and to start afresh. Reform in this field is not a matter of making good what is bad, but of making better what is good already.

The present system has its origins deep in the history of the country's social services. Broadly, it is the product of the last hundred years, though some of its elements go much farther back. But most of the impetus has been gathered in the last generation or two, and it was left to the present century to develop most of the personal health services as they are now known . . .

The main reason for change is that the Government believe that, at this stage of social development, the care of personal health should be put on a new footing and be made available to everybody as a publicly sponsored service. Just as people are accustomed to look to public organisation for essential facilities like a clean and safe water supply or good highways, accepting these as things which the community combines to provide for the benefit of the individual without distinction of section or group, so they should now be able to look for proper facilities for the care of their personal health to a publicly organised service available to all who want to use it – a service for which all would be paying as taxpayers and ratepayers and contributors to some national scheme of social insurance.

In spite of the substantial progress of many years and the many good services built up under public authority and by voluntary and private effort, it is still not true to say that everyone can get all the kinds of medical and hospital service which he or she may require. Whether people can do so still depends too much upon circumstances, upon where they happen to live or work, to what group (e.g. of age, or vocation) they happen to belong, or what happens to be the matter with them. Nor is the care of health yet wholly divorced from ability to pay for it, although great progress has already been made in eliminating the financial barrier to obtaining most of the essential services. There is not yet, in short, a comprehensive cover for health provided for all people alike. That is what it is now the Government's intention to provide.

To take one very important example, the first-line care of health for everyone requires a personal doctor or a family doctor, a general medical practitioner available for consultation on all problems of health and sickness. At present, the National Health Insurance scheme makes this provision for a large number of people; but it does not give it to the wives and the children and the dependants. For extreme need, the older Poor Law still exists. For some particular groups there are other facilities. But for something like half the population, the first-line health service of a personal medical adviser depends on what private arrangements any particular person can manage to make.

Even if a person has a regular doctor – and this is not now assured to all – there is no guaranteed link between that doctor and the rest of necessary medical help. The doctor, both in private practice and in National Health Insurance practice, has to rely on his own resources to introduce his patient to the right kinds of special treatment or clinic or hospital – a great responsibility in these days of specialised medicine and surgery – or the patient has to make his own way to whatever local authority or other organisation happens to cater for his particular need.

When a hospital's services are needed, it is far from true that everyone can get all that is required. Here it is not so much a question of people not being eligible to get the service which they need, as a matter of the practical distribution of those services. The hospital and specialist services have grown up without a national or even an area plan. In one area there may be already established a variety of hospitals. Another area, although the need is there, may be sparsely served. One hospital may have a long waiting list and be refusing admission to cases which another hospital not far away could suitably accommodate and treat at once. There is undue pressure in some areas on the hospital out-patient departments – in spite of certain experiments which some of the hospitals have tried (and which should be encouraged) in arranging a system of timed appointments to obviate long waiting. Moreover, even though most people have access to a hospital of some kind, it is not necessarily access to the right hospital. The tendency in the modern development of medicine and surgery is towards specialist centres – for radiotherapy and neurosis, for example – and no one hospital can be equally equipped and developed to suit all needs, or to specialise equally in all subjects. The time has come when the hospital services have to be thought of, and planned, as a wider whole, and the object has to be that each case should be referred not to one single hospital which happens to be 'local' but to whatever hospital concentrates specially on that kind of case and can offer it the most up-to-date technique.

Many services are also rendered by local authorities and others in special clinics and similar organisations, designed for particular groups of the population or for particular kinds of ailment or medical care. These are, for the most part, thoroughly good in themselves, and they are used with advantage by a great many people in a great many districts. But, owing to the way in which they have grown up piecemeal at different stages of history and under different statutory powers, they are usually conducted as quite separate and independent services. There is no sufficient link either between these services themselves or between them and general medical practice and the hospitals.

In short, general medical practice, consultant and specialist opinion, hospital treatment, clinic services for particular purposes, home nursing, midwifery and other branches of health care need to be related to one another and treated as many aspects of the care of one person's health. That means that there has to be somewhere a new responsibility to relate them, if a service for health is to be given in future which will be not only comprehensive and reliable but also easy to obtain.

Last, but not least, personal health still tends to be regarded as something to be treated when at fault, or perhaps to be preserved from getting at fault, but seldom as something to be positively improved and promoted and made full and robust. Much of present custom and habit still centres on the idea that the doctor and the hospital and the clinic are the means of mending ill-health rather than of increasing good health and the sense of well-being. While the health standards of the people have enormously improved, and while there are gratifying reductions in the ravages of preventable disease, the plain fact remains that there are many men and women and children who could be and ought to be enjoying a sense of health and physical well-being which they do not in fact enjoy. There is much subnormal health still, which need not be, with a corresponding cost in efficiency and personal happiness.

These are some of the chief deficiencies in the present arrangements which, in the view of the Government, a comprehensive health service should seek to make good . . .

The scope of a 'comprehensive' service

The proposed service must be 'comprehensive' in two senses – first, that it is available to all people and, second, that it covers all necessary forms of health care. The general aim has been stated at the beginning of this Paper. The service designed to achieve it must cover the whole field of medical advice and attention, at home, in the consulting room, in the hospital or the sanatorium, or wherever else is appropriate – from the personal or family doctor to the specialists and consultants of all kinds, from the care of minor ailments to the care of major diseases and disabilities. It must include ancillary services of nursing, of midwifery and of the other things which ought to go with medical care. It must secure first that everyone can be sure of a general medical adviser to consult as and when the need arises, and then that everyone can get access – beyond the general medical adviser – to more specialised branches of medicines or surgery. This cannot all be perfected at a stroke of the pen, on an appointed day; but nothing less than this must be the object in view, and the framing of the service from the outset must be such as to make it possible.

From: *A National Health Service*, Ministry of Health, Cmd 6502, HMSO (1944), pp. 6-9

Document four
THE CHADWICK PRESCRIPTION FOR PUBLIC HEALTH

ON THE COSTS OF PREVENTABLE ILL HEALTH

It appears that fever, after its ravages amongst the infant population, falls with the greatest intensity on the adult population in the vigour of life. The periods at which the ravages of the other diseases, consumption, smallpox, and measles take place, are sufficiently well known. The proportions in which the diseases have prevailed in the several counties will be found deserving of peculiar attention.

A conception may be formed of the aggregate effects of the several causes of mortality from the fact, that of the deaths caused during one year in England and Wales by epidemic, endemic, and contagious diseases, including fever, typhus, and scarlatina, amounting to 56,461, the great proportion of which are proved to be preventible, it may be said that the effect is as if the whole county of Westmorland, now containing 56,469 souls, or the whole county of Huntingdonshire, or any other equivalent district, were entirely de-populated annually, and were only occupied again by the growth of a new and feeble population living under the fears of a similar visitation. The annual slaughter in England and Wales from preventible causes of typhus which attacks persons in the vigour of life, appears to be double the amount of what was suffered by the Allied Armies in the battle of Waterloo . . .

ON THE CAUSES OF ILL-HEALTH

First, as to the extent and operation of the evils which are the subject of the inquiry: That the various forms of epidemic, endemic, and other disease caused, or aggravated, or propagated chiefly amongst the labouring classes by atmospheric impurities produced by decomposing animal and vegetable substances, by damp and filth, and close and overcrowded dwellings prevail amongst the population in every part of the kingdom, whether dwelling in separate houses, in rural villages, in small towns, in the larger towns – as they have been found to prevail in the lowest districts of the metropolis.

That such disease, wherever it attacks are frequent, is always found in connexion with the physical circumstances above specified, and that where those circumstances are removed by drainage, proper cleansing, better ventilation, and other means of diminishing atmospheric impurities, the frequency and intensity of such disease is abated; and where the removal of the noxious agencies appears to be complete, such disease almost entirely disappears . . .

Secondly. As to the means by which the present sanitary conditions of the labouring classes may be improved:
The primary most important measures, and at the same time the most practicable, and within the recognized province of public administration, are drainage, the removal of all refuse of habitations, streets, and roads, and the improvement of the supplies of water . . .

That for the protection of the labouring classes and of the ratepayers against inefficiency and waste in all new structural arrangements for the protection of the public health, and to ensure public confidence that the expenditure will be beneficial, securities should be taken that all new local public works are devised and conducted by responsible officers qualified by the possession of the science and skill of civil engineers . . .

The advantages of uniformity in legislation and in the executive machinery, and of doing the same things in the same way (choosing the best), and calling the same officers, proceedings, and things by the same names, will only be appreciated by those who have observed the extensive public loss occasioned by the legislation for towns which makes them independent of beneficent, as of what perhaps might have been deemed formerly aggressive legislation.

From: Edwin Chadwick, *Report on the Sanitary Conditions of the Labouring Population of Great Britain* (1842), 1965 edn by M. W. Flinn, Edinburgh University Press, p. 78

Document five
THE HEALTH OF THE POPULATION, 1901

Increase in numbers is commonly regarded as a sign of national progress, and as evidence of the soundness of the State. Recent growth of population in the United Kingdom, however, is actually a symptom of political decline. A vast population has been created by the factory and industrial systems, the majority of which is incapable of bearing arms.

Spectacled school-children hungry, strumous, and epileptic, grow into consumptive bridegrooms and scrofulous brides, and are assured beforehand of the blessing of the Church, the aid of the compassionate, and such solace as hospitals provided wholesale by unknown donors can supply. If a voice be raised in protest against the unhealthy perversion of the command, 'Be ye fruitful and multiply' it is drowned in a chorus of sickly emotion . . .

In the Manchester district 11,000 men offered themselves for war service between the outbreak of hostilities in October 1899 and July 1900. Of this number 8000 were found to be physically unfit to carry a rifle and stand the fatigues of discipline. Of the 3000 who were accepted only 1200 attained the moderate standard of muscular power and chest measurement required by the military authorities. In other words, two out of every three men willing to bear arms in the Manchester district are virtually invalids.

From: Arnold White, *Efficiency and Empire*, Methuen (1901), pp. 100–3

Document six
HEALTH AND HEALTH SERVICES IN THE 1930s: THE REPORT FROM POLITICAL AND ECONOMIC PLANNING

WHAT IS HEALTH?

Health means more than not being ill. A new attitude is needed, involving not so much a departure from the old as a more thorough grasp of the different elements in health policy. Many people are at any given moment suffering from defects, injuries or sickness so pronounced as to make them unable to carry on ordinary occupations and leisure activities. These are the 'cases' with which a large part of the organised health services mainly deal. But in addition there are far larger numbers of people suffering temporarily or permanently from less acute defects, injuries or inadequacies which are not sufficient to unfit them for work or play, and may not even be noticed at all, but nevertheless suffice to place them in an unnecessarily weak position for creating and maintaining good physique, energy, happiness or resistance to disease. Provided that the argument is not pushed too far it is useful to bear in mind a distinction between the mass of socially and economically incapacitating disabilities usually treated as cases of ill-health and the even larger mass of deficiencies and disabilities which do not incapacitate and are often unrecognised or not thought serious. No contemporary health policy can be considered adequate which does not deal with the second group as well as the first.

   Until recently medicine was inevitably confined largely to work of a salvage nature. Neither knowledge, nor imagination, nor physical resources were adequate to pass the stage of patching up ill-health and to create boldly and consciously the conditions in which a healthy population could grow and flourish. While efforts at effecting the cure of diseases cannot be relaxed, efforts at prevention of ill-health can and must be increased. The aspect of raising standards of nutrition and of fitness should be given much more prominence. Health must come first: the mere state of not being ill must be recognised as an inacceptable substitute, too often tolerated or even regarded as normal. We must, moreover, face the fact that while immense study has been lavished on disease no one has intensively studied and analysed health, and our ignorance of the subject is still so deep that we can hardly claim scientifically to know what health is. To the extent that health is a positive element mere negative attempts to palliate or even to cure specific diseases cannot be regarded as a solution to the problem.

In the first and most important range of health-creating services come those activities which provide more and better food, housing, recreation, and social and economic security, and which stimulate the knowledge and will to make use of these facilities. The really essential health services of the nation are the making available of ample safe fresh milk to all who need it, the cheapening of other dairy products, fruit and vegetables, new accommodation to replace slums and relieve overcrowding, Green Belt schemes, playing-fields, youth hostels and physical education, social insurances which relieve the burden of anxiety on the family and advances in employment policy which improve security of tenure or conditions of work and, finally, education in healthy living through training and propaganda. Health problems are frequently the result of social and industrial conditions, and the attempt to deal with these problems piecemeal results in a lopsided development of the health services. It is necessary to remember that there are often two alternative policies for dealing with ill-health – either to treat the cases or to deal with the social and economic conditions producing the cases.

Personal health services, whether preventive or curative, can only deal effectively with limited numbers of persons, and they can hardly be made satisfactory so long as the numerical burden of cases thrown upon them is excessively inflated by wholesale failures in education or in essential social and economic provision. The more careless about health the community is, and the more often its members need serious doctoring, the worse doctoring they are likely to get, because the cases coming up for attention will be too many and at too late a stage.

The report concludes:

What does the Report show? To sum it up, it describes how a bewildering variety of agencies, official and unofficial, have been created during the past two or three generations to work for health mainly by attacking specific diseases and disabilities as they occur, and by maintaining the sufferers. To a much more limited extent attempts have successfully been made to find out and to eradicate the social and economic causes of sickness and disability such as bad housing, sanitation and water supply, and dangerous or unhealthy working conditions.

Although all these efforts have had remarkable results they have failed to give the nation an acceptable measure of good health or to reduce the economic burden of sickness and accidents. Perhaps the most fundamental defect in the existing system is that it is overwhelmingly preoccupied with manifest and advanced diseases or disabilities and is more interested in enabling the sufferers to go on functioning in society somehow than in studying the nature of health and the means of producing and maintaining it. From this it naturally follows that millions of pounds are spent in looking after and trying to cure the victims of accidents and illnesses which need never have occurred if a fraction of this amount of intelligence and money had been devoted to tracing the social and economic causes of the trouble and making the necessary readjustments. While everyone knows that cholera, bubonic plague, malaria, scurvy and other scourges have been eliminated by the engineer or through raising the standard of living rather than by medical treatment, we are all too apt to think of health in terms of curing and treating disease, and to ignore or underrate the extent to which habits of life, the layout of our towns and buildings, labour management, transport, food manufacturing and distribution and so forth can and must be brought into the campaign for fitness. Basically health is a problem of knowledge and education. The type of survey as we have attempted should be carried out much more thoroughly as an essential and continuous function of government. There should be men and women constantly tracing back into the factory, the office, the traffic system and the home the origins of defects and diseases which are a burden on the nation. There should also be in the universities and the schools men and women evolving and conveying to the new generation an attitude of life based on healthy minds and bodies and prepared to face the implications, instead of stopping short, as we still do, at the stage of lip service.

From: *Report on the British Health Services*, Political and Economic Planning (1937)

THE BEVERIDGE REPORT AND THE ROLE OF A HEALTH SERVICE

ASSUMPTION B. COMPREHENSIVE HEALTH AND REHABILITATION SERVICES

426. The second of the three assumptions has two sides to it. It covers a national health service for prevention and for cure of disease and disability by medical treatment; it covers rehabilitation and fitting for employment by treatment which will be both medical and post-medical. Administratively, realisation of Assumption B on its two sides involves action both by the departments concerned with health and by the Ministry of Labour and National Service. Exactly where the line should be drawn between the responsibilities of these Departments cannot, and need not, be settled now. For the purpose of the present Report, the two sides are combined under one head, avoiding the need to distinguish accurately at this stage between medical and post-medical work. The case for regarding Assumption B as necessary for a satisfactory system of social security needs little emphasis. It is a logical corollary to the payment of high benefits in disability that determined efforts should be made by the State to reduce the number of cases for which benefit is needed. It is a logical corollary to the receipt of high benefits in disability that the individual should recognise the duty to be well and to co-operate in all steps which may lead to diagnosis of disease in early stages when it can be prevented. Disease and accidents must be paid for in any case, in lessened power of production and in idleness, if not directly by insurance benefits. One of the reasons why it is preferable to pay for disease and accident openly and directly in the form of insurance benefits, rather than indirectly, is that this emphasises the cost and should give a stimulus to prevention. As to the methods of realising Assumption B, the main problems naturally arise under the first head of medical treatment. Rehabilitation is a new field of remedial activity with great possibilities, but requiring expenditure of a different order of magnitude from that involved in the medical treatment of the nation.

427. The first part of Assumption B is that a comprehensive national health service will ensure that for every citizen there is available whatever medical treatment he requires, in whatever form he requires it, domiciliary or institutional, general, specialist or consultant, and will ensure also the

provision of dental, ophthalmic and surgical appliances, nursing and mid-wifery and rehabilitation after accidents. Whether or not payment towards the cost of the health service is included in the social insurance contribution, the service itself should

(i) be organised, not only by the Ministry concerned with social insurance, but by Departments responsible for the health of the people and for positive and preventive as well as curative measures;

(ii) be provided where needed without contribution conditions in any individual case.

Restoration of a sick person to health is a duty of the State and the sick person, prior to any other consideration. The assumption made here is in accord with the definition of the objects of medical service as proposed in the Draft Interim Report of the Medical Planning Commission of the British Medical Association:

(a) to provide a system of medical service directed towards the achievement of positive health, of the prevention of disease, and the relief of sickness;

(b) to render available to every individual all necessary medical services, general and specialist, and both domiciliary and institutional.

From: *Report on Social Insurance and Allied Services* (Chairman: Sir W. Beveridge), Cmd 6404, HMSO London (1942), paras 426–7

Document eight
OBJECTIVES OF THE NHS, 1979

The Merrison Commission outlined the objectives of the NHS in the following way:

ENCOURAGING AND ASSISTING INDIVIDUALS TO REMAIN HEALTHY

We consider it legitimate and positively desirable to devote public resources to the maintenance and promotion of personal as well as public health, not only by the constraints of law but also by offering exhortation, education and incentives. The NHS cannot cover the whole field. Though protracted unemployment and poor social conditions may impair the quality of life and health, it is the responsibility of other organs of government to promote employment and to care for the environment. The encouragement and advancement of good personal health is vitally important . . . It is a proper objective of the NHS to keep the individual in good health.

EQUALITY OF ENTITLEMENT

We consider, like the framers of the original legislation, that the NHS should be available without restriction by age, social class, sex, race or religion to all people living in the UK.* We are in no doubt that one of the most significant achievements of the NHS has been to free people from fear of being unable to afford treatment for acute or chronic illness, but we regret that they must often wait too long for such treatment.

A BROAD RANGE OF SERVICES OF A HIGH STANDARD

This is perhaps the most difficult matter we have to discuss and it is at the heart of our terms of reference. We deal with it more fully in Part II of the report, but our definition of this objective includes health promotion, disease prevention, cure, care and after care. The NHS was, from the first, designed to be a comprehensive service. The 1944 White Paper said:

> The proposed service must be 'comprehensive' in two senses – first, that it is available to all people and, second, that it covers all necessary forms of health care.

The impossibility of meeting all demands for health services was not anti-cipated. Medical, nursing and therapeutic techniques have been developed to levels of sophistication and expense which were not foreseen when the NHS was introduced.

Standards of cure and care within a given level of resources are in practice largely in the hands of the health professions. They are nevertheless of the greatest concern to the patient. The aim must always be to raise standards in areas where there are deficiencies, but not at the expense of places where services are already good. The NHS has achieved much. It should remain an objective of a national health service to see that it has an active role in disseminating high standards. Sir George Godber, Chief Medical Officer at the Department of Health and Social Security 1960–73, puts the point thus:

> The burden upon the NHS is that of generalization from the example of the best and the result of having such a national service should be the more rapid development of improved services available to all.

EQUALITY OF ACCESS

It is unrealistic to suppose that people in all parts of the United Kingdom can have equal ease of access to all services of an identical standard. Access to the highest standard of care will be limited by the numbers of those who can provide such care. There are parts of the country which are better or worse provided with services than others. We draw attention . . . to the special problems of rural areas and declining urban areas . . . Nonetheless, a fundamental purpose of a national service must be equality of provision so far as this can be achieved without an unacceptable sacrifice of standards . . .

A SERVICE FREE AT THE TIME OF USE

Charges for services within the NHS have always been a matter of controversy, and have led on occasion to the resignation of ministers . . . there are three points to be made here. First, the purpose of charges may be to raise revenue, or discourage the frivolous use of the service, or both. Second, charges may be made for a service which, though provided by or through the NHS, is not essential to the care or treatment of patients – for example, amenity beds in NHS hospitals. Third, in any consideration of charges, it is important to stress that 'free at the time of use' is quite different from 'free'. We do not have a free health service; we have a service to which all taxpayers, employees and employers contribute, regardless of the use they make of it. The effect of this is that those members of the community who do not require extensive use of the NHS help to pay for the care of those who do. It is worth remembering that about 60% of the total expenditure of the NHS goes on children, the old, the disabled, the mentally ill and the mentally handicapped.

SATISFYING REASONABLE EXPECTATIONS

This objective can be considered from the point of view of the individual patient, or more generally. Most patients lack the technical knowledge to make informed judgments about diagnosis and treatment. Ignorance may as easily be a reason for a patient being satisfied with his treatment as for his being dissatisfied. One aspect of care on which he will be reliable, however, is whether he has been humanely treated. While doctors are properly deferred to as experts on the technical aspects of medicine, options, when they exist, should be carefully explained and wherever feasible the choice of treatment left to the patient and his relatives. Maximum freedom of choice seems to us an important aspect of this objective although we recognise that there may sometimes be practical limitations on complete freedom of choice for patients. A patient, or potential patient, who is capable of deciding for himself, should be free to:

consult a doctor, dentist, or other health professional;
change his practitioner;
choose a particular hospital or unit with the help of his general practitioner; and
refuse treatment or advice where the health or safety of others would be endangered.

More generally, it is important for any health service to carry its users with it, given that it can never satisfy all the demands made upon it. It is misleading to pretend that the NHS can meet all expectations. Hard choices have to be made. It is a prime duty of those concerned in the provision of health care to make it clear to the rest of us what we can reasonably expect.

A NATIONAL SERVICE RESPONSIVE TO LOCAL NEEDS

Health services meet different situations in different parts of the country. The range, speed of development and pattern of service delivery will need to vary. Some services can best be provided on a national or regional basis; specialised treatment may require complicated equipment and a higher degree of expertise than can be provided in every community. But if inflexibility is to be avoided, health authorities should implement national policy in the context of their particular geographical and demographic constraints.

* . We propose no change in policy towards providing treatment to non-residents of the UK. It is right that those who fall ill while they are in this country should continue to receive treatment under the NHS but that unless there is a reciprocal agreement with a particular country a charge should be made if treatment is specifically sought in the UK.

From: *Report of the Royal Commission on the National Health Service* (Chairman: Sir Alec Merrison), Cmnd 7615, HMSO London (1979), p. 9–12

Document nine
KEITH JOSEPH'S RATIONALE FOR THE PROPOSED REORGANISATION IN 1974

NATIONAL HEALTH SERVICE REORGANISATION: ENGLAND

Foreword

For two years I have been responsible for the National Health Service – and for the personal social services.

Throughout this time my respect for the achievements of the National Health Service has steadily grown. Whatever its defects we would be utterly wrong to take for granted the massive performance of this remarkable network of services and the ease of mind that it has brought to all the people of this country. I am sure that they feel a deep sense of gratitude to all those involved: to the members of the governing authorities; to the men and women who make their careers in the service, whether in direct contact with patients or in supporting services; and to the voluntary workers.

But at the same time I have come to recognise, as many others have, that while this good work will continue, nothing like its full potential can be realised without changes in the administrative organisation of the service.

Hence this White Paper. It is about administration, not about treatment and care. But the purpose behind the changes proposed is a better, more sensitive, service to the public. Administration is not of course an end in itself. But both the patients and those who provide treatment and care will gain if the administration embodies both a clear duty to improve the service and the facilities for doing so.

Let me illustrate this. Everyone is aware of gaps in our health services. Even for acute illness, where we provide at least as good a service for our whole population as any country in the world, there are some respects in which we achieve less than we could. On the non-acute side the service for the elderly, for the disabled, and for the mentally ill and the mentally handicapped have failed to attract the attention and indeed the resources which they need – and all the more credit to the staff who have toiled so tirelessly for their patients despite the difficulties.

It is well understood now, moreover, that the domiciliary and community services are under-developed – that there is a need for far more home helps, home nurses, hostels and day centres and other services that support people outside hospital. Often what there is could achieve more if it were better co-ordinated with other services in and out of hospital. It is well understood too that there must be more emphasis on prevention – or at the least on early detection and treatment.

For the imblances and the gaps Governments must take their share of the responsibility. Resources were and still are stretched. The acute services had a legitimate priority. But the shortcomings were not rational. They did not result from a calculation as to the best way to deploy scarce resources. They just happened.

Why did they just happen? Because it has never been the responsibility – nor has it been within the power – of any single named authority to provide for the population of a given area of a comprehensible size the best health service that the money and skills available can provide. There has been no identified authority whose task it has been, in co-operation with those responsible for complementary services, to balance needs and priorities nationally and to plan and provide the right combination of services for the benefit of the public.

It is to enable such an authority to operate in each area, with the best professional advice, that the Government proposes to reorganise the administration of the National Health Service as explained in this White Paper.

The National Health Service is one of the largest civilian organisations in the world. Its staff is growing rapidly. It contains an ever-growing multitude of skills that depend on and interact with each other. It serves an ever-growing range of health needs with ever more complex treatments and techniques. And though the Government has made substantial additions to a programme of expenditure which was already planned to grow at an above-average rate, there is never enough money – and never likely to be – for everything that ideally requires to be done. Nor, despite the great increase since 1948, are there ever enough skilled men and women.

Real needs must therefore be identified, and decisions must be taken and periodically reviewed, as to the order of priorities among them. Plans must be worked out to meet these needs and management and drive must be continually applied to put the plans into action, assess their effectiveness and modify them as needs change or as ways are found to make the plans more effective.

Effective for what? – to improve the service for the benefit of all. The plans must therefore be effective in providing what patients need: primarily, treatment and care in hospital; support at home; diagnosis and treatment in surgery, health centre or out-patient clinic; or day care.

Furthermore they must include arrangements whereby the public can express their wishes and preferences, and know that notice will be taken of them. That is why I attach great importance to the establishment of strong community health councils, and to improved methods for enquiring into complaints, including the appointment of a health ombudsman.

The health services depends crucially on the humane planning and provision of the personal social services, and therefore on effective and understanding collaboration with local government. No doubt arguments will continue about the theoretical advantages of making both health and social services the responsibility of a single agency. But the formidable practical difficulties, which have been fully argued elsewhere, rule this out as a realistic solution, and require us to concentrate instead on ensuring that the two parallel authorities – one local, one health – with their separate statutory responsibilities shall work together in partnership for the health and social care of the population. This White Paper demonstrates the Government's concern to see that arrangements are evolved under which a more coherent and smoothly interlocking range of services will develop for all the needs of the population.

The doctor and other professional workers will gain too. The organisational changes will not affect the professional relationship between individual patients and individual professional workers on which the complex of health services is so largely built. The professional workers will retain their clinical freedom – governed as it is by the bounds of professional knowledge and ethics and by the resources that are available – to do as they think best for their patients. This freedom is cherished by the professions and accepted by the Government. It is a safeguard for patients today and an insurance for future improvements.

But the organisational changes will also bring positive gains to the professional worker. He – or she – will have the opportunity of organising his or her own work better and of playing a much greater part than hitherto in the management decisions that are taken in each area. At the same time the more systematic and comprehensive analysis of needs and priorities that will lie behind the planning and operations of each area will help professional workers to ensure their skills bring the greatest possible benefit to their patients.

We are issuing a White Paper and promoting legislation about the administration of the National Health Service, solely in order to improve the health care of the public. Administrative reorganisation within a unified health service that is closely linked with parallel local government services will provide a sure foundation for better services for all.

KEITH JOSEPH
Secretary of State for Social Services

From: *National Health Service Reorganisation: England*, Cmnd 5055, HMSO London (1972), pp. v–vii

Document ten
MAIN ACTIVITIES UNDERTAKEN AT NHS REGION, AREA AND DISTRICT FROM 1974

RHA (1)	AREA HQ (2)	DISTRICT (3)
1. Regional planning and policy making	1. Area planning and policy making	1. Managing health facilities and services not reserved to Area HQ
2. Allocation of resources between AHAs	2. Allocation of resources between Districts	2. Planning of District services within Regional and Area guidelines
3. Monitoring performances of AHAs	3. Monitoring performances of Districts	3. Formulation of District budgets
4. Developing and implementing regional personnel (including education and training) policies	4. Developing and implementing area personnel (including education and training) policies; formal employment of all AHA staff	4. Personnel work for District staff
5. Developing regional supply policies and making regional contracts	5. Developing area supply policies and making Area contracts	5. Undertaking building and engineering and grounds maintenance
6. Implementing major capital building programme and providing to AHAs a design service and professional advice on works matters	6. Undertaking selected capital building works delegated by RHAs; a programme of minor works; specialised maintenance and day to day property management	
7. Property management	7. Managing ambulance services in non-metropolitan counties	

RHA (1)	AREA HQ (2)	DISTRICT (3)
8. Managing ambulance services in metropolitan counties	8. Collaboration with local authorities including arranging for certain staff to be made available to local authorities	
9. Managing the Blood Transfusion Service	9. Managing community dental and hospital pharmaceutical services	
10. Providing management services (including computer services, OR, statistical and information services) to Areas and Districts	10. Child Health (including school health) services	
11. Employment of regional staff and of medical and dental consultants and senior registrars (except in teaching Areas)	11. Determining financial policies and those financial services to be provided from Area	
12. Managing the research programme for the Region	12. Managing health education	
13. Determination of matters reserved to RHAs (eg approval of schemes of management directions on extra-territorial management)	13. In teaching Areas, the provision of substantial clinical teaching facilities and the employment of consultants and senior registrars	
14. Public relations services		
15. Legal services		

From: DHSS, NHS Reorganisation Circular HRC (74) 18, HMSO, London (1974), p.6

THE GROWTH OF HEALTH AND PERSONAL SOCIAL SERVICE EXPENDITURE 1956/7–1976/7

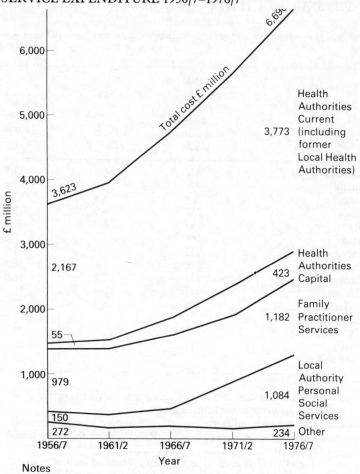

Notes

1. Expenditure is shown at November 1976 prices.

2. Over the years there have been variations in the nature and coverage of the services. The chart therefore shows the broad trend only.

3. Separate accounts were not kept for England and Wales before 1967/8. This chart is on an England and Wales basis over the whole period in order to present a consistent picture.

From: DHSS, *Annual Report 1977*, HMSO London (1978)

A COMPARATIVE ANALYSIS OF HEALTH SERVICE 'INPUTS' AND 'OUTPUTS'

Health Service resources and results: international comparisons 1974 or near date[1]

Country	Per capita total expenditure on health US $[2]	% Trend GDP[3]	Doctors (per 10,000 1974)
Australia	308	6.5	13.9
Canada	408	6.8	16.6
Finland	265	5.8	13.3
France	352	6.9	13.9
Italy	191	6.0	19.9
Japan	166	4.0	11.6
Netherlands	312	7.3	14.9
Norway	270	5.6	16.5
Sweden	416	7.3	16.2
USA	491	7.4	16.5
W. Germany	336	6.7	19.4
England and Wales			13.1
Scotland	212	5.2	16.1
N. Ireland			15.3

Notes: 1. There are a number of caveats concerning the figures in this table. Details are given in the sources listed.

2. The column is indicative rather than definitive: it has been derived by multiplying per cent of *trend* GDP spent on health care by *actual* GDP adjusted for purchasing power differences.

3. Trend GDP is used to avoid the influence of cyclical business fluctuations on the level of output, which could distort the measured share of health expenditure in that output. For details see OECD, *Public Expenditure on Health*, Paris, 1977, p. 9

Nurses (per 10,000 1974)	Life expectancy at age 1		Perinatal mortality (per 1,000 live births)	Maternal mortality (per 100,000 births)
	M	F		
54.1	68.5	75.4	22.4	11.3
57.8	69.7	77.0	17.7	10.8
46.0	66.8	75.5	17.1	10.6
23.7	69.5	77.1	18.8	24.0
7.8	70.0	76.0	29.6	42.4
16.1	70.8	76.0	18.0	38.3
22.5	71.2	76.9	16.4	10.3
46.4	71.4	77.7	16.8	3.3
58.6	72.0	77.4	14.1	2.7
40.4	68.0	75.6	24.8	15.2
27.6	68.6	74.9	23.2	45.9
33.7	69.5	75.6	21.3	13.0
45.6	67.7	74.0	22.7	21.5
36.6	67.0	73.6	25.9	17.1

Sources: Organisation for Economic Co-operation and Development, *Public Expenditure on Health*, Paris, 1977, Table 1.

McKinsey & Co, *International Comparisons of Health Needs and Health Services*, 1978.

Irving B. Kravis, Alan W. Heston and Robert Summers, 'Real GDP per capita for more than one hundred countries', *Economic Journal*, June 1978, Table 4.

From: *Report of the Royal Commission on the National Health Service* (Chairman: Sir Alec Merrison), Cmnd 7615, HMSO London (1979), p. 23

NHS GROSS EXPENDITURE – PROPORTION SPENT ON EACH SERVICE

	Hospital services	Pharma- ceutical services	General medical services	General dental services
1950	54.9	8.4	10.1	9.9
1951	55.7	9.7	9.5	7.8
1953	55.7	9.7	15.8	5.9
1953	55.5	9.5	10.8	5.5
1954	56.7	9.4	10.6	5.9
1955	57.2	9.5	10.2	6.3
1956	57.4	9.8	9.9	6.3
1957	56.8	9.7	9.7	6.4
1958	57.5	10.0	9.8	6.5
1959	57.1	10.2	9.2	6.5
1960	57.2	10.1	10.0	6.3
1961	57.0	9.8	9.6	6.2
1962	59.0	9.7	8.5	6.0
1963	60.1	10.1	8.3	5.7
1964	60.3	10.2	7.9	5.5
1965	60.4	11.1	7.8	5.1
1966	60.8	11.2	7.5	5.2
1967	61.3	10.9	8.1	5.1
1968	60.9	10.4	8.0	4.9
1969[3]	64.3	10.6	8.1	5.0
1970	65.2	10.2	8.7	5.0
1971	66.6	10.0	8.3	5.0
1972	67.2	9.9	8.1	4.6
1973	67.4	9.6	7.5	4.5
1974[4]	66.6	8.6	6.5	4.3
1975	63.4	8.6	6.2	4.1
1976	61.7	9.1	6.2	3.9
1977	61.5	10.0	6.1	3.7
1978	61.1	10.4	6.0	3.6
1979	62.6	10.1	6.3	3.9
1980[5]	62.7	9.4	6.2	3.9

General ophthalmic services	Community health services[1]	Other[2]	Total
5.2	7.8	3.7	100.0
2.8	8.5	6.0	100.0
2.1	8.7	2.1	100.0
2.2	8.8	7.7	100.0
2.5	8.7	6.2	100.0
2.5	8.9	5.4	100.0
2.3	8.9	5.4	100.0
2.2	8.8	6.4	100.0
2.1	8.9	5.2	100.0
2.1	9.1	5.8	100.0
2.0	9.1	5.3	100.0
1.8	9.3	6.3	100.0
1.7	9.8	5.3	100.0
1.6	10.0	4.2	100.0
1.7	10.0	4.4	100.0
1.6	10.3	3.7	100.0
1.5	10.2	3.6	100.0
1.5	10.7	2.4	100.0
1.4	10.5	3.9	100.0
1.5	7.9	2.6	100.0
1.4	7.1	2.4	100.0
1.3	7.1	1.7	100.0
1.2	6.9	2.1	100.0
1.1	7.0	2.9	100.0
1.0	5.7	7.3	100.0
1.2	6.4	9.9	100.0
1.2	6.1	11.8	100.0
1.2	6.2	11.3	100.0
1.1	6.1	11.7	100.0
1.0	6.3	9.7	100.0
0.9	6.2	10.7	100.0

Notes

Figures may not add up to totals because of rounding

1. Figures prior to 1974 refer to former Local Health Authority Services.
2. Includes headquarters administration (RHAs, AHAs, Health Boards and Boards of Governors), central administration, ambulance services, mass radiography services etc, and centrally financed items such as laboratory, vaccine and research and development costs, etc, not falling within the finance of any one service. Figures from 1974 onwards are not strictly comparable with earlier years.
3. Change in definition of NHS. Certain local health authority services transferred from NHS to Social Services.
4. Reorganisation of NHS. Administration of certain NHS community health services transferred from local authorities to new AHAs. School health services formerly administered by the Department of Education and Science also transferred to the NHS.
5. Estimated.

From: Office of Health Economics, *Compendium of Health Statistics 1981*, Office of Health Economics (1982), Table 1.3

Document fourteen

RESOURCE ALLOCATION – THE NATURE OF THE
PROBLEM – DEFINITIONS AND DISTINCTIONS: THE 2ND
RAWP REPORT OUTLINES THE BASIS FOR ALLOCATING
RESOURCES

INTRODUCTION AND BACKGROUND

1.1   There is ample evidence to demonstrate that demand for health care throughout the world is rising inexorably. England has no immunity from this phenomenon. And because it can also be shown that supply of health care actually fuels further demand, it is inevitable that the supply of health care services can never keep pace with the rising demands placed upon them. Demand will always be one jump ahead. This is a problem for Government and society in general and not, fortunately, one to which the Working Party was called upon to address its mind. We mention it at the beginning of this Report, however, to emphasize two points. Firstly that the resources available to the NHS are bound to fall short of requirements as measured by demand criteria and secondly that supply of facilities has an important influence on demand in the locality in which they are provided.

1.2   Supply of health facilities is, in England as elsewhere, also variable and very much influenced by history. The methods used to distribute financial resources to the NHS have, since its inception, tended to reflect the inertia built into the system by history. They have tended to increment the historic basis for the supply of real resources (e.g. facilities and manpower); and, by responding comparatively slowly and marginally to changes in demography and morbidity, have also tended to perpetuate the historic situation.

1.3   This led us in our Interim Report to interpret the underlying objective of our terms of reference as being to secure, through resource allocation, that there would eventually be equal opportunity of access to health care for people at equal risk. We reaffirm this view. It has involved us in seeking criteria which are broadly responsive to relative need, not supply or demand, and to employ those criteria to establish and quantify in a relative way the differentials of need between different geographical locations. For practical purposes these geographic locations must correspond with those into which the NHS is organized to administer the delivery of health care, viz, Regions, Areas and Districts.

1.4   In searching for criteria which are responsive in this way, we have had perforce to consider only those criteria, the supporting statistical data for which are readily available and reliable at all three levels of disaggregation required. We have further taken as an aim the desirability of keeping the methods proposed as simple as possible, consistent with the overall objective. The degree of refinement necessary is to some extent a matter of judgment, but we have not by any means regarded perfection in this context as an aim. On the contrary, we have rejected many approaches which might have made the criteria more sensitive, but which on examination would have led to much greater complexity with little significant change in the result.

1.5   *Resource allocation is concerned with the distribution of financial resources which are used for the provision of real resources. In this sense it is concerned with the means rather than the end. We have not regarded our remit as being concerned with how the resources are deployed.* This must be a matter for the administering Authorities and is essentially part of their policy-making, planning and decision-making functions in response to central guidelines on national policies and priorities. Resource allocation will clearly have an important influence on the discharge of those functions and be the most critical guideline within which they have to be discharged. This serves, however, to emphasize the importance, as our terms of reference direct, of ensuring that the availability of the finite resource at the NHS's disposal should be determined in relation to criteria of need.

CRITERIA OF NEED

Size of Population

1.6   Health care is for people and clearly the primary determinant of need must be the size of the population. This must therefore be the basic divisor used to distribute the resource available to each level required.

Population Make-up

1.7   The make-up of the population is, however, critical. People do not have identical needs for health care. For example, the elderly (men and women aged 65 and over) form about 14% of the total population, yet they occupy more than half the non-psychiatric hospital beds (excluding maternity). Women have needs different from men, and children too are heavy users of health care facilities. Similarly, patterns of morbidity are different between the sexes at different ages. Thus the age/sex make-up of the population needs to be taken into account as well as its size.

Morbidity

1.8   Even when differences due to age and sex are fully accounted for, populations of the same size and make-up display different morbidity characteristics. The reasons are simple enough to guess but harder to quantify; environment, social circumstances, heredity, occupation etc all play a part. But a population-based measure of need which takes no account of different patterns of morbidity would ignore geographic variations which, on the data available, are significant.

Cost

1.9   The costs of providing care in response to need are also variable. Some conditions are very expensive to treat, others less so. It is not enough to use criteria which predict the likely incidence of the more expensive forms of care, unless at the same time some account is taken of the differential cost involved. Furthermore, the costs of exactly the same form of care may vary from place to place depending on local variations in market forces. A clear example of this is the weighting paid to staff employed in the London area.

Health Care Across Administrative Boundaries

1.10   The populations for which the administering Authorities are responsible for delivering health care are primarily those who reside within their geographic boundaries. In some cases these responsibilities are adjusted to take account of people residing in overlap areas – by means of formal agency or extra-territorial management arrangements. For resource allocation purposes the population needs to be that for which the Authority exercises a management responsibility.

1.11   But these arrangements do not take account of patients who receive cars outside the managed area of their particular Authority. Patient flows across boundaries result from the fact that few Areas and Districts are entirely self-sufficient in terms of the services they provide. In some cases these 'deficiencies' are planned, e.g. Regional specialties, in others they are unplanned and are often the inevitable consequence of new and arbitrary administrative boundaries not matching established patterns of health care delivery. To a large extent unplanned patient flows are also a measure of geographical disparity in health care provision. Whether patient flows are from choice or necessity, the populations used for revenue allocations need to be adjusted to take account of the movement. And such adjustment ought also to reflect the different costs of care involved.

Medical and Dental Education

1.12   The NHS has a responsibility to provide clinical facilities for the teaching of students qualifying through the University Medical Schools. Service facilities which are used for medical and dental education are more costly to provide. The incidence of these costs is, however, unrelated either to the size or to the needs of the populations served by the hospitals where medical and dental education is undertaken. Means must therefore be found of identifying the additional costs necessarily involved and protecting those costs from the effects of allocation processes based upon population and service need criteria.

Capital Investment

1.13 Health services require considerable capital investment in buildings, plant and equipment. Whilst the need for capital investment may to a considerable extent be measurable by criteria similar to those used for determining need for current expenditure, there is one significant difference. As mentioned earlier in this chapter, the distribution of capital stock is still very much influenced by the historic patterns of health care delivery. There are not only geographic inequalities in the quantity of stock available but also in its age and condition. Nor do these factors of quantity and quality go hand in hand. Regions which are well provided in quantitative terms may, for the same historic reasons, have a large proportion of ageing stock. Furthermore, the effects of population movement, demographic change and the redefinition of administrative boundaries have all exacerbated the 'mislocation' problem.

From: DHSS, *Sharing Resources for Health in England*, Report of the Resource Allocation Working Party, HMSO London (1976), p. 7–10

Document fifteen

A LIST OF GOVERNMENT POLICY DOCUMENTS AND REPORTS ON THE CARE AND TREATMENT OF DEPENDENT GROUPS

Royal Commission on Mental Illness and Mental Deficiency, HMSO 1957

DHSS, *Better Services for the Mentally Handicapped*, Cmnd 4683, HMSO 1971

DHSS, *Better Services for the Mentally Ill*, Cmnd 6233, HMSO 1975

Report of the Committee of Enquiry into Mental Handicap Nursing and Care (Chair: Peggy Jay), HMSO 1979

DHSS, *Reports of the Development Team for the Mentally Handicapped*. First Report 1976/77, HMSO, 1978; Second Report 1978/79, HMSO, 1980

DHSS, *Mental Handicap: Progress, Problems and Priorities*, HMSO 1980

DHSS, *Report of a Working Group on Organisation and Management Problems of Mental Illness Hospitals*, 1980

DHSS, *A Happier Old Age*. A discussion document on Elderly People in our Society, HMSO 1978

DHSS, *Growing Older*, White Paper on the Elderly, Cmnd 8173, HMSO 1981

DHSS, *Report of a Study on the Respective Roles of the Acute, General and Geriatric Sectors in the Care of the Elderly Hospital Patient*, 1981

DHSS, *Report of a Study on Community Care*, 1981

DHSS, *Care in the Community*, a Consultative Document on Moving Resources for Care in England, 1981

HEALTH ADVISORY SERVICE, *The Rising Tide, Developing Services for Mental Illness in Old Age*, NHS Advisory Service, 1982

Document sixteen
ELDERLY PEOPLE IN GREAT BRITAIN

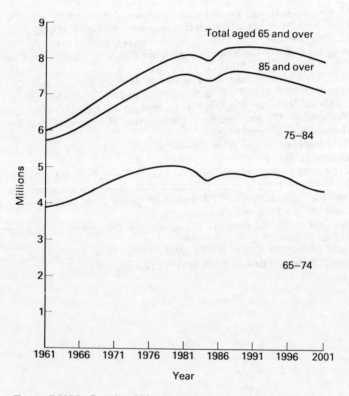

From: DHSS, *Growing Older*, HMSO, London (1981), Chart A

Document seventeen
THE CONCEPT OF COMMUNITY CARE: A DHSS WORKING PARTY'S APPROACH

COMMUNITY CARE: A DESCRIPTION OF SERVICES OR A POLICY OBJECTIVE?

Possibly the most important source of confusion over the term community care arises from switches between its use as a *description* of what services/resources are involved (e.g. community care is those services provided outside of institutions . . .) and *statements of objectives* (e.g. community care for the mentally ill is minimising disruption of ordinary living . . .). It may be useful to look at each of these separately.

Used *descriptively*, community care sometimes means those services provided by local authority social services departments rather than the NHS. This shorthand stems from the policy thrust, stressed particularly in the late 1960s and early 1970s, of shifting the main responsibility for some people, particularly some long-stay hospital patients, from the NHS to the PSS. However, it has always been recognised that this was something of an over simplification since community health services – general practitioners, district nurses, health visitors and so on – are a core element of community care. They contribute to community-based packages of services, provided as alternatives to long-term hospital care, as well as dealing with about 90 per cent of illness presented without any recourse to in-patient services. Moreover, personal social services staff often exclude residential care when they use the term community care. Frequently, therefore, community care is used to mean all services/support provided outside of institutions, regardless of which agency (NHS, PSS or voluntary) provides them. But even this is not quite such a water-tight distinction as it may first appear – are hostels or group homes covered by the institutional umbrella or not? And what about community-based packages of care which in relation to the mentally ill might include short spells of acute psychiatric care in hospital or, in relation to elderly people, a short acute episode (e.g. a hip replacement) which may enable the elderly person to continue to live at home, possibly with continuing domiciliary support (e.g. from district nurses or meals on wheels). A further complicating dimension is a growing tendency to equate community care with support provided by individuals in a given community to its own most vulnerable members and to exclude formally provided services, whether from statutory agencies or the organised voluntary sector.

If, on the basis of paragraph above, it would seem that on a description level there is no one predominant concept, the problem is further complicated when we turn to community care defined in terms of its *objectives*. The range includes:

- to treat conditions which do not require in-patient services and to select for referral those cases requiring secondary care;
- to facilitate early discharge of acute in-patients;
- to provide back-up for day surgery or out-patient treatment;
- to provide an alternative for some of those people currently cared for long-term in hospital or residential homes;
- to enable an individual to remain in his own home wherever possible rather
- than have him cared for long-term in a hospital or residential home;
- to give support and/or relief to informal carers (family, friends and neighbours) so that they can cope with the stress of caring for a dependent person;
- the delivery of appropriate help, by the means which cause the least possible disruption to ordinary living, in order to relieve an individual, family or neighbourhood of the stresses and strains contributing to or arising in consequence of physical or emotional disorder;
- to provide the most cost-effective package of services given the needs and wishes of the person being helped;
- to integrate all the resources of a geographical area in order to support the individuals within it. These resources might include informal carers, NHS and personal social services and organised voluntary effort but also sheltered housing, the local social security office, the church, local clubs and so on.

It will be noted that the objectives, explicit or implicit in statements about community care, range from the very specific to all encompassing approaches to care giving. The client group in relation to which objectives are set is perhaps the most important variable. But the nature of the resources available and current practice patterns in a given locality also help fashion objectives. It therefore seems likely that the concept of community care will continue to elude a definitive statement and that aspects of the various definitions described above, either descriptive or in terms of objectives, will be given prominence at different times.

From: DHSS, *Report of a Study on Community Care*, DHSS, London (1981), p. 7–9

FOREWORD TO *PATIENTS FIRST*

Patrick Jenkin, Secretary of State for Social Services, outlines the intentions of the 1982 reorganisation.

1.   We have been studying the working of the National Health Service for nearly four years, first in Opposition and more recently in Government, and we have reached the firm conclusion that the structure and management arrangements of the Service introduced in 1974 do not provide the best framework for the effective delivery of care to patients. The Royal Commission on the NHS which reported on the 18th of July has confirmed us in our view. It put forward a great many proposals which the Government will consider and judge in their proper time. It is, however, fundamental to making a national health system work well in response to patients' needs that the structure and management of the service should be right. That is what this consultative paper is about.

2.   The greater part of it is concerned with the need for structural change in England. As is explained in paragraphs 46 and 47 there is not the same need in Wales, but our broad philosophy of simplifying management arrangements in the National Health Service applies throughout England and Wales.

3.   Our approach stems from a profound belief that the needs of patients must be paramount. Whatever structure and management arrangements are devised must be responsive to those needs. The closer decisions are taken to the local community and to those who work directly with patients, the more likely it is that patients' needs will be their prime objective.

4.   It is doctors, dentists and nurses and their colleagues in the other health professions who provide the care and cure of patients, and promote the health of the people. It is the purpose of management to support them in giving that service. The efficient management of the Service is therefore of the highest importance, not least when resources are tight. The more economical it can be, the more resources there will be for patient care. On the quality of management will depend the effective planning and day-to-day operation of the National Health Service.

5.   We are determined to see that as many decisions as possible are taken at the local level – in the hospital and in the community. We are determined to

have more local health authorities, whose members will be encouraged to manage the Service with the minimum of interference by any central authority, whether at region or in central government departments. We ask that our proposals should be judged by whether they achieve these aims.

6.   The NHS is only one part of our welfare services. Families may need help from the services of local government – the social services, education and housing. We attach high importance to the NHS working together with these services, but we have come to the conclusion that this does not necessarily mean that they need to do this within common administrative boundaries. What is necessary, and what will, we know, be readily forthcoming, is the will to work together.

7.   Over the last few years – indeed ever since the 1974 reorganisation – there has been discussion about the need for further change. We now have the report of the Royal Commission which points the way forward. We believe that Ministers must now give a firm lead, and this is what we are doing. We do, however, want the views of those concerned and we look forward to receiving these by the end of next April, so that we can take final decisions and get the necessary changes moving from the middle of the year.

8.   It is no part of our purpose to make change for change's sake. Much that exists is good and should be kept. Where change is needed, it should accord with the local needs of local communities. Therefore there must be flexibility, both on what changes are made and on the timing of change. We must balance the need for change with the need for stability, for the sake of patients and staff alike. The area health authorities have done much for the patient; in modifying the structure, we must build on what they have done. The regional health authorities have had an important role, and will continue to have it in effecting the changes within their region. But their role may change; and it will be right that they should see themselves responding to the needs and challenges of the future. Those who work in the national Health Service, at every level and in every aspect of its care for patients, have played a full and honourable part; and we are confident that they will adapt themselves to the changing needs of patient care.

9.   We must never forget that it is people, not organisations, who have the care and cure of patients in their charge. Just as the needs of patients will change over the years, so will the needs of those who care for them. The pattern we propose therefore in this consultative paper must not be seen as a final and rigid blueprint to last for all time. On the contrary, it will fail if it does not embody within itself the ability to respond flexibly and positively to the future needs of the people.

PATRICK JENKIN
Secretary of State for Social Services
Nicholas Edwards
Secretary of State for Wales

From: DHSS, *Patients First. Consultative Paper on the Structure and Management of the National Health Service in England and Wales*, HMSO London (1979), p. 1–3

LETTER FROM THE SECRETARY OF STATE FOR SOCIAL SERVICES PREFACING CARE IN ACTION

OUTLINING POLICIES AND PRIORITIES

To the Chairman and Members of District Health Authorities   February 1981

Dear Chairman,

Although they are addressed to the chairmen and members of the new district health authorities, I want this letter and handbook to be widely available. There are messages I want everyone to heed. The handbook reminds us that we all have a personal responsibility for our own health. We also have a duty to help one another – a message stressed in chapter 3 on 'The Voluntary Sector'.

The handbook sets out the main policies and priorities which Ministers will look to you to follow in running the services for which you are responsible. We want to give you as much freedom as possible to decide how to pursue policies and priorities in your own localities. Local initiatives, local decisions, and local responsibility are what we want to encourage. This is the main purpose of the current reorganisation of the structure and management of the National Health Service.

You have therefore a wider opportunity than your predecessors to plan and develop services in the light of *local* needs and circumstances. But a National Health Service must also have regard to *national* policies and priorities, and I must ask you to take account of them, as set out in this handbook, in making your plans and decisions.

You will see that I am not asking district health authorities to make any abrupt changes of direction. The main emphasis of our priorities continues to be along the lines on which your predecessors were already working, and includes giving a high priority both to the prevention of ill health and to the so-called 'Cinderella' services for people who are mentally ill or handicapped, and those who are elderly. A White Paper on the elderly will shortly be published, covering not only health and personal social services but also social security, housing, transport and other matters.

You will see I have referred to health and social services together. Although run by different authorities, they are part of the broad spectrum of care, stretching from the acute and emergency hospital services, through to domiciliary care and support in the community. I want to see as close a collaboration between health authorities and local government as possible. How this should be done must be for you and your colleagues in local government to decide in the light of local circumstances. I also attach importance to the theme of collaboration with the voluntary services and with the private sector.

I am sure you do not need reminding that the Government's top priority must be to get the economy right; for that reason, it cannot be assumed that more money will always be available to be spent on health care. You will find that clinicians and others working in the health services are anxious to make the best use of resources, to cut out waste and to find ways (through, for instance, local budgeting) to use money more effectively. I hope that you will feel it right to give them every encouragement.

The provision of these services at a time of economic difficulty presents a challenge to Ministers, to you as chairmen and members of authorities, and to all who serve the public, whether in the statutory or in the voluntary services or in the private sector. It is my hope that the policies and priorities set out in this handbook will help us all to meet that challenge.

From: DHSS, *Care in Action. A Handbook of Policies and Priorities for the Health and Personal Social Services in England*, HMSO (1981)

CASES ILLUSTRATING THE DIFFICULTY OF DISTINGUISHING BETWEEN CLINICAL AND POLICY DECISIONS IN HEALTH CARE

CASE 1: OBSTETRICS

The major teaching hospital in the West Midlands Region has exceptional skills and resources to detect potential abnormalities among prospective mothers and their babies. It has a dual role: first, it serves the Region as a centre of excellence, taking referrals from other hospitals in the Region; second, it has a district general hospital maternity role with respect to the District within which it is situated. Upon examination of the way in which this latter role is actually carried out, some interesting facts emerge. Women living in the four electoral wards of the District where there are low perinatal mortality rates have ten times the chance of having their babies in this hospital as women living in parts with high perinatal mortality rates. In the worst electoral ward in the District, the perinatal mortality rate (over a five-year period) is 35.8 per 1,000 live births. Women living there have a one in thirty chance of being delivered in the centre of excellence on their doorsteps. The best electoral ward has a perinatal mortality rate of 17.22: women living there have a one in two chance of being delivered there. Two alternative conclusions may be drawn from these figures. If perinatal mortality is regarded as principally the consequence of social and economic deprivation, as implied by the work of the National Perinatal Epidemiology Unit in Oxford, then it may be argued that the hospital ought to be directing its efforts simply to cope with the situation on a remedial and short-term basis, while leaving the causes to be dealt with elsewhere. Thus, the hospital should admit a higher proportion of women from wards with high perinatal mortality rates. If, however, it is argued that the figures show that, where the hospital does a great deal of work, perinatal mortality is lower (as a result of the hospital's effective work), then surely any *additional* resources for the hospital should be tied to increased workloads in wards where those perinatal mortality rates are at present relatively high. But this has not happened. Instead, substantial additional funds have been allocated for nurse staffing, with the aim of increasing the hospital's annual throughput by 1,000 births, without any conditions being attached. Thus funding is in no way linked to specific desired outcomes. The pattern of obstetric care, says the Authority, is a matter properly to be determined by consultant staff, although it is their booking policies which are at the root of the problem. Clinical freedom is thereby extended beyond the care of the individual patient, to the realms of resource allocation and political decision-making . . .

CASE 2: EYES

Recent development in the technology of ophthalmology have enabled consultants to perform extremely sophisticated operations which take a great deal of time. In consequence, waiting lists for relatively simple operations, such as the removal of cataracts, have built up. Sometimes the equipment that consultants are using to enable them to perform more intensive work has been obtained outside the NHS, by voluntary and public donation. This is likely to be the case especially where there is a strong industrial tradition and numbers of industrialists prepared to act philanthropically. Additionally, of course, the revenue consequences of such acquisitions or gifts are rarely met by the original donors, and thereby become a burden on the service. Now it *may* be that the public, if asked, would wish this more intensive ophthalmic work to be carried out, in preference to larger numbers of cataract operations. But the question is never put. It is not the kind of issue considered by health authorities. Prior to 1974, public discussion, too, was non-existent. Now, in a limited way, such issues are beginning to arise in local media, through the work of CHCs. Once again, the boundaries of clinical freedom have been extended to allow consultant medical staff to determine just how the Service will operate and to subvert substantially the NHS planning system, and with it any sense of priorities determined in a quasi-democratic way through the health authorities' deliberations.

From: Burkeman, S., 'A consumer's response to Merrison and Patients First', *The Yearbook of Social Policy in Britain, 1979*, M. Brown and S. Baldwin (eds.), Routledge and Kegan Paul, London (1980), p. 129–30

Document twenty-one
THE 'MEDICAL' MODEL

Probably the most important model is that which we have called the 'medical' model. It seems to have two major components: the *disease* component and the *engineering* component. Typically, the disease component holds that illness, as manifested in signs and symptoms, is due to pathological processes in the biochemical functions of the body. Specific pathogens cause specific diseases which are, as it were, 'hosted' by the patient's body. The emphasis on specific, individual etiology leads to emphasis on individual specific cures. Newer, multicausal theories of disease do not fundamentally question the basics of the disease approach which emphasises the disease rather than the patient, cure rather than prevention, and individuals rather than populations. These emphases on illness rather than health imply the engineering component by which diseases, their detection and treatment become increasingly technical. This engineering approach is summarised by McKeown thus:

> . . . Medical education begins with the study of the structure and function of the body, continues with examination of disease processes, and ends with clinical instruction on selected sick people; medical service is dominated by the image of the acute hospital where the technological resources are concentrated; and medical science reflects the mechanistic concept, for example in the attention given to the chemical basis of inheritance and the immunological response to transplanted organs. These researches are strictly in accord with the physical model, the first being thought to lead ultimately to control of gene structure and the second to replacement of diseased organs by normal ones. (T. McKeown, 'A Historical Appraisal of the Medical Task' in G. McLachlan and T. McKeown (eds.), *Medical History and Medical Care*, OUP, 1971, p. 30.)

From: Illsley, R., 'Everybody's Business? Concepts of Health and Illness' in *Health and Health Policy. Priorities for Research*, Social Science Research Council, June 1977, Appendix 4, p. 3

Document twenty-two
THE COURT REPORT'S VIEW OF 'THE SOCIAL
DIMENSION': ILL-HEALTH AND DISABILITY IN
CHILDREN

We have already had occasion to refer repeatedly to the correlation between
social class and the prevalence of ill-health and disability in children. As we
pass from the children of professional families to those of unskilled workers
there is a significant increase in bedwetting, squint, stuttering, dental disease
and non-infective seizures, and bronchitis and pneumonia and infective
diarrhoea are more frequent and more severe. Disease does not occur in a bodily
system but in a child, a member of a particular family living in a particular
community. Illness in childhood cannot be fully understood without reference
to the child's development and social circumstances. Conventional classifi-
cations fail to reveal the adverse social factors that may lie behind a diagnostic
label and contribute to the form, management and outcome of the illness.
Poverty, inadequate housing and unemployment are still with us; and
although the majority of parents care for their children faithfully and well,
many are hindered from doing so by physical or mental illness, or instability in
their personal relationships.

The effect of environment can also be seen in growth. In one group of urban
children at 15 children in social classes I and II were on average 4.5 cm taller
and 4.4 kg heavier than children in social classes IV and V. In a national
study,* when all adverse factors were compounded, the 'social' difference in
height was nearly 14 cm. In a study** of all short children (below the third
centile), in a northern city at the age of 10, 82% were normal in terms of
freedom from disease. The majority of their families however belonged to
social classes IV and V and the children had been brought up in poor
conditions. In at least a third of these 'normal' children the adverse social
conditions were considered the cause of their deficient growth. Short stature
can be normal; it can also be a disease of the social environment and an
important pointer to a group of socially deprived children. *There is now
extensive evidence that an adverse family and social environment can retard
physical, emotional and intellectual growth, lead to more frequent and more serious
illness and adversely affect educational achievement and personal behaviour.*

Infant deaths 1964 England and Wales, number and rate per 1,000 legitimate live births – social class

	I & II		III		IV & V
1,714	(12.8)	7,101	(17.2)	4,931	(20.8)

Children 1–14, 1959–63, England and Wales, numbers of deaths (and rates per 100,000 per year) – social class

Age	I	II	III	IV	V
1–4	436 (69.0)	1,329 (73.4)	6,147 (88.7)	2,324 (93.3)	1,521 (154.0)
5–9	209 (32.8)	818 (35.1)	3,243 (41.1)	1,234 (41.4)	744 (66.6)
10–14	173 (29.6)	823 (28.8)	2,771 (31.3)	1,091 (30.3)	555 (41.4)

A special analysis of the 1959–63 child deaths shows that the death rate for children aged 1–4 and 5–9 in Social Class V was approximately twice that in Social Classes I and II and more than 50% higher than that for Social Class IV. The differences for children aged 10–14 are less striking, but nevertheless the death rate in Social Class V was a third higher than that for Social Class IV. The difference in deaths from respiratory diseases is particularly noticeable. For children aged 1–4 the death rate from pneumonia in Social Class V was 25.2 per 100,000 compared with 13.9 for Social Class IV and 10.0 for Social Class I. Children in Social Class V experienced considerably higher death rates from accidents, poisonings and violence. Although these figures relate to a period 15 years ago and the death rate from disease and accident has fallen appreciably since then it is unlikely that the large social class differences have been eliminated. They are a sad commentary on avoidable deaths in childhood.

* Davis, R., Butler, N., and Goldstein, H., (1972). *From Birth to Seven*, Second Report of the National Child Development Study. Longman in association with the National Children's Bureau.
Lacey, K. A., and Parkin, M. J., (1974). 'The normal short child', *Arch. Dis. Child* **49, 417–24.

From: *Fit for the Future. Report of the Committee on Child Health Services* (Chair: Donald Court), Cmnd 6684, HMSO, Vol. 1, p. 50

Document twenty-three

DEATHS PER 100,000 POPULATION – MAJOR CAUSES BY
AGE AND SEX GREAT BRITAIN

| | *Males* | | | | | *Females* |
	1950–53 average	1961	1974	1950–53 average	1961	1974
Ages under 1 year						
Infective, etc diseases	249	75	67	199	71	51
Pneumonia	527	320	149	416	254	108
Cogenital anomalies	460	460	403	430	455	401
All causes	3,293	2,450	1,883	2,554	1,920	1,419
Ages 1–14						
Infective, etc diseases	15	4	3	14	3	2
Cancer, including leukaemia	8	8	6	7	7	5
Pneumonia	7	6	3	7	5	3
Motor vehicle accidents	11	9	7	5	5	5
All other accidents	13	12	8	7	5	4
All causes	85	62	45	67	44	34
Ages 15–34 years						
Infective, etc diseases	26	3	1	33	3	1
Cancer, including leukaemia	15	15	13	13	12	11
Motor vehicle accidents	19	31	28	3	6	7
All other accidents	21	16	15	3	3	4
Suicide	6	8	8	3	4	4
All causes	136	108	96	105	59	47
Ages 35–44 years						
Infective, etc diseases	42	9	3	27	6	3
Cancer, including leukaemia	58	53	46	71	68	64
Heart diseases	54	68	78	34	27	21
Motor vehicle accidents	11	15	13	2	4	4

	Males			Females		
	1950–53 average	1961	1974	1950–53 average	1961	1974
All other accidents	21	20	18	4	4	8
Suicide	12	15	12	7	9	7
All causes	288	248	227	228	180	158
Ages 45–74 years						
Infective, etc diseases	89	27	10	26	10	5
Cancer, including leukaemia	350	384	380	266	271	300
Heart diseases	417	484	563	196	179	181
Cerebrovascular diseases	115	109	91	121	96	75
Bronchitis	114	113	63	26	21	20
All causes	1,439	1,412	1,343	848	759	742
Ages 65–74 years						
Infective, etc diseases	126	71	23	34	18	11
Cancer, including leukaemia	1,053	1,186	1,348	655	620	658
Heart diseases	1,924	1,912	1,945	1,204	1,072	909
Cerebrovascular diseases	724	678	551	653	579	428
Pneumonia	184	236	256	108	136	154
Bronchitis	461	549	389	158	117	69
All causes	5,487	5,530	5,190	3,462	3,145	2,685

From: Central Statistics Office, *Annual Abstract of Statistics*, in West, P. A., *The Nation's Health and the NHS*, Kings Fund Project Paper RC14, Kings Fund (1980), p. 43

Document twenty-four
THE USE OF HEALTH SERVICES BY SOCIAL CLASS

Table A. Social class and use of health services (1970–72)

| | | *Percentage of those under 7 years who have never* | | |
| | | | *Been immunised against* | |
Social class	*Visited a dentist*	*Smallpox*	*Polio*	*Diphtheria*
I	16	6	1	1
II	20	14	3	3
IIIN	19	16	3	3
IIIM	24	25	4	6
IV	27	29	6	8
V	31	33	10	11

Table B

| | *General practitioner index*[1] | | *Hospital OPD index*[2] | |
Social Class	*Male*	*Female*	*Male*	*Female*
I	1.2	2.0	1.3	1.6
II	1.0	1.3	1.0	1.1
IIIN	0.9	1.3	1.0	1.1
IIIM	0.8	1.2	0.9	0.8
IV	0.8	0.8	0.7	0.6
V	0.6	0.7	0.6	0.5

1. Ratio of prevalence of chronic handicapping illnesses among adults to general practitioners' consultation rates.
2. Ratio of prevalence of chronic handicapping illnesses among adults to hospital out-patient consultation rates.

From: *Report of a Research Working Group on Inequalities in Health*, DHSS 1981, p. 106, and Blaxter, M., 'Social Class and Health Inequalities,' in Carter C. O. and Peel, J. (eds), *Equalities and Inequalities in Health*, Academic Press (1976).

Document twenty-five
WORK AND HEALTH

1.   Engels, who came to live in England in 1842, in his account 'The Conditions of the Working Class in England' drew attention to ill health due to working conditions. In Engels' view many disorders were a consequence of the physical demands of industrialism. He discussed curvature of the spine, deformities of the lower extremities, flat feet, varicose veins, and leg ulcers as manifestations of work demands that required long periods of time in an upright posture. Engels commented on the health effects of posture, standing, and repetitive movements.

> All these affections are easily explained by the nature of factory work . . . The operatives . . . must stand the whole time. And one who sits down, say upon a window-ledge or a basket, is fined, and this perpetual upright position, this constant mechanical pressure of the upper portions of the body upon spinal column, hips, and legs, inevitably produces the results mentioned. This standing is not required by the work itself . . .

He also commented on the conditions in cotton mills which led to 'brown lung' or byssinosis.

> In many rooms of the cotton and flax-spinning mills, the air is filled with fibrous dust, which produces chest affections, especially among workers in the carding and combing-rooms . . . The most common effects of this breathing of dust are blood-spitting, hard, noisy breathing, pains in the chest, coughs, sleeplessness – in short, all the symptoms of asthma . . .

Engels discussed pulmonary disorder among coal miners. He reported that unventilated coal dust caused both acute and chronic pulmonary inflammation that frequently progressed to death. Engels observed that 'black spittle' – the syndrome now called coal miners' pneumoconiosis, or black-lung – was associated with other gastrointestinal, cardiac, and reproductive complications. By pointing out that this lung disease was preventable, Engels illustrated the contradiction between profit and adequate health conditions in capitalist industry.

Every case of this disease ends fatally . . . in all the coal-mines which are properly ventilated this disease is unknown, while it frequently happens that miners who go from well to ill-ventilated mines are seized by it. The profit-greed of mine owners which prevents the use of ventilators is therefore responsible for the fact that this working-men's disease exists at all.

From: *The Condition of the Working Class in England*, Engels, F. (first published 1845), Progress Publishers, Moscow (1973), pp. 190–3, 279

2. Ruth Cavendish in her account of working with women on a production line also comments on work conditions and their effects on health.

The speed of the line affected your whole body. Constant physical pressure for eight hours left you tensed up. We all felt the same. I don't know whether assembly line workers suffer from stress diseases more than other types of worker, but it wouldn't surprise me. Arlene had recently started seeing 'a butterfly' in front of her eyes and the doctor said she had high blood pressure. Many women were taking Valium and Librium for 'nerve trouble'. They all looked older than their age, pale, tired and drawn. They thought I was about eight years younger than I was and I thought them ten years older. Even the 20-year olds had deep lines round their eyes.

My diary was full of days when I was 'bursting inside', 'gone over my physical limit', 'whirring', or had 'pains in the chest and felt faint'. It must be bad for the heart to push yourself so hard, and work at a pace much faster than is normal for the body.

It certainly took years off their lives. Apart from looking worn out, they thought fifty was old and didn't expect to live much after sixty or retirement age. That was realistic statistically, given that manual workers have a much lower life expectancy than professional workers. The two labourers who died while I was there were just under sixty, and three other men were said to have dropped dead from heart attacks on the shopfloor during the past year. On my last day, one of the progress chasers, in his mid-forties, had a heart attack. Alice thought the fact it was only men who dropped dead at work proved that 'we women are much stronger'. But the older women did look really haggard and some had difficulty keeping up with the speed.

You also suffered from various aches and pains. Sitting in the same position all day was almost unbearable – it made me feel like a stiff slug that couldn't even stretch. Backache and neckache were common, and excruciatingly painful.

From: Cavendish, R., *Women on the Line*, Routledge and Kegan Paul (1982), p. 118

Document twenty-six
UNEMPLOYMENT AND HEALTH IN FAMILIES

Fagin and his associates carried out a study of 22 families where the male breadwinner had been unemployed for at least 16 weeks and came to the general conclusions shown below:

Our interviews with the families revealed close associations in time between changes in health and the experience of unemployment. As we have described, health changes were not restricted to the male breadwinner; his wife and children often reported fluctuations. Health did not necessarily worsen after unemployment; some families actually reported less health problems. And often the recurrence or marked worsening of a previous illness, and not the emergence of a new illness, co-incided with the event of unemployment.

The following are summaries of what we think are the main areas of concern about health and unemployment that appeared in the families we interviewed.
1. Following the onset of unemployment, spouses with previous histories of poor health suffer relapses and an aggravation of their previous illnesses. This is usually more marked in the male breadwinner, especially if his disability or handicap had neither prevented him from keeping a job nor caused his unemployment. The deterioration in the wife's health, in particular if they were not working, could have been associated with the insecurity accompanying unemployment and the emotional and physical changes in her husband.
2. Male breadwinners with previous records of ill-health may improve following the onset of unemployment. We observed this when ill-health was a manifestation of unhappiness, instability, or high stress at the work place.
3. For men with previous poor health records, returning to work may be associated with fewer reported health problems. This could be due to the threat of losing the job through illness and further long term unemployment.
4. The wife of a man who cannot return to work because of health problems may also report fewer health difficulties than before her husband lost his job, especially if she has to work and the family relies on her income.
5. The loss of a job can set in motion psychological changes which in some male breadwinners result in clinical depression, with feelings of sadness, hopelessness and self-blame, lethargy, lack of energy and loss of self-esteem, insomnia, withdrawal and poor communication, loss or gain of weight, sui-

cidal thoughts, impulsive, sometimes violent outbursts, and an increased use of tobacco or alcohol. These men are often treated by their General Practitioners with medication (mild tranquillisers and anti-depressants), especially if the men's confidence and self-esteem depended to a large extent on their jobs. If the depression occurs immediately after the loss of the job, anxiety and agitation pre-dominate; but if it occurs after many months of unsuccessful job search, it is characterised particularly by lethargy, resignation and withdrawal. The wives of these men, especially if they are not employed, may also become depressed.

6.   The job loss may also be accompanied by physical symptoms of a kind usually considered to be precipitated by psychological mechanisms. These symptoms include asthmatic attack, skin lesions such as psoriasis, backaches and headaches. These occur mainly in the male breadwinners.

7.   Health problems or an established illness in the unemployed male breadwinner relieves the tension he experiences when he cannot regain employment. The dictum that 'it is better to be sick and unemployed, than healthy and unemployed' seems to be true for a jobless man in our society.

8.   The return to employment is not necessarily associated with fewer reports of health problems. A wife who expected her life-style to change when her husband returned to work was disappointed, and developed a depression which required expert help. Health problems in the male breadwinner may be associated with the extra strain he experiences trying to avoid losing his job again. One young man in our sample had a mild coronary a few months after finding a job.

9.   Unemployment can affect children's health. The younger children of men who were out of work for longer periods commonly had disturbances in feeding habits, were prone to accidents, sleeping difficulties, behaviour problems and other ailments.

10. The unemployed man's prior relationship to his job, his perception of society's attitude to his joblessness, his chances of regaining employment, the strength of the marital and family relationships, his wife's employment status, the degree of financial stress imposed by his unemployment, the power of the sick-role in his family, and his ability to fill his empty time with other activities, interests or marginal employment: all these contribute to the final outcome of physical and mental wellbeing in the families of the unemployed.

From: Fagin, L., *Unemployment and Health in Families*, DHSS London (1981), pp. 114–17

THE BLACK REPORT ON INEQUALITIES IN HEALTH

The Black Report as a result of its concern for inequalities in health spread its remit well beyond the health service. The following are its recommendations for changes in policy outside the NHS:

First we have attempted to pay heed to those factors which are correlated with the *degree* of inequalities. Secondly, we have tried to confine ourselves to matters which are immediately practicable, in political, economic and administrative terms, which will nonetheless, properly maintained, exert a long-term structural effect. And thirdly, we have continued to feel it right to give priority to young children and mothers, disabled people and measures concerned with prevention. Above all we consider that the *abolition of child poverty should be adopted as a national goal for the 1980s.* We recognise that this requires a redistribution of financial resources far beyond anything achieved by past programmes, and is likely to be very costly. Our recommendations here are presented as a modest first step which might be taken towards this objective.

i. As an immediate goal the level of child benefit should be increased to 5½% of average gross male industrial earnings, or £5.70 at November 1979 prices.

ii. Larger child benefits should be progressively introduced for older children, after further examination of the needs of children and consideration of the practice in some other countries.

iii. The maternity grant should be increased to £100.

iv. We recommend the introduction of an infant care allowance over a 5 year period, beginning with all babies born in the year following a date to be chosen by the Government.

Beyond these initial elements of an anti-poverty strategy, a number of other steps need to be taken.

v. Provision of meals at school should be regarded as a right. Representatives of local authorities and community dieticians should be invited to meet representatives of parents and teachers of particular schools at regular intervals during the year to seek agreement to the provision and quality of meals. Meals in schools should be provided without charge.

vi. The Health Education Council should be provided with sufficient funds to mount child accident prevention programmes in conjunction with the Royal Society for the Prevention of Accidents. These programmes should be particularly directed at local authority planners, engineers, and architects.

vii. A comprehensive disablement allowance for people of all ages should be introduced by stages at the earliest possible date beginning with people with 100 per cent disablement.

viii. Representatives of the DHSS and DE, HSE, together with representatives of the trade unions and CBI, should draw up minimally acceptable and desirable conditions of work.

ix. Government Departments, employers and unions should devote more attention to preventive health through work organisation, conditions and amenities, and in other ways. There should be a similar shift of emphasis in the work and functions of the Health and Safety Commission and Executive, and the Employment Medical Advisory Service.

x. Local Authority spending on housing improvements under the 1974 Housing Act should be substantially increased.

xi. Local authorities should increasingly be encouraged to widen their responsibilities to provide for all types of housing need which arise in their localities.

xii. Policies directed towards the public and private housing sectors need to be better co-ordinated.

xiii. Special funding, on the lines of joint funding, for health and local authorities should be developed by the Government to encourage better planning and management of housing, including adaptations and provision of necessary facilities and services for disabled people of all ages by social service and housing departments.

Our recommendations reflect the fact that the reduction of health inequalities depends upon contributions from within many policy areas, and necessarily involving a number of government departments. Our objectives will be achieved *only* if each department makes its appropriate contribution. This in turn requires a greater degree of co-ordination than exists at present.

xiv. Greater co-ordination between Government Departments in the administration of health related policies is required, by establishing inter-departmental machinery in the Cabinet Office under a Cabinet sub-committee along the lines of that established under the Joint Approach to Social Policy (JASP), with the Central Policy Review staff also involved. Local counterparts of national co-ordinating bodies also need to be established.

xv. A Health Development Council should be established with an independent membership to play a key advisory and planning role in relation to a collaborative national policy to reduce inequalities in health.

From: *Report of a Research Working Group on Inequalities in Health* (Chairman: Sir Douglas Black), DHSS London (1981), pp. 348–50

Document twenty-eight
DEFINITION OF PREVENTION

INTRODUCTION

Prevention in relation to health is either an attempt to prevent disease or disability before it occurs (primary prevention), the early detection and treatment of conditions with a view to returning the patient to normal health (secondary prevention), or the continuing treatment of disease or disability to avoid needless progression or complications (tertiary prevention).

Prevention permeates virtually all aspects of the health services, not simply those which are normally regarded as mainly or wholly preventive. Moreover, a great deal of vital preventive activity takes place outside the National Health Service in such fields as education, housing, transport, employment, social services and environmental planning; and there are yet other fields at both national and local level which also offer important opportunities for prevention, for example, in the areas of taxation, prices and consumer protection, food hygiene and the provision of leisure and recreational facilities.

PRIMARY PREVENTION

This is action which prevents the occurrence of certain diseases or disabilities. Immunisation and vaccination are specific forms of primary prevention which have been particularly effective in recent years in helping to eradicate many of the major infectious diseases. Improved sanitation, safe water supplies, better housing and nutrition are all examples of primary prevention which have saved the lives of millions and improved the quality of life for all.

In the National Health Service, services mainly or wholly concerned with primary prevention include health education, fluoridation, immunisation and vaccination, family planning, health visiting and some aspects of ante- and post-natal care; but primary prevention is an important aspect of many other health services.

Examples of primary prevention outside the National Health Service are clean air and anti-pollution controls, motorcycle crash helmet and car seat belt legislation and much of the work of the factory inspectorate and the environmental health services.

SECONDARY PREVENTION

Secondary prevention is the early detection of a condition which, if appropriately treated, would be cured – so returning the patient to normal health. This form of preventive activity usually takes the form of screening techniques and periodic medical examinations. In general, though not invariably, a selective approach to screening has been adopted in this country, screening efforts being concentrated on 'high risk' groups for particular conditions. In child and school health especially, medical examinations are becoming increasingly selective.

Outside the National Health Service wide secondary prevention is carried out in the Employment Medical Advisory Service and the occupational health services in screening workers at risk of industrial diseases.

TERTIARY PREVENTION

This is concerned with minimising disability arising out of existing disease or injury. The continuing treatment of established disease to arrest its progress is a form of tertiary prevention. So too are those methods of treatment aimed at the rehabilitation of the patient who has recovered from an acute attack of disease or in whose case the disease process has been wholly or partially arrested. Tertiary prevention is a function of a wide range of health services and is particularly important in the care of sufferers from chronic diseases or conditions such as diabetes mellitus, epilepsy, mental disorder, spinal injury and deformities of the feet.

In addition to services provided by the NHS, educational, occupational and social services agencies frequently have important roles to play in tertiary prevention and the rehabilitation of individual patients.

From: DHSS/DES, *Prevention and Health*, HMSO London (1977), p. 82

THE COMPLEXITY OF AGENCIES INVOLVED IN THE CARE OF THE IMPAIRED

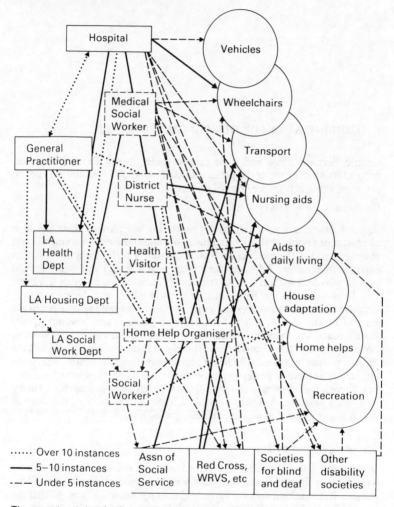

The actual weight of referrals, in one sample of 200 impaired people, for services to help with daily living in the community.

From: Blaxter, M., *Principles and Practice in Rehabilitation*, Royal Commission on the NHS, Cmnd 7615, HMSO, London (1979)

Document thirty
TWO VIEWS OF THE DOCTOR

1. THE LIMITATIONS OF THE MEDICAL PROFESSION

George Bernard Shaw had some caustic things to say about the medical profession when he wrote the preface to *The Doctor's Dilemma* in 1911. Below are some extracts from the original preface.

On the character of doctors . . .

Again I hear the voices indignantly muttering old phrases about the high character of a noble profession and the honor and conscience of its members. I must reply that the medical profession has not a high character; it has an infamous character. I do not know a single thoughtful and well-informed person who does not feel that the tragedy of illness at present is that it delivers you helplessly into the hands of a profession which you deeply mistrust, because it not only advocates and practises the most revolting cruelties in the pursuit of knowledge, and justifies them on grounds which would equally justify practising the same cruelties on yourself or your children, or burning down London to test a patent fire extinguisher, but, when it has shocked the public, tries to reassure it with lies of breath-bereaving brazenness. That is the character the medical profession has got just now. It may be deserved or it may not; there it is at all events: and the doctors who have not realised this are living in a fool's paradise. As to the honor and conscience of doctors, they have as much as any other class of men, no more and no less.

On our dependence on doctors . . .

If mankind knew the facts, and agreed with the doctors, then the doctors would be in the right; and any person who thought otherwise would be a lunatic. But mankind does not agree, and does not know the facts. All that can be said for medical popularity is that until there is a practicable alternative to blind trust in the doctor, the truth about the doctor is so terrible that we dare not face it. Moliere saw through the doctors; but he had to call them in just the same. Napoleon had no illusions about them; but he had to die under their treatment just as much as the most credulous ignoramus that ever paid sixpence for a bottle of strong medicine. In this predicament most people, to save themselves from unbearable mistrust and misery, or from being driven by their conscience into actual conflict with the law, fall back on the old rule that if you cannot have what you believe in you must believe in what you have. When your child is ill or your wife dying, and you happen to be very fond of them, or even when, if you are not fond of them, you are human enough to forget every personal grudge before the spectacle of a fellow creature in pain or peril, what you want is comfort, reassurance, something to clutch at, were it but a straw. This the doctor brings you. You have a wildly urgent feeling that something must be done; and the doctor does something. Sometimes what he does kills the patient; but you do not know that; and the doctor assures you that all that human skill could do has been done. And nobody has the brutality to say to the newly bereft father, mother, husband, wife, brother, or sister, 'You have killed your lost darling by your credulity.'

On the difficulty of judging standards of practice . . .

Fortunately for the doctors, they very seldom find themselves in this position [of being accused of malpractice], because it is so difficult to prove anything against them. The only evidence that can decide a case of malpractice is expert evidence; that is, the evidence of other doctors; and every doctor will allow a colleague to decimate a whole countryside sooner than violate the bond of professional etiquet by giving him away. It is the nurse who gives the doctor away in private, because every nurse has some particular doctor whom she likes; and she usually assures her patients that all the others are disastrous noodles, and soothes the tedium of the sick-bed by gossip about their blunders. She will even give a doctor away for the sake of making the patient believe that she knows more than the doctor. But she dare not, for her livelihood, give the doctor away in public. And the doctors stand by one another at all costs.

Thus everything is on the side of the doctor. When men die of disease they are said to die from natural causes. When they recover (and they mostly do) the doctor gets the credit of curing them. In surgery all operations are recorded as successful if the patient can be got out of the hospital or nursing home alive, though the subsequent history of the case may be such as would make an honest surgeon vow never to recommend or perform the operation again. The large range of operations which consist of amputating limbs and extirpating organs admits of no direct verification of their necessity. There is a fashion in operations as there is in sleeves and skirts; the triumph of some surgeon who has at last found out how to make a once desperate operation fairly safe is usually followed by a rage for that operation not only among the doctors, but actually among their patients. There are men whom the operating table seems to fascinate: half-alive people who through vanity, or hypochondria, or a craving to be the constant objects of anxious attention or what not, lose such feeble sense as they ever had of the value of their own organs and limbs. They seem to care as little for mutilation as lobsters or lizards, which at least have the excuse that they grow new claws and new tails if they lose the old ones. Whilst this book was being prepared for the press a case was tried in the Courts, of a man who sued a railway company for damages because a train had run over him and amputated both his legs. He lost his case because it was proved that he had deliberately contrived the occurrence himself for the sake of getting an idler's pension at the expense of the railway company, being too dull to realize how much more he had to lose than to gain by the bargain even if he had won his case and received damages above his utmost hopes . . .

As a matter of fact, the rank and file of doctors are no more scientific than their tailors; or, if you prefer to put it the reverse way, their tailors are no less scientific than they. Doctoring is an art, not a science: any layman who is interested in science sufficiently to take in one of the scientific journals and follow the literature of the scientific movement, knows more about it than those doctors (probably a large majority) who are not interested in it, and practise only to earn their bread. Doctoring is not even the art of keeping people in health (no doctor seems able to advise you what to eat any better than his grandmother or the nearest quack): it is the art of curing illnesses. It does happen exceptionally that a practising doctor makes a contribution to science (my play describes a very notable one); but it happens much oftener that he draws disastrous conclusions from his clinical experience because he has no conception of scientific method, and believes, like any rustic, that the handling of evidence and statistics needs no expertness. The distinction between a quack doctor and a qualified one is mainly that only the qualified one is authorized to sign death certificates, for which both sorts seems to have about equal occasion.

THE SOLUTION

Shaw looked to public health doctors as the kinds of doctors who could best deal with ill-health . . .

The Public Doctor

What then is to be done?

Fortunately we have not to begin absolutely from the beginning; we already have, in the Medical Officer of Health, a sort of doctor who is free from the worst hardships, and consequently from the worst vices, of the private practitioner. His position depends, not on the number of people who are ill, and whom he can keep ill, but on the number of people who are well. He is judged, as all doctors and treatments should be judged, by the vital statistics of his district. When the death-rate goes up his credit goes down. As every increase in his salary depends on the issue of a public debate as to the health of the constituency under his charge, he has every inducement to strive towards the ideal of a clean bill of health. He has a safe, dignified, responsible, independent position based wholly on the public health; whereas the private practitioner has a precarious, shabby-genteel, irresponsible, servile position, based wholly on the prevalence of illness.

. . . and in conclusion . . .

let me sum up my conclusion as dryly as is consistent with accurate thought and live conviction.

1. Nothing is more dangerous than a poor doctor: not even a poor employer or a poor landlord.

2. Of all the anti-social vested interests the worst is the vested interest of ill-health.

3. Remember that an illness is a misdemeanor; and treat the doctor as an accessory unless he notifies every case to the Public Health Authority.

4. Treat every death as a possible and, under our present system, a probable murder, by making it the subject of a reasonably conducted inquest; and execute the doctor, if necessary, *as* a doctor, by striking him off the register.

5. Make up your mind how many doctors the community needs to keep it well. Do not register more or less than this number; and let registration constitute the doctor a civil servant with a dignified living wage paid out of public funds.

6. Municipalize Harley Street.

7. Treat the private operator exactly as you would treat a private executioner.

8. Treat persons who profess to be able to cure diseases as you treat fortune tellers.

9. Keep the public carefully informed, by special statistics and announcements of individual cases, of all illnesses of doctors or in their families.

10. Make it compulsory for a doctor using a brass plate to have inscribed on it, in addition to the letters indicating his qualifications, the words 'Remember that I too am mortal'.

11. In legislation and social organization, proceed on the principle that invalids, meaning persons who cannot keep themselves alive by their own activities, cannot, beyond reason, expect to be kept alive by the activity of others. There is a point at which the most energetic policeman or doctor, when called upon to deal with an apparently drowned person, gives up artificial respiration, although it is never possible to declare with certainty, at any point short of decomposition, that another five minutes of the exercise would not effect resuscitation. The theory that every individual alive is of infinite value is legislatively impracticable. No doubt the higher the life we secure to the individual by wise social organization, the greater his value is to the community, and the more pains we shall take to pull him through any temporary danger or disablement. But the man who costs more than he is worth is doomed by sound hygiene as inexorably as by sound economics.

12. Do not try to live for ever. You will not succeed.

13. Use your health, even to the point of wearing it out. That is what it is for. Spend all you have before you die; and do not outlive yourself.

14. Take the utmost care to get well born and well brought up. This means that your mother must have a good doctor. Be careful to go to a school where there is what they call a school clinic, where your nutrition and teeth and eyesight and other matters of importance to you will be attended to. Be particularly careful to have all this done at the expense of the nation, as otherwise it will not be done at all, the chances being about forty to one against your being able to pay for it directly yourself, even if you know how to set about it. Otherwise you will be what most people are at present: an unsound citizen of an unsound nation, without sense enough to be ashamed or unhappy about it.

From: The Preface to *The Doctor's Dilemma: A Tragedy*, G. B. Shaw (first published 1911), Constable & Co Ltd, London, 1932 (standard edn), pp. 4–5, 10, 11, 12, 64, 77–8

2. THE QUALITIES OF A 'GOOD' DOCTOR

John Berger discusses a country doctor . . .

He is acknowledged as a good doctor. The organization of his practice, the facilities he offers, his diagnostic and clinical skill are probably somewhat under-rated. His patients may not realize how lucky they are. But in a sense this is inevitable. Only the most self-conscious consider it lucky to have their elementary needs met. And it is on a very basic, elementary level that he is judged a good doctor.

They would say that he was straight, not afraid of work, easy to talk to, not stand-offish, kind, understanding, a good listener, always willing to come out when needed, very thorough. They would also say that he was moody, difficult to understand when on one of his theoretical subjects like sex, capable of doing things just to shock, unusual.

How he actually answers their needs as a doctor is far more complicated than any of these epithets imply. To understand this we must first consider the special character and depth of any doctor-patient relationship.

The primitive medicine-man, who was often also priest, sorcerer and judge, was the first specialist to be released from the obligation of procuring food for the tribe. The magnitude of this privilege and of the power which it gave him is a direct reflection of the importance of the needs he served. An awareness of illness is part of the price that man first paid and still pays for his self-consciousness. This awareness increases the pain or disability. But the self-consciousness of which it is the result is a social phenomenon and so with this self-consciousness arises the possibility of treatment, of medicine.

We cannot imaginatively reconstruct the subjective attitude of a tribesman to his treatment. But within our culture today what is our own attitude? How do we acquire the necessary trust to submit ourselves to the doctor?

We give the doctor access to our bodies. Apart from the doctor, we only grant such access voluntarily to lovers – and many are frightened to do even this. Yet the doctor is a comparative stranger.

The degree of intimacy implied by the relationship is emphasized by the concern of all medical ethics (not only ours) to make an absolute distinction between the roles of doctor and lover. It is usually assumed that this is because the doctor can see women naked and can touch them where he likes and that this may sorely tempt him to make love to them. It is a crude assumption, lacking imagination. The conditions under which a doctor is likely to examine his patients are always sexually discouraging.

The emphasis in medical ethics on sexual correctness is not so much to restrict the doctor as to offer a promise to the patient: a promise which is far more than a reassurance that he or she will not be taken advantage of. It is a positive promise of physical intimacy without a sexual basis. Yet what can such intimacy mean? Surely it belongs to the experiences of childhood. We submit to the doctor by quoting to ourselves a state of childhood and simultaneously extending our sense of family to include him. We imagine him as an honorary member of the family.

In cases where the patient is fixated on a parent, the doctor may become a substitute for this parent. But in such a relationship the high degree of sexual content creates difficulties. In illness we ideally imagine the doctor as an elder brother or sister.

Something similar happens at death. The doctor is the familiar of death. When we call for a doctor, we are asking him to cure us and to relieve our suffering, but, if he cannot cure us, we are also asking him to witness our dying. The values of the witness is that he has seen so many others die. (This, rather than prayers and last rites, was also the real value which the priest once had.) He is the living intermediary between us and the multitudinous dead. He belongs to us and he has belonged to them. And the hard but real comfort which they offer through him is still that of fraternity.

It would be a great mistake to 'normalize' what I have just said by concluding that quite naturally the patient wants a *friendly* doctor. His hopes and demands, however contradicted by previous experience, however protected they may be by scepticism, however undeclared even to himself, are much more profound and precise.

In illness many connexions are severed. Illness separates and encourages a distorted, fragmented form of self-consciousness. The doctor, through his relationship with the invalid and by means of the special intimacy he is allowed, has to compensate for these broken connections and reaffirm the social content of the invalid's aggravated self-consciousness.

When I speak of fraternal relationship – or rather of the patient's deep, unformulated expectation of fraternity – I do not of course mean that the doctor can or should behave like an actual brother. What is required of him is that he should recognize his patient with the certainty of an ideal brother. The function of fraternity is recognition.

This individual and closely intimate recognition is required on both a physical and psychological level. On the former it constitutes the art of diagnosis. Good general diagnosticians are rare, not because most doctors lack medical knowledge, but because most are incapable of taking in all the possibly relevant facts – emotional, historical, environmental as well as physical. They are searching for specific conditions instead of the truth about a man which may then suggest various conditions. It may be that computers will soon diagnose better than doctors. But the facts fed to the computers will still have to be the result of intimate, individual recognition of the patient.

On the psychological level recognition means support. As soon as we are ill we fear that our illness is unique. We argue with ourselves and rationalize, but a ghost of the fear remains. And it remains for a very good reason. The illness, as an undefined force, is a potential threat to our very being and we are bound to be highly conscious of the uniqueness of that being. The illness, in other words, shares in our own uniqueness. By fearing its threat, we embrace it and make it specially our own. That is why patients are inordinately relieved when doctors give their complaint a name. The name may mean very little to them; they may understand nothing of what it signifies; but because it has a name, it has an independent existence from them. They can now struggle or complain *against* it. To have a complaint recognized, that is to say defined, limited and depersonalized, is to be made stronger.

The whole process, as it includes doctor and patient, is a dialectical one. The doctor in order to recognize the illness fully – I say fully because the recognition must be such as to indicate the specific treatment – must first recognize the patient as a person: but for the patient – provided that he trusts the doctor and that trust finally depends upon the efficacy of his treatment – the doctor's recognition of his illness is a help because it separates and depersonalizes that illness.

From: J. Berger, *A Fortunate Man. The Story of a Country Doctor*, Penguin, London (1969) pp.62–74

Document thirty-one

DIAGRAM ILLUSTRATING THE SHIFT IN EMPHASIS IN THE CONCEPTUALISATION OF HEALTH AND ILLNESS

(The shift has occurred from left to right.)

Illness	Health
Treatment	Prevention
Cure	Care
Disease	Behaviour producing disease
Individual	Population as unit of treatment
Illness as concern of medical profession	Health as business of everybody, biocrats, social services
Right to treatment	Duty to remain healthy

From: Illsley, R., *Health and Health Policy. Priorities for Research,* Social Science Research Council (1977), Appendix 4, p. 15

ILLICH AND THE LIMITS OF MEDICINE

Illich, in The Limits of Medicine presents an extreme statement of the effects of medicalisation. He argues that institutionalised medicine has become a threat to health through social, clinical and structural iatrogenesis. This has been a consequence of industrialisation, bureacratization and professionalisation of medicine. Iatrogenesis, 'damage done by the provider', has according to Illich occurred on three levels: the clinical, the social and the structural. Clinical iatrogenesis occurs when pain, sickness and death result from the provision of medical care. Illich recounts a tale of the illness caused by the effect of drugs; and 'fashionable operations', operations which are at best effective, at worst damage the patient; irksome, painful, time-consuming diagnostic procedures. In summary, 'a professional and physician-based health must produce clinical damage which outweighs its practical benefits'.

DOCTOR-INFLICTED INJURIES OR CLINICAL IATROGENESIS

Unfortunately, the futility of medical care is the least of the torts a proliferating medical enterprise inflicts on society. The impact of medicine constitutes one of the most rapidly expanding epidemics of our time. The pain, dysfunction, disability and even anguish which result from technical medical intervention now rival the morbidity due to traffic, work and even war-related activities. Only modern malnutrition is clearly ahead.

The technical term for the new epidemic of doctor-made disease, *Iatrogenesis* is composed of the Greek words for 'physician' (*iatros*) and for 'origin' (*genesis*). Iatrogenic disease comprises only illness which would not have come about unless sound and professionally recommended treatment had been applied. Within this definition, a patient can sue his therapist if the latter, in the course of his treatment, has not applied a recommended treatment and thus risked making him sick.

In a more general and more widely accepted sense, clinical iatrogenic disease comprises all clinical conditions for which remedies, physicians or hospitals are the pathogens or 'sickening' agents. I will call this plethora of therapeutic side-effects *clinical-iatrogenesis*.

Medicines have always been potentially poisonous, but their unwanted side-effects have increased with their effectiveness and widespread use. Every 24 to 36 hours, from 50% to 80% of adults in the US and UK swallow a medically prescribed chemical. Some take a wrong drug, others get a contaminated or old batch, others a counterfeit, others take several drugs which are dangerous, or take them in dangerous combinations, others receive injections with improperly sterilized syringes or brittle needles. Some drugs are addictive, other mutilating, others mutagenic, although perhaps only in synergy with food colouring or insecticide. In some patients, antibiotics alter the normal bacterial flora and induce super-infection, permitting more resistant organisms to proliferate and invade the host. Other drugs contribute to the breeding of drug-resistant strains of bacteria. Subtle kinds of poisoning thus have spread even faster than the bewildering variety and ubiquity of nostrums. Unnecessary surgery is a standard procedure. Disabling non-diseases result from the medical treatment of non-existent diseases and are on the increase: the number of children disabled in Massachusetts from cardiac non-disease exceeds the number of children under effective treatment for cardiac disease.

Doctor-inflicted pain and infirmity have always been a part of medical practice. Professional callousness, negligence and sheer incompetence are age-old forms of malpractice. With the transformation of the doctor from an artisan exercising a skill on personally known individuals into a technician applying scientific rules to classes of patients, malpractice acquired a new anyonymous, almost respectable status. What had formerly been considered an abuse of confidence and a moral fault can now be rationalized into the occasional breakdown of equipment and operators. In a complex technological hospital, negligence becomes 'random human error', callousness becomes 'scientific detachment', and incompetence becomes a 'lack of specialized equipment'. The depersonalization of diagnosis and therapy has turned malpractice from an ethical into a technical problem.

In 1971, between 12,000 and 15,000 malpractice suits were lodged in US courts. However, doctors are vulnerable in court only to the imputation of having acted against the medical code, of having been guilty of the incompetent performance of prescribed treatment, or of dereliction out of greed or laziness. Most of the damage inflicted by the modern doctor does not fall into any of these categories. It occurs in the ordinary practice of well-trained men who have learned to bow to prevailing professional judgement and procedure, even though they know (or could and should know) what damage they do.

The US Department of Health calculates that 7% of all patients suffer compensatable injuries while hospitalized, though few of them do anything about it. Moreover, the average frequency of reported accidents in hospitals was higher than in all industries but mines and high-rise construction. A national survey indicates that accidents were the major cause of death in US children, and that these accidents occurred more often in hospitals than in any other kind of place. One in 50 children admitted to a hospital suffered an accident which required specific treatment. University hospitals are relatively more pathogenic, or, in blunt language, more sickening. It has been established that one out of every five patients admitted to a typical research hospital acquires an iatrogenic disease, sometimes trivial, usually requiring special treatment, and in one case in thirty leading to death. Half of these episodes resulted from complications of drug therapy; amazingly, one in ten came from diagnostic procedures. Despite good intentions and claims to public service, with a similar record of performance a military officer would be relieved of his command, and a restaurant or amusement centre would be closed by the police . . .

SOCIAL AND STRUCTURAL IATROGENESIS

On a second level, medical practice sponsors sickness by reinforcing a morbid society that not only industrially preserves its defectives, but also exponentially breeds demand for the patient role. On the one hand defectives survive in increasing numbers and are fit only for life under institutional care, while on the other hand, medically certified symptoms exempt people from destructive wage-labour and excuse them from the struggle to reshape the society in which they live. Second level iatrogenesis finds its expression in various symptoms of social over-medicalization . . .

STRUCTURAL IATROGENESIS

On a third level, the so-called health professions have an even deeper, structurally health-denying effect insofar as they destroy the potential of people to deal with their human weakness, vulnerability and uniqueness in a personal and autonomous way. Structural iatrogenesis . . . is the ultimate backlash of hygienic progress and consists in the paralysis of healthy responses to suffering. It strikes when people accept health management designed on the engineering model, when they conspire in an attempt to produce something called 'better health' which inevitably results in the heteronomous, managed maintenance of life on high levels of sub-lethal illness. This ultimate backlash of medical 'progress' must be clearly distinguished from both clinical and social iatrogenesis.

From: Illich, I., *Medical Nemesis: The Expropriation of Health*, Marion Boyars, London (1975), pp. 21–7

THE TUC'S COMMENT ON THE BLACK REPORT

According to the *Black Report*, health differences between classes and inequalities of life-chances can be traced through all stages of a person's life. This can be effectively illustrated if we take the case of two hypothetical families – the Jones's and the Smythe's.

Mr Smythe is the financial director of a large company. Mrs Smythe does not work and she is soon to give birth to her third child. They live in a pleasant suburb on the edge of the green belt with their two children, Emily aged five, and Rodney aged 10. They own their own home and the area where they live is mainly populated by professional people. There are plenty of recreational and sporting facilities, good schools and a brand new health centre in the locality.

Mr Jones is an unskilled labourer at a factory. His wife supplements the family income by working as an office cleaner. They live in a high rise block of flats in the centre of the city. The flats were built in the late fifties and are poorly serviced with play areas and parks. The Jones's also have two children, Janet aged five and John aged 10. Mrs Jones's is also expecting her third child. The family is registered with a local GP whose list of patients is already oversubscribed.

These two imaginary families are at opposite ends of the social scale in terms of occupation, and income. In between there are different shades of grey, but how are these two different families likely to fare under the existing National Health Service arrangements? Based on the *Black Report* these are some of the likely outcomes.

There is a 60 per cent probability that Mrs Jones will not have consulted an obstetrician by the fifth month of her pregnancy. By that time it may be too late to diagnose congenital abnormalities like spina bifida or blood disorders in her unborn baby.

Mrs Jones's poorer living standards will probably mean her standard of nutritional diet is poor. She is nearly twice as likely as Mrs Smythe to die in childbirth, or her baby to be still-born or die within the first few months of life.

If her baby is a boy and survives birth, he is still four times more likely to die before his first birthday than Mrs Smythe's new born son.

Like his brother John, the new-born Jones boy is ten times more likely to die, before he is 14, through an accident involving fire, a fall or drowning, than his counterpart Rodney Smythe. John is seven times more likely to be knocked down and killed in a road accident.

Similar disadvantages will follow him into adult life. In only one case – asthma – is Rodney more likely to die than John at an early age.

Though statistics show that Janet Jones is not as likely to be an accident victim as her brother, her individual health and life expectancy will tend to follow the pattern of her mother and maternal grandmother.

Mr Jones's health and life expectancy is also considerably poorer than that of Mr Smythe – and if his son also becomes a manual worker his health is likely to follow a similar pattern too.

Although the actual health of all families has improved since the setting up of the NHS, the relative gap between professional and unskilled manual workers has actually widened.

Contrary to popular belief, Mr Jones is much more likely to die of lung cancer or duodenal ulcer than Mr Smythe. He is twice as likely to die of a disease affecting the nervous system; three times as likely to suffer and die from a parasitic disease; four times as likely to incur a mental disorder, or a respiratory disease and die.

In contrast, the Smythe family are more likely to follow a nutritionally satisfactory diet, to consult preventive services such as dentists, chiropodists and opticians. Mrs Smythe is more likely to have planned her family than Mrs Jones, or to have been screened to test if she might have treatable breast or cervical cancer. The *Black Report* comments that health facilities tend to be geared towards the middle-class consumer rather than the working class.

Also the high-density urban areas where working-class people live tend to have a lower per-capita expenditure than the suburban areas which are not so densely populated. The Smythe family are likely to have frequent medical check-ups as a matter of course – the Jones are more likely to use their GP after illness has set in, and consequently visit him more often.

The unavoidable inference from the *Black Report* is that the people whose health is at greatest risk are those with the lowest incomes, and worst living conditions. Families like the Jones are the ones most at risk – they are also getting the worst deal out of the NHS.

This evidence must lead to the inevitable conclusion that the NHS is not doing its job as well as it might, and the current run-down into a two-tier system of private care and state care envisaged by the Government will make matters worse.

But of even greater concern, the establishment of an efficient health service alone would not be enough. It is living standards rather than health-care services which determine the overall state of people's health. The living standards of many ordinary working people are so low that their health and life span are severely affected.

From: Trades Union Congress, *The Unequal Health of the Nation: A TUC Summary of the Black Report*, TUC, London (1981)

LIST OF REPORTS AND STATUTES

1858	Medical Act
1902	Midwives Act
1911	National Insurance Act
1918	Maternity and Child Welfare Act
1919	Nurses Registration Act
1920	The Ministry of Health. Consultative Council on Medical and Allied Services. Interim Report on the future provision of Medical Services and Allied Services. (Dawson Report) HMSO
1921	Ministry of Health Report on the Finance of Voluntary Hospitals (The Cave Committee). HMSO
1926	Report of the Royal Commission on National Health Insurance. Cmd 2596, London, HMSO
1928	National Health Insurance Act
1936	National Health Insurance Consolidating Act
1937	PEP Report on the British Health Services. Political and Economic Planning
1938	British Medical Association (BMA). A General Medical Service for the Nation
1944	Ministry of Health. A National Health Service. (Coalition government White Paper). Cmd 6502, HMSO
1946	National Health Service Act. 1946
1956	Report of a Committee of Inquiry into the Cost of the National Health Service. (Guillebaud Report). Cmd 9663, HMSO
1959	Report of the Committee on Maternity Services. (Cranbrook Report). HMSO
1959	Mental Health Act
1960	Royal Commission Report on Doctor's and Dentist's Remuneration. (Pilkington Report). Cmnd 939, HMSO

1962	Ministry of Health. A Hospital Plan for England and Wales. Cmnd 1604, HMSO
1962	Medical Services Review Committee. A Review of the Medical Services in Great Britain. (Porritt Report). 1962
1963	Ministry of Health. The Field of Work of the Family Doctor. (Gillie Report). HMSO
1966	Report of the Committee on Senior Nursing Staff Structure. (Salmon Report). HMSO
1967	Report of the Committee of Enquiry into ths Relationship of the Pharmaceutical Industry with the National Health Service 1965–1967. (Sainsbury Report). Cmnd 3410, HMSO
1968	Ministry of Health. The Administrative Structure of Medical and Related Services in England and Wales. 1st Green Paper. HMSO
1968	Royal Commission on Medical Education. (Todd Report). Cmnd 3569, HMSO
1968	Department of Health and Social Security formed
1968	Health Service and Public Health Act 1968. HMSO
1969	DHSS. The Functions of the District General Hospital. (Bonham-Carter Report). HMSO.
1970	Report of the Committee on Local Authority and Allied Personal Social Services. (Seebohm Report). Cmnd 3703, HMSO
1970	Social Services Act
1970	DHSS. The Future Structure of the National Health Service. 2nd Green Paper. HMSO
1971	DHSS. The National Health Service Reorganisation: Consultative Document. HMSO
1972	Department of Employment. Safety and Health at Work: Report of the Committee 1970–1972. (Chair: Lord Robens). Cmnd 5034, HMSO
1972	National Health Service Reorganisation: England. Cmnd 5055, HMSO
1972	DHSS. Management Arrangements for the Reorganised National Health Service. (The Grey Book). HMSO
1972	Report of the Committee on Nursing. (Briggs Report). Cmnd 5115, HMSO
1973	The National Health Service Reorganisation Act. HMSO

1973	DHSS. Report of the Committee on Hospital Complaints Procedure. (Davies Report). HMSO
1974	Safety and Health at Work Act
1974	DHSS. Democracy in the National Health Service. HMSO
1975	Report of the Committee of Enquiry into the Regulation of the Medical Profession. (Merrison Report). Cmnd 6018, HMSO
1976	DHSS. Sharing Resources for Health in England: Report of the Resource Allocation Working Party. HMSO
1976	DHSS. Report of the Committee on Child Health Services. Fit for the Future. (Court Report). HMSO
1976	DHSS. Priorities for Health and Social Services in England.
1976	DHSS. Prevention and Health: Everybody's Business: A Reassessment of Public and Personal Health. HMSO
1977	DHSS. Priorities in the Health and Social Services: The Way Forward. HMSO
1977	National Health Service Act.
1978	DHSS. Medical Manpower – The Next Twenty Years: A Discussion Paper. HMSO
1979	Royal Commission on the National Health Service. (Merrison Report). Cmnd 7615, HMSO
1979	DHSS. Patients First. A Consultative Paper. HMSO
1980	Health Services Act
1980	DHSS. The Future Pattern of Hospital Provision in England – A Consultative Paper. HMSO
1980	House of Commons Social Services Committee. Second Report. Perinatal and Neonatal Mortality. Session 1979/80. HMSO
1980	House of Commons Social Services Committee. The Government's White Papers on Public Expenditure: the Social Services. Third Report, Session 1979/80. HC 702, HMSO
1981	DHSS. Care in Action. A Handbook of Policies and Priorities for the Health and Personal Social Services in England. HMSO
1981	House of Commons Social Services Committee. Public Expenditure on the Social Services. Third Report, Session 1980/81. HC 324, HMSO
1981	House of Commons Committee of Public Accounts.

	Financial Control and Accountability in the National Health Service. Seventeenth Report, Session 1980/81. HMSO
1981	DHSS. Health Services in England: Review of the NHS Planning System. A Consultative Document HMSO
1981	Care in the Community. A Consultative Document on Moving Resources for Care in England HMSO
1982	House of Commons Committee of Public Accounts. Financial Control and Accountability in the National Health Service. Seventeenth Report, Session 1981/82. HMSO
1983	DHSS. Health Care and its Costs: The Development of the National Health Service in England. HMSO (See also Document 15 for reports on dependent groups)

LIST OF HEALTH MINISTERS 1919–1981

1919–21	Dr Christopher Addison
1921–22	Sir Alfred Mond
1922–23	Sir Arthur Griffith-Boscawen
1923	Neville Chamberlain
1923–24	Sir William Joynson-Hicks
1924	John Wheatley
1924–29	Neville Chamberlain
1929–31	Arthur Greenwood
1931	Neville Chamberlain
1931–35	Sir E Hilton-Young
1935–38	Sir Kingsley Wood
1938–40	Walter Elliot
1940–41	Malcolm MacDonald
1941–43	Ernest Brown
1943–45	Henry Willink
1945–51	Aneurin Bevan
1951	Hilary Marquand
1951–55	Iain MacLeod
1955–57	Hugh Turton
1957	Dennis Vosper
1957–60	Derek Walker-Smith
1960–63	Enoch Powell
1963–64	Anthony Barber
1964–68	Kenneth Robinson

SECRETARIES OF STATE FOR SOCIAL SERVICES

1968–70	Richard Crossman
1970–74	Sir Keith Joseph
1974–76	Barbara Castle

SELECT BIBLIOGRAPHY

ABEL-SMITH, B., *The Hospitals 1800–1948*, Heinemann, London (1964)

ABEL-SMITH, B., *The National Health Service: The First Thirty Years*, HMSO, London (1978)

ABEL-SMITH, B., *A History of the Nursing Profession*, Heinemann, London (1960)

ABEL-SMITH, B., *Value for Money in Health Services*, Heinemann, London (1976)

ALFORD, R., *Health Care Politics*, University of Chicago, Chicago (1975)

ATKINSON, P., DINGWALL, R. and MURCOTT, A., *Prospects for the National Health Service*, Croom Helm, London (1979)

BARNARD, K., and LEE, K., *Conflicts in the NHS*, Croom Helm, London (1977)

BARRETT, S. and FUDGE, C., (eds.), *Policy and Action: Essays on the Implementation of Public Policy*, Methuen, London (1981)

BEVAN, A., *In Place of Fear*, MacGibbon & Kee, London (1981)

BLACK, D. and THOMAS, G. P., *Providing Health Services*, Croom Helm, London (1978)

BLAXTER, M., *The Health of Children. A review of research on the place of health in cycles of disadvantages*, Heinemann, London (1981)

BOSANQUET, N., (ed.), *Industrial Relations in the NHS: The Search for a System*, King Edwards Hospital Fund for London, London (1979)

BROWN, R. G. S., *The Management of Welfare*, Fontana, London (1975)

BROWN, R. G. S., *Reorganising the National Health Service*, Robertson, Oxford (1979)

BROWN, R. G .S., *New Bottles: Old Wine?*, Institute for Health Studies, Hull (1974)

BROWN, G., and HARRIS, T., *The Social Origins of Depression*, Tavistock, London (1978)

BUTLER, J., *Family Doctors and Public Policy*, Routledge & Kegan Paul, London (1973)

CARTWRIGHT, A.,*Patients and their Doctors*, Routledge & Kegan Paul, London (1967)

CARTWRIGHT, A., and ANDERSON, R., *Patients and their Doctors*, Institute for Social Studies in Medical Care, Royal College of General Practitioners, Occasional Paper No. 8, London (1979)

CARTWRIGHT, A., *Human Relations and Hospital Care*, Routledge & Kegan Paul, London (1964)

CARTWRIGHT, F. E., *A Social History of Medicine*, Longman, London (1977)

CASTLE, B., *The Castle Diaries 1974–76*, Weidenfeld & Nicholson (1980)

COCHRANE, A., *Effectiveness and Efficiency. Random Reflections on Health Services*, Nuffield Provincial Hospitals Trust (1971)

CROSSMAN, R. G. H., *The Diaries of a Cabinet Minister. Vol. 3: Secretary of State for Social Services 1968–1970*, Hamilton and Cape, London (1977)

CROSSMAN, R. G. H., *A Politician's View of Health Service Planning*, University of Glasgow (1972)

DAVIS, A. and HOROBIN, G., *Medical Encounters; the experience of illness and treatment*, Croom Helm, London (1977)

DONNISON, J.,*Midwives and Medical Men: a history of interprofessional rivalry and women's rights*, Heinemann, London (1977)

DOYAL, L., *The Political Economy of Health*, Pluto Press, London (1979)

DOYAL, L., *The Migrant Worker in the NHS*, North London Polytechnic, London (1980)

DRAPER, P., BEST, G. and DENNIS, J.,, *Health Money and the National Health Service*, Unit for the Study of Health Policy, London (1976)

ECKSTEIN, H., *Pressure Group Politics: the case of the British Medical Association*, Allen & Unwin, London (1980)

ECKSTEIN, H., *The English Health Service: its origins, structure and achievements*, Oxford University Press, London (1959)

EPSTEIN, S.,*The Politics of Cancer*, Doubleday, New York (1979)

FELDSTEIN, M. S., *Economic Analysis for Health Service Efficiency*, North Holland (1967)

FINLAYSON, A., and MCEWAN, J.,*Coronary Heart Disease and Patterns of Living*, Croom Helm, London (1977)

FOOT, M., *Aneurin Bevan*, Vol. 2, Davis Poynter, London (1973)

FORSYTH, G., *Doctors and State Medicine*, Pitman, London (1971)

FREIDSON, F., *The Profession of Medicine: a study of the sociology of applied knowledge*, Dodd, Meade & Co, New York (1970)

FUCHS, V., *Who Shall Live? Health Economics and Social Choice*, Basic Books Inc., New York (1974)

HAM, C., *Policy Making in the National Health Service. A Case Study of the Leeds Regional Hospital Board*, Macmillan, London (1981)

HAM, C., *Health Policy in Britain*, Macmillan, London (1982)

HAYWOOD, S. C., *Managing the Health Service*, Allen & Unwin, London (1974)

HAYWOOD, S., and ALASZEWSKI, A., *Crisis in the Health Service*, Croom Helm, London (1980)

HAYWOOD, S., and ELCOCK, H., *The Buck Stops Where? Accountability and Control in the National Health Service*, Institute of Health Studies, Hull (1980)

HECLO, H., and WILDAVSKY, A., *The Private Government of Public Money*, Macmillan, New York (1974)

HELLER, T., *Restructuring the Health Service*, Croom Helm, London (1978)

HENLEY, A., *Asian Patients in Hospital and at Home*, King Edward's Hospital Fund, London (1979)

HICKS, D., *Primary Health Care: a review*, DHSS, HMSO, London (1976)

HODGKINSON, R., *The Origins of the National Health Service*, The Wellcome Historical Medical Library, London (1967)

HONIGSBAUM, F., *The Division of Labour in British Medicine: a history of the separation of general practice from hospital care 1911–1968*, Kogan Page, London (1979)

JACKSON, J. A., (ed.), *Professions and Professionalism*, Cambridge University Press (1970)

JOHNSON, T., *Professions and Power*, Macmillan, London (1972)

JONES, K., *A History of the Mental Health Services*, Routledge & Kegan Paul, London (1972)

JONES, K., *et al.*, *Opening the Door*, Routledge & Kegan Paul, London (1975)

KLEIN, R., *Inflation and Priorities*, Centre for Studies in Social Policy, London (1975)

KLEIN, R., and LEWIS, J., *The Politics of Consumer Representation: a study of Community Health Councils*, Centre for Studies in Social Policy, London (1976)

KOGAN, M., *et al.*, *The Working of the National Health Services*, Royal Commission on the NHS. Research Paper No. 1, HMSO (1978)

LEESON, J., and GRAY, J., *Women in Medicine*, Tavistock, London (1978)

LE GRAND, J., *Strategies of Equality: Redistribution and the Social Services*, Allen & Unwin, London (1982)

ILLICH, I., *Limits to Medicine: Medical Nemesis: The Expropriation of Health*, Marion Boyars, London (1976). First edition entitled *Medical Nemesis: The Expropriation of Health* (1975)

INGLE, S. and TETHER, P., *Parliament and Health Policy*, Gower Publishing Allen & Unwin, London (1982)

LEVITT, R., *The People's Voice*, King Edward's Hospital Fund for London, London (1980)

LEVITT, R., *The Reorganisation of the NHS*, Martin Robertson (3rd edn). Oxford (1980)

LLEWELYN DAVIES, M., *Maternity: Letters from Working Women*, Virago, London (1978)

LINDSEY, A., *Socialised Medicine in England and Wales*, University of North Carolina Press, Chapel Hill (1962)

MACKENZIE, W. J. M., *Power and Responsibility in Health Care*, Oxford University Press, Oxford (1979)

MCCARTHY, M., *Epidemiology and Policies for Planning I*, King Edward's Hospital Fund for London, London (1982)

MCKEOWN, T., *The Role of Medicine. Dream, Mirage or Nemesis?*, Blackwell, Oxford (1979)

MAXWELL, R., *Health Care – the Growing Dilemma*, McKinsey, New York (1974)

MAXWELL, R. J., *Health and Wealth: an international study of health care*, Lexington Books, Mass., Toronto (1981)

MINISTRY OF NATIONAL HEALTH AND WELFARE. (CANADA). *A New Perspective on the Health of the Canadians* (The Lalonde Report), Ottawa (1974)

NAVARRO, V., *Medicine under Captialism*, Croom Helm, London (1974)

NAVARRO, V., *Class Struggle, the State and Medicine*, Robertson, Oxford (1978)

OAKLEY, A., *Women Confined: towards a sociology of childbirth*, Robertson, Oxford (1980)

OWEN, D., *In Sickness and in Health*, Quartet Books, London (1976)

PARRY, N., and PARRY, J., *The Rise of the Medical Profession*, Croom Helm, London (1976)

PARSTON, G., *Planners, Politics and Health Services*, Croom Helm London (1980)

PATER, J. E., *The Making of the National Health Service*, King's Fund Historical Series I, King Edward's Hospital Fund for London (1981)

PERRIN, J., *et al.*, *Management of Financial Resources in the National Health Service*, Research Paper No. 2. Royal Commission on the NHS, HMSO (1979)

POLITICS OF HEALTH GROUP, *Going Private*, available from 9 Poland Street, London W1 (1981)

POWELL, J. E., *A New Look at Medicine and Politics*, Pitman, London (1966)

RADICAL STATISTICS HEALTH GROUP, *The Unofficial Guide to Official Health Statistics*, available from 9 Poland Street, London W1, London (1980)

ROBINSON, D., and HENRY, S., *Self Help and Health*, Robertson, Oxford (1977)

STEVENS, R., *Medical Practice in Modern England*, Yale University Press (1966)

STACEY, M. *et al.*, *Health and the Division of Labour*, Croom Helm, London (1977)

STACEY, M. *et al.*, (eds.), *Health Care and Health Knowledge*, Croom Helm, London (1979)

STACEY, M. (ed.), *The Sociology of the NHS*, Sociological Review Monograph 22, University of Keele (1976)

STIMSON, G., and WEBB, B., *Going to See Doctor: the consultation process in general practice*, Routledge & Kegan Paul, London (1975)

TOWNSEND, P., and DAVIDSON, N., *Inequalities in Health*, Pelican, London (1982)

WATKIN, B., *Documents on Health and Social Services. 1834 to the Present day*, Methuen, London (1975)

WATKIN, B., *The National Health Service: the first phase*, Allen and Unwin, London (1978)

WIDGERY, D., *Health in Danger: the crisis in the NHS*, Macmillan, London (1979)

WILLOCKS, A. J., *The Creation of the National Health Service*, Routledge & Kegan Paul, London (1967)

WILLIAMSON, J. D., *Self-Care in Health*, Croom Helm, London (1978)

WOODWARD, J. and RICHARDS, D., (eds.), *Health Care and Popular Medicine in 19th Century England*, Croom Helm, London

INDEX